D1226654

Mastering Medicine

PROFESSIONAL SOCIALIZATION IN MEDICAL SCHOOL

Robert H. Coombs

 THE FREE PRESS
A Division of Macmillan Publishing Co., Inc.
NEW YORK

Collier Macmillan Publishers
LONDON

CARNEGIE LIBRARY
LIVINGSTONE COLLEGE
SALISBURY, N. C. 28144

Copyright © 1978 by The Free Press
        A Division of Macmillan Publishing Co., Inc.

All rights reserved. No part of this book may be reproduced or
transmitted in any form or by any means, electronic or mechanical,
including photocopying, recording, or by any information storage and
retrieval system, without permission in writing from the Publisher.

The Free Press
A Division of Macmillan Publishing Co., Inc.
866 Third Avenue, New York, N.Y. 10022

Collier Macmillan Canada, Ltd.

Library of Congress Catalog Card Number: 77–85351

Printed in the United States of America

printing number

1 2 3 4 5 6 7 8 9 10

Library of Congress Cataloging in Publication Data

Coombs, Robert H
    Mastering medicine.

    Bibliography: p.
    Includes index.
    1. Medical education--Social aspects--United States.
2. Medical students--United States. 3. Professional
socialization. I. Title.
R745.C935   610.73'69   77-85351
ISBN 0-02-906640-9

610.7369
C 775

To
Carol Jean

106690

Contents

Preface

THIS BOOK IS THE PRODUCT of a decade's research concerning the professional socialization of young men and women training to become physicians in medical school. Made possible by grants from the National Institute of Mental Health and the National Fund for Medical Education, it is the culmination of an intensive longitudinal analysis of an entire class of medical students, from the time they were accepted into medical school until they had graduated and were eventually involved in residency training programs.

In order to examine the transition whereby incumbents of one status (college student) progressively advance to another (physician) and to explore the dynamic processes of professional socialization that make this status passage possible, I have conducted a panel analysis involving sequential measurement at seven points in time—the first, during the summer prior to the freshman year; the second, during orientation week; and again near the end of each school year; and a final inquiry, a mailed questionnaire about specialty choice, which was completed during the first weeks of residency training.

Although the literature on professional socialization contains many theory fragments and diverse empirical studies that deal with delimited aspects of the total subject, a comprehensive generic framework that analyzes the interplay of changing personality and social structure has rarely been applied to a specific case study. To achieve such a goal has been my ambition.

The conceptual framework utilized in studying the personal effects of medical socialization consists of the following components: first, the *socializees*, the recruits who comprise the trainee clientele; second, the *social organization* as socializing environment; third, the *socializing process*, the evolving engagement of individual socializees in the workings of the socializing system; and, finally, the *socialization outcome*, the developmental personality changes that occur as a result of participation in the socializing system. In this regard I have benefited from Daniel Levinson's

(1967) insightful essay entitled "Medical Education and the Theory of Adult Socialization."

The study design utilizes time, that is, stages of medical training, as the sole independent or antecedent variable. All other measures, such as the many attitudes, values, and experiences that are amenable to change, are analyzed in temporal perspective.

In conducting this research, I have tried to combine methods of field-work with individual case analyses. Among the study population, for example, I personally conducted and tape-recorded 229 (of a possible 239) open-ended interviews (lasting from one and one-half to three hours), administered serially a battery of standardized psychological tests and attitude scales, and collected field notes as a participant observer.

In exploring the psychosocial interior of medical professionalization, I have depended largely upon the perceptions of those undergoing the experience. To capture an emotional feel of this training adventure, as well as an intellectual understanding, I tried to immerse myself in the inner world of the medical student, to perceive and feel as he or she does. While this approach may have beneficial results from both a practical and a theoretical standpoint, it does present a partisan view of social reality, a view which may at times differ markedly from that of the administration and faculty.

At the same time, however, I tried to sensitize myself to the faculty viewpoint by inviting leading administrators and educators from each medical school in the United States and Canada to attend a week-long conference on the topic "Psychosocial Aspects of Medical Training." My study has profited from the shared experiences of the 97 participants who represented 60 medical schools.

Although it depicts a case study in a particular institution, a medical school in the Eastern United States, the book benefits from insights gained in supplemental interviews with medical trainees at a West Coast medical school—especially with women and ethnic/racial minorities who, unfortunately, were in short supply in my study population—and from practicing physicians who offered retrospective views.

In undertaking this ambitious project, however, my motives have not been solely academic; practical considerations have also propelled me. By studying the ways students adjust to medical school and how their personalities are affected—and changed—by that training, I hope to chart for prospective students a clear and realistic assessment of training vicissitudes. That is, I wish to keep them from falling victim to the ever-present romantic hyperbole.

The medical profession has for generations been enveloped in a romantic aura. Since the early days of the nineteenth century, the popular image of the medical doctor has been that of a stalwart and dedicated person who would travel miles to patients through storm and dark of night—by horse and buggy if roads were passable, on foot if not. He (for in those days a doctor was, almost without exception, male) was believed to be an individual of steel who was never bothered by the sleep he did not get or the pay he did get in the form of setting hens or sacks of turnips or merely promises and appreciation. He was perceived as gentle and comforting and uncomplaining.

The physical surroundings of this stereotyped American idol have been modernized, and women are entering the field of medicine in increasing numbers, but the basic concept is much the same. Television has been particularly active in perpetuating the stereotype of a god-like super-human who performs miracles in antiseptic edifices with technology constantly deepening the pool of available knowledge.

It is true that physicians do accomplish miracles with the aid of steadily improving diagnostic tools and new techniques. And they *are* for the most part dedicated, hard-working people. However, the glamour and heroics of a doctor's life, as portrayed by television, folklore, and other means, are exaggerated, while the struggle to become a physician, at times almost overwhelmingly difficult for many students, is understated or ignored. It is a disservice to beginning medical students to allow them to start their careers with unrealistic expectations about the years that lie between the undergraduate degree and the coveted title of "doctor." Many idealistic medical students become perplexed and disillusioned while trying to adjust from what they expected to what *is*. My own study supports this statement. The enthusiasm expressed at the onset of training by the medical students comprising my study population was soon replaced by varying degrees of disenchantment.

Throughout the past five decades, an average of about 5 to 10 percent of all students have dropped out of medical school each year, a process costly to all concerned (Gough and Hall, 1975). Although there is less attrition from American medical schools now than in former years, more than 700 students currently withdraw each year (Crowley, 1975b). Since this country is suffering from a shortage of trained doctors, any reduction in this number could have great practical significance. If reading this book causes a few would-be students to realize in advance that they are unsuited for a medical career, or, conversely, encourages them to press onward, it will have performed a valuable service.

Representative studies indicate that another 20 to 30 percent of medical students who do not drop out of school continue at the expense of their emotional, physical, or marital health. These students are seen by a staff psychiatrist at some point during their training, and there are undoubtedly many others who could benefit from professional counseling. Even among those who complete medical school without apparent serious problems, most are not strangers to feelings of self-doubt, inferiority, and insecurity. They are, in short, human.

Beginning students perceive physicians as an elite group possessing superior qualities of intellect and personality. They also view their class-mates—especially those who have earned graduate degrees—as mental giants. This feeling is intensified when it is pointed out in the dean's traditional welcoming speech, as it often is, that their class is the most highly qualified of any class ever admitted. To cover up their own feelings of inferiority, students try to impress one another with their brilliance and medical aptitude. Unfortunately, this role-playing reinforces their anxieties and sometimes paralyzes their learning processes. By the time students gain sufficient perspective to understand that many problems they encounter are not the direct result of their personal deficiencies, it is some-times too late.

Because I am writing not only for the social scientist interested in professional socialization but also for the prospective medical student and others interested in medical education, I have tried to avoid technical jargon and have relegated most statistical data to footnotes. Both to en-hance readability and to keep the narrative close to the reality of the socialization experience, I have incorporated many quotations and illustra-tive materials.

It is my hope that all who read this book will find in it something of value and interest—whether they be academicians, students, or the public that is ultimately to be served. Medical trainees are, after all, the future guardians of the people's health, and it is they who will determine the quality of health care in our rapidly changing world. Therefore, none can discount the significance of the journey through medical school nor watch with disinterest the intriguing process whereby students who struggle to master medicine are transformed into physicians.

Acknowledgments

DURING THE YEARS required to complete this study, I have benefited greatly from colleagues and staff who have generously provided helpful suggestions, administrative support, and technical assistance.

First, I acknowledge the agencies that provided the initial financial support via research grants—the National Institute of Mental Health (grants MH 15454 and MH 19292) and the National Fund for Medical Education (grant 884-348). Later assistance came from the California Department of Health and the University of California, Los Angeles. Executives of the latter agencies were consistently supportive; in this regard I thank Herbert Dörken, Marshall R. Hanson, Louis Jolyon West, Ransom J. Arthur, Charles V. Keeran, Michael T. McGuire, and Ralph W. Glorioso. During the planning and implementation stage Robert L. Tuttle and Lucille W. Hutaff were particularly helpful.

A superb staff has facilitated the many technical aspects of the project. Blake P. Boyle, Lois S. Starr, and Michael P. Compton did a lion's share of the coding, tabulating, and preliminary data analyses. Editing and proofing were accomplished by Catherine Jackson, P. Jeri Walsh, Katherine K. Haydock, and Lou L. Hartney. Melvin C. Oathout provided library services and double-checked the accuracy of references. Indexing was completed by Lou L. Hartney. Rachael Lowder, Jerold J. Barentsen, and Katherine K. Haydock handled myriad business details. Interview transcriptions were completed by Lorraine M. Turnbull, who also typed the many revised drafts to perfection. I am deeply appreciative of the efficiency and congeniality that have consistently characterized these associates.

Louis P. Stein, Lawrence J. Goldman, and Pauline S. Powers each assisted in obtaining important ancillary data that immeasurably strengthened three of the chapters. An additional chapter benefited from the technical help of Harrison G. Gough and Wallace B. Hall, who, at the Institute of Personality Assessment and Research, University of California at Berkeley, interpreted results of the California Psychological Inventory.

Donald M. Hayes, Douglas R. Coombs, Gary Greenberg, and Blake P. Boyle read earlier drafts of the manuscript and made helpful suggestions. William Glance has been generous in providing technical information about the study institution, and Robert P. Liberman has been gracious in offering answers to my inquiries about technical features of medical practice.

Finally, my thanks to the medical students who for several years completed research forms, answered seemingly endless questions, and tolerated my participant observations. For their friendship and willingness to give precious time and share intimate feelings and experiences, I owe them an enormous debt.

PART I

MEDICAL SOCIALIZATION:
A CASE STUDY

1. Studying the Socialization of Medical Students

Going through medical school is like getting your hand caught in a meat grinder. It just keeps grinding and scooping up more of you as it goes. You gradually get bundled up into a processed package and pop out as a doctor. (A senior)

THIS IS THE STORY of an entire class of students who were training to become physicians at a medical school in the Eastern United States. Besides sharing professors, courses, and clinical events, they also experienced together a myriad of changing views and outlooks as the dynamic processes of medical professionalization took place. It is this status passage, through which untrained students are transformed into doctors, that I, as a sociologist with a lively interest in professional socialization, followed closely for several fascinating years.

STUDY SETTING

As is the case with most medical schools, the institution at which I conducted my longitudinal study is associated with a university and a teaching hospital. There a large variety of medical problems are presented by the more than 20,000 patients admitted annually, and the outpatient clinic treats an additional 100,000 patients each year. Affiliations with other community health services also strengthen specific training programs within the medical center.

In content and length, the curriculum at this institution resembles the model utilized at most medical colleges—approximately two years of basic medical sciences followed by two years devoted to the clinical specialties of medicine. As in many other medical schools, however, revisions are con-

stantly being implemented to meet the demands of students and society.[1] *
Fifteen departments, each chaired by a professor, share in the curriculum
(e.g., anatomy, physiology, psychiatry, surgery). In addition to the full-time
teaching staff of physicians and surgeons, private practitioners from the
entire state volunteer their services to clinical departments. An attending
staff of more than 300 physicians participates in patient care and teaching
programs. Straight and mixed internship programs [2] are available at the
hospital, and the medical center offers 17 training programs for residents
(e.g., neurosurgery, otolaryngology, urology).

Each applicant to the medical school must take the Medical College
Admission Test (MCAT) sponsored by the Association of American Medical Colleges. Written evaluations by previous instructors and personal
interviews at the medical school are also taken into consideration by the
Committee on Admissions, in addition to the applicant's academic performance and MCAT scores. The degree of Doctor of Medicine is conferred upon those who satisfactorily complete four years of study in the
medical sciences and who have passed Parts I and II of the examination
given by the National Board of Medical Examiners.

MY ROLE

My first exposure to medical school came when I, with nine other
nonmedical behavioral scientists and two physicians, was awarded a postdoctoral fellowship to explore ways in which our subject expertise could be
incorporated into the medical curriculum. For six weeks we attended
orientation lectures delivered by 25 different medical specialists, and also
accompanied a variety of physicians and fourth-year medical students as
they went about their clinical activities. This intensive exposure to the
inner world of clinical practice and training, the busy wards, the surgery
and delivery rooms, and the private clinics, stimulated many more questions
than could readily be answered.

The opportunity to pursue answers to these questions came when I was
later offered a faculty position at the medical center. This position kept me
in close physical proximity to medical personnel and made me privy to
inside information about the inner workings of medical education.

My first task was to become thoroughly acquainted with previous research in the field of medical education. Consequently, I spent much of
the next year in reading about this subject and in lecturing to medical
students and becoming better acquainted with them. What I read and

* Numbered notes appear at the end of each chapter.

what I observed seemed worlds apart. Most of the research papers contained a good deal of data, but appeared to lack "feel" or affect. It seemed clear that a systematic study of the subjective aspects in medical training was needed if I were to understand fully the evolution of layman to physician. I therefore elected to carry out such a study with one class of medical students, observing them through all four years of their training. Unofficially, I had prepared for this study for a year; officially, it began in the summer of 1967, when members of the entering class of 1971 received my welcoming letter and attitude scales designed to assess their expectations of medical school.

In undertaking this study, I had several advantages: As a member of the faculty, I had the cooperation of the administration and the faculty, yet I was far enough removed from their daily affairs to maintain a detached perspective; and I had already established amiable relationships with students in the previous class, thus forming a basis of support for my study population. As a junior member of the faculty in a nontraditional department (Behavioral Sciences), I played only a minor role in the students' training experience.

I launched my study with full awareness of the difficulties inherent in establishing and maintaining rapport with a large group over a lengthy period of time. I did not anticipate immediate problems, for students are usually idealistic and eager to please during the first weeks of medical school. But I knew, from observing their predecessors, that it would not take long for them to acquire a defensive, resistant attitude.[3]

In dealing with students as research subjects, I tried to keep them from feeling pressured. If one failed to respond to my invitation for an interview, I asked only once more. I also made certain students knew that their particular responses would not be identified even though their views and experiences would be reflected in my writings.

I tried to make sure that all participating students benefited from our interactions. To this end, I let them know that I was available at any time for personal counseling or other help. I wrote letters of recommendation, arranged extracurricular learning experiences for them to share, and tried to be helpful in other ways. Most important, I made certain that they knew how much I appreciated their cooperation in helping me prepare a book that might benefit future medical students. As a result, some came to view this project as theirs as much as mine, and most were congenial and co-operative throughout the entire study.

Especially during the first two years, they seemed to enjoy the interview experience. By providing anxious students an opportunity to unwind emotionally—or, as one expressed it, "to vent my spleen"—I apparently was able, through these interviews, to meet their need to release pent-up feelings and anxieties. In later years, when the need to ventilate was less urgent, students continued to cooperate largely because of the personal relationship established during those difficult early years of adjustment.

For the senior-year interviews, I repeated the same battery of psychological tests that were taken during freshman orientation—tests requiring four to five hours of tedious paperwork. It was rewarding when nearly 80 percent of the seniors took part in this final phase. When I finally taped my last personal interviews with the members of the class and collected lengthy test data, I realized how much these students had enriched my life, personally and professionally.

DESIGN OF THE STUDY

Objectives and Approach

Since my initial aim was to obtain emotional as well as intellectual understanding of what students undergo in medical school, it was clear that the principal sources of information could not be paper-and-pencil data. Research subjects, especially students, who are veterans of many "tests," are not likely to reveal their anxieties, feelings, and thoughts in response to a written questionnaire. To gain a comprehensive view of their attitudes and feelings, I realized that it would be necessary to allow senses, intellect, and emotions to become thoroughly immersed in a relationship with the research subjects over an extended period of time.[4]

In addition to wanting to know how students adjust to medical school, I also wished to learn more about the changes in attitudes, values, and behavioral styles associated with their status transition. My goal was akin to that of the entomologist studying the transformation of caterpillars into butterflies. Although the developmental changes among students are social and psychological rather than biological, they are no less fascinating. An adequate perspective on such an evolutionary process obviously requires systematic and repeated observations of the same individuals over a period of time; so my study was necessarily a longitudinal one.[5]

A further objective was to report the socialization process from the viewpoint of those undergoing the experience. As such, the study has a phenomenological emphasis, one that seeks to portray the realities of medical training as seen by students. My investigation was designed to avoid structuring student views. That is, I did not want to fit their views and comments into response categories previously developed by myself or others. So the interview schedule was set up to insure a systematic coverage of topics, but it contained very few preset response categories. Instead, I asked leading open-ended questions and probed until I understood both what the students thought and how intense their feelings were.* Verbal responses were tape recorded.

My final objective was to study the interpersonal dynamics among the principal actors in this drama. Although I could have traced the development of specific individuals in the class more easily, the unit of analysis I chose for this study was the group—one entire class which shared a common experience of entering and passing through a formal socialization system that had predetermined stages designed to change the participants into physicians.[6]

An entering class of medical students is not dissimilar to a military company whose members must depend upon one another for well-being. Since they sometimes feel that they are behind enemy lines, these students share a unique and intense group experience. The resulting situational adjustments and long-term personality developments are intimately entwined with their group experiences—and to overlook these experiences is to miss the flavor of medical socialization.

My approach to studying an entire class of medical students has been to try to understand the student culture or the collective conscience of the group; [7] to discover, if possible, the patterns of thinking and behaving that are common to the class at its various stages and under varying circumstances. While this approach obviously raises logistic problems in collecting and presenting the data, these problems are offset by the more comprehensive view of the socialization experience, a view that is not available in the existing literature on medical socialization.

Collecting Data

Personal interviews with the students supplied most of the information for this book, but, as previously mentioned, additional information came from the attitude scales and psychological tests and from my field notes as a participant observer.

Attitude Scales and Standardized Psychological Tests

When I mailed all members of the incoming class letters indicating my desire to follow their class in a systematic study throughout its entire

---

* The lack of preset responses undoubtedly affected the numerical results. Given a similar population, a larger number of respondents will no doubt identify a known trait when specifically prompted by a printed questionnaire, for instance, than when simply asked an open-ended and general question. An example is the question, "What type of person is attracted to surgery?" Had the students been asked to complete a printed checklist of descriptive features, it is likely that a significantly larger number of respondents would have indicated "action- and result-oriented," for example. It is probably safe to assume that identification of the same trait by a few students through unstructured probing carries as much weight as identification of that trait by a larger number of persons prompted by a questionnaire.

sojourn in medical school, I enclosed a copy of Hutchins' *Medical College Environment Index* (n.d.), listing 69 descriptive statements about medical school. I asked that each student respond to the MCEI statements as he or she imagined medical school to be. In addition, I enclosed two scales developed by Leonard Eron (1955) to measure cynicism and humanitarianism. Nearly all of the study group completed these tests.[8]

During orientation sessions held soon after their arrival, I asked students to complete a battery of standardized psychological tests including the *California Psychological Inventory* (Gough, 1967), *Study of Values* (Allport, Vernon, and Lindzey, 1960), *Survey of Interpersonal Values* (Gordon, 1960), *Adjective Check List* (Gough and Heilbrun, 1965), and *The Social Insight Test* (Chapin, 1967). This test battery, which requires four or five hours to complete, was repeated at the end of the senior year, as was previously mentioned. The Eron and Hutchins tests were administered at the end of each school year. The percentage of students who participated in these tests each year is shown in Table 1-1.

Interviews

Each member of the class was interviewed toward the latter part of each academic year. (The interviews were conducted at this time so that students would have experienced the full variety of courses and clinical services offered during the year.) Since students were probed on more than 200 items of information and elaborated a good deal, the tape-recorded interviews varied in length from one and one-half to three hours. The interviews were guided by the use of pertinent questions that had been categorized and arranged into topical categories—such as student–faculty relations. Over the four years, 229 interviews out of a possible 239 (95.8 percent) were successfully completed. All but two of the interviews were personally conducted by me.

Since the initial interviews revealed that students were inclined to give rational rather than subjective responses, I tried to wean them from their exam-taking mentality by stressing that I was interested only in their experiences and their feelings about medical school and was in no way testing the extent of their knowledge. I also emphasized that they should not feel inhibited or reserved, but should feel free to respond openly, as though they were chatting with an understanding friend.

For the most part the interviews appeared to be successful in probing the affective component, and students' responses seemed to me to be genuine and spontaneous. Participants appeared to be generally relaxed except when certain topics (for example, psychosexual problems) made them uncomfortable or carried overtones of personal failure. At these times, students would sometimes sidestep my questions or give conventional responses so as to look good or normal in my eyes. Not wanting to struc-

TABLE 1-1. Percentage of Students Participating in Tests Each Year.

Test Name		Test Year			
	Pre-freshman (N = 62)	Freshman (N = 62)	Sophomore (N = 59)	Junior (N = 59)	Senior (N = 59)
Medical College Environment Index	95.2	96.8	84.7	71.2	72.9
Cynicism	95.2	98.3	84.7	76.3	76.3
Humanitarianism	95.2	98.3	84.7	76.3	76.3
California Psychological Inventory	95.2	—	—	—	71.2
Study of Values	93.5	—	—	—	71.2
Survey of Interpersonal Values	90.3	—	—	—	76.3
Adjective Check List	93.5	—	—	—	76.3
Social Insight Test	95.2	—	—	—	76.3

ture their responses to fit my expectations,[9] I tried *nonverbally* to show that I sympathized with their values and attitudes, and when it was necessary to make a comment, I tried to be supportive of what they were saying.

Participant Observation

In addition to the interview data and the written tests, I made my own observations as an involved participant, a neophyte faculty member at the medical school. The commonplace of medical school was new to me. Only in this regard can I claim any measure of personal objectivity. Certainly my own impressions color the presentation and interpretation of findings, since the interview materials are necessarily filtered through my own psychological set. Thus this book portrays not only the students' perceptions of medical school realities but also my perceptions of their perceptions.

Although I have tried to be cautious and rigorously methodological, conducting an antiseptic investigation as a detached observer was not my goal. Such an approach would cause me to miss the affective components of student adjustment and professional development and would probably hamper my efforts to achieve the rapport necessary for a longitudinal survey of this nature.[10]

But personal involvement also has disadvantages. Since I was an integral part of the study environment, my attitudes and values may be reflected in some of the responses given by students. I do not mean to imply, however, that I had any significant impact upon their training, for as a junior member of the faculty, I had no real authority in the inner workings of the medical center, even though I was acutely aware of what was going on.

Other observational data were also contributed by two medical students who, during the summer months, assisted me as research fellows. Following his sophomore year, Lawrence J. Goldman took extensive field notes concerning his own feelings and attitudes as he adjusted to his initial clinical experiences in the hospital's Intensive Care Unit (ICU). There he was exposed for the first time to seriously ill, postoperative, and dying patients. Each day he observed and recorded how he and others working in the ICU reacted to and coped with these emotionally stressful experiences.[11]

The other student, Louis P. Stein, made lengthy field notes during his fourth year on the inner workings of medical student culture. These notes, dealing with the informal social structure and dynamics that pervaded the class throughout the entire four years, were acquired by Stein during informal group discussions with his classmates.[12]

Processing and Analyzing Data

Students frequently asked me how I was going to make anything out of all the data I was acquiring. At times I asked myself the same question, because the sheer bulk of the information threatened to inundate me.[13] A variety of methods were used for processing and analyzing these materials, and with each step, new perspectives unfolded.

The material tape-recorded during the interviews was transcribed onto the standard-format forms I had used as the interview schedule. My notes about the students' nonverbal responses were also penciled on these forms. These transcripts were coded with identification numbers; no names appeared.

Code categories were constructed on the basis of an inductive content analysis of all responses to a particular question—like sorting out similar playing cards from a deck. As previously mentioned, I avoided fitting student responses to a priori constructs because I wanted to create a picture of what was in their minds.

My guidelines required that each set of code categories pertaining to a given interview question be both exhaustive and mutually exclusive. This meant that every response had to fit unambiguously into only one category of the set. The coding was complicated by the fact that the same student often gave more than one response to a given question. For example, a participant might name a variety of characteristics in describing persons who select surgery as a specialty. Thus one student described surgeons as "an egotistical bunch, but they don't like sitting on their asses the way internal medicine people do." Since this comment was judged to fit two response categories, it was coded under both: (1) action- and result-oriented; and (2) egotistical.[14]

To assure high coding reliability, every response recorded during the first two years was coded independently by three different people. Whenever a fourth person, the coding supervisor,[15] agreed with all three coders on any response, the coding decision was considered 100-percent reliable, and a score of 1.0 was given. One dissenting opinion among the three coders was ignored if the coding supervisor solidly agreed with the other two. In such instances, the disagreeing coder was simply assumed to be in error. Stated another way, a coding reliability of 0.75 was considered acceptable. If any two disagreed with the other two, all were asked to check for error by independently recoding the response. If the reliability was still less than 0.75, the code categories were assumed to be ambiguous and were revised; coding then began anew.

This method allowed us to obtain high coding reliability: 0.88 in the freshman year and 0.93 in the sophomore year. Coding reliability was equally high during the third and fourth years when it was checked on every fifth response, even though only one seasoned coder and the coding supervisor verified the code categories during this time.

Because the same questions were repeated each year, changes in student attitudes are observable. In order to analyze patterns in student development, responses have been quantified and tabulated. These patterns are described in the text. Although the typical patterns are generally emphasized, minority views are sometimes discussed at length because of the unique insights they provide. For journalistic reasons, I have tried to avoid tabular display; but for those interested, basic statistics are presented in footnotes.

To avoid weighing down the text with myriad numbers, I have generalized by using the conventional words *few*, *some*, *many*, and *most*. They may be interpreted as follows:

Few—not more than 10 percent of the respondents.
Some—more than 10 percent but less than 25 percent.
Many—more than 25 percent but less than 50 percent.
Most—more than 50 percent; a majority.
Typically—used interchangeably with "most."

Limitations of Study

Naturally, this study, like all others, has its limitations. Although four consecutive interviews were held with each participant, a more comprehensive view of medical socialization would ideally have had two additional interviews—one before the beginning of medical school and another during the internship year; but this was not feasible within the time limitations of the study.*

It became apparent during the senior-year interviews that although students would soon have the doctor status, their developmental process was not yet complete. They had made great strides but were not yet full-fledged doctors, psychologically speaking. Although I felt that the study should continue for at least another year, I finally had to reject the idea as being impractical. I did manage, however, to stay in touch with the study population by mail until all had completed their internships and were accepted into residency training programs.[16]

Another limitation of the study is the scant attention given to the views and experiences of minority populations. Minimal representation of women and racial/ethnic minorities in the class I studied made it difficult to generalize about their unique problems and experiences. Before completing this book, however, I tried to sensitize myself to these students and their views by interviewing minority representatives from each class at a large medical school on the West Coast. Fortunately, others have recently writ-

---

* As our paper-and-pencil test data indicate, some of the most profound challenges and changes occur during the first weeks of school. But several months of intensive work were required to interview the entire class, and the new arrivals were accessible only for a brief period before they began their course work. Also, to hire an interviewing staff would have required funds that were not yet available and would also have prevented me from developing a personal rapport with the students that would last throughout the ensuing four years.

ten about the medical training of minority populations, and I refer the reader to these sources.[17]

Because the findings of this study are derived from a relatively small class in only one of the more than 100 medical schools that existed in the United States at the time of this study, the limitations of the case-study method apply to these findings. Obviously an intensive case study of one particular class of students has advantages for in-depth analysis. But the peculiarities of one medical school may not exist at another; thus one must use caution in generalizing these results. Even within the same school, furthermore, particular classes may have distinctive "personalities" of their own.[18]

The medical curriculum in various schools has undergone more changes in the past few years than during the previous half century.[19] Nevertheless, personal conversations with faculty and students from numerous medical schools and my reading on this subject cause me to believe that there are many more cultural uniformities than unique features among the various schools in the United States and Canada.[20] Although each school may have its peculiarities, medical schools in the United States seem very similar in basic social structure, so it is likely that most students have a similar experience. Faculty members frequently move from one medical school to another with the result that a cross-fertilization and standardization of ideas takes place. So, while I do not wish to imply that the particular findings in this study population match in detail those that might be obtained at other medical schools, it appears that the basic features of medical student experiences throughout the country are not strikingly dissimilar.[21]

CONCEPTUAL BACKGROUND FOR THE STUDY

In addition to having practical value for medical students and their teachers and administrators, this book, as I have mentioned, is intended to contribute to an understanding of the psychosocial dynamics of professional socialization, particularly the processes whereby students develop the necessary attitudes and skills for assuming the weighty responsibilities and challenges of the medical role. The concepts discussed in this section provide a background for analyzing the social system that shapes students into doctors.

Socialization

In sociopsychological (as opposed to political) parlance, the term "socialization" refers to the social conditioning of the human personality, as contrasted with physical maturation.[22] It pertains to the process whereby a person internalizes the knowledge, skills, values, and behaviors deemed appropriate by socializing agents, those who instruct or influence (parents, teachers, etc.). In other words, socialization is the process of transforming a human being into a self who possesses a sense of identity and is endowed with appropriate attitudes, values, and ways of thinking, and with other personal yet social attributes.

The familiar concepts of *status*, *role*, and *self-image* are basic for understanding socialization processes. By *status* I mean a social position (doctor, for example) that is set in the structure of a group before a given individual comes along to occupy it. By contrast, a *role* is that which a person in a given status is expected to do. Perceiving oneself as an incumbent of a particular status (doctor) and feeling comfortable in the enactment of the appropriate role (diagnosing illness, prescribing remedies, etc.) is, of course, a social, not a biologic, derivative. This *self-image*, acquired through interaction with others, determines one's feelings of personal adequacy in the performance of the expected role.

Informal Socialization Process

The internalization of status and role definitions, as well as basic values, attitudes, and behavioral traits associated with self-identities, often comes not by formal instruction or conscious design but through informal processes, such as imitation and identification, and is reinforced by social sanctions (rewards and punishments). These informal and sometimes unconscious processes begin, of course, in childhood through interaction with significant others such as parents.

Although an infant has no conception of sex status, for example, his parents see the world as composed of two basic types of people—male and female—and they expect different behavior from each type (Coombs, 1968b). Parents pass on these differential role expectations, acquired through a lifetime of experience, in much the same manner as they received them. Thus, once a male child recognizes his own status, he observes and imitates the role behavior of others who have similar status. When he learns that his actions affect the attitudes of others toward him, he becomes sensitive to what they think. His concept of self consists, then, of status definitions that he imagines others have of him; thus, he views himself as he imagines significant others see him. To enhance his own self-esteem and to gain the approval of others, he behaves as he believes others expect a person of his status to behave. The resulting self-concept, which consists of internalized status definitions, is the unifying feature of personality and the end result of successful socialization. If one has learned to play successfully a role that corresponds to a particular status with which he identifies himself, he naturally feels comfortable with that status and role.

Formally Organized Socialization

Although personalities are significantly shaped by such informal social-ization processes, especially during infancy and early childhood, formally organized approaches (schools, for example) also prepare persons for future roles.[23] After the age of five or six, considerable learning takes place in formal organizations explicitly designed to change people.

Like organizations that process things, the organizations that process people have a point of entry, a series of movements or advancements through the system, and a point of exit. Their goal, of course, is to turn out a product that has greater social worth than it had at entry. Schools, for instance, seek to develop the potentialities of those who pass through the system, and mental hospitals and prisons try to change people by teach-ing them more appropriate roles than those with which they enter.[24] The formal responsibility of such agencies is to influence participants so that they leave the setting with different attitudes, values, and skills from those they had initially. Socialization agents, those persons who act on behalf of the organization, educate, train, or modify the recruits. Their task is to change people, to prepare them for new positions by teaching the appro-priate skills and attitudes required of persons in these positions.

Some socialization organizations have serial patterns while others have disjunctive ones (Brim and Wheeler, 1966). In serial patterns, organiza-tional recruits (freshmen, for example) are preceded by others who have already been through the same process (for example, sophomores and up-perclassmen) and who can therefore help the neophytes to adjust to the socialization experience (for instance, by pointing out ways to "beat the sys-tem"). In this way these predecessors can have a major impact on the recruits and can significantly influence the socializing system. In the dis-junctive pattern (for example, a summer training institute), recruits do not follow in the footsteps of their predecessors. Clearly, the medical school pattern fits the serial rather than the disjunctive pattern.

Another distinguishing trait of people-changing agencies pertains to whether they process recruits individually or collectively. When a group or cohort, such as a class of medical students, is the target, the socialization process may be significantly enriched or otherwise altered because recruits can arrive at collective solutions to their problems. This collective action provides emotional support for recruits when they are threatened or other-wise confronted with difficulty by socializing agents (for example, faculty). The peer group may also contribute significantly to the learning process. In professional schools, for example, students may learn as much from each other as they do from the faculty.

Formalized entrance requirements exist in socialization organizations, so that recruits usually have in common a standard basis for their recruit-ment. Because of this, they are often similar in social background and lifestyle. Much of the flavor of recruits' interactions is provided by this similarity or occasional lack of it, and this can also influence their socialization experiences and the outcome of such experiences. The informal social network that spontaneously emerges among the recruits provides a context for dealing with the formal socialization experience. This collective consciousness or social climate, then, sets the overall feeling and tone through which formal socialization objectives are accomplished.

The Medical School as a Socializing Agency

In sociological terms, the medical school is a formal socializing organization whose mission is to process medical aspirants so that they can function effectively and confidently in their new status as physicians. Recruits have a specified time in which to enter and exit, and, within this time, they move through clearly delineated processing stages. Each stage is designed to expose participants to designated experiences that help them acquire the appropriate skills, attitudes, and behavioral dispositions required for success in their future status. During each stage recruits are molded to fit the predetermined objectives of the socialization agents (the faculty) whose mandate it is to prepare future doctors. Since the pattern is both serial and collective, however, classmates and other students may also play a significant role in how learning is experienced and interpreted.

In less technical terms, our objective is to understand the intricate workings of this social machinery which, as the senior says in the epigram at the beginning of the chapter, keeps grinding away at students until eventually each one gets "bundled up into a processed package and pops out as a doctor." By studying an entire class of medical students from the time they were accepted for admission until they exit as physicians, I seek to foster an understanding of the psychosocial dynamics of this socializing system, both formally (how it is designed to work) and informally (how it actually works within the context of interpersonal relationships that spontaneously emerge). By examining the views and feelings of an entire class during its total medical school experience, I hope to illuminate the subtleties inherent in this fascinating social evolution.

Previous Studies of Medical Socialization

The sociology of medical professionalization was born when Robert K. Merton published his classical essay, "Some Preliminaries to a Sociology of Medical Education" (Merton, 1957), and related introductory studies (Merton, Reader, and Kendall, 1957). Earlier research had focused primarily on practical issues relating to student selection and achievement. Little consideration was given to the processes whereby such students acquire the professional role (Bloom, 1965).

Since then, two divergent yet complementary research approaches have stimulated interest in the attitudinal changes occurring in medical school and the events that produce them (Bloom, 1963). The first approach utilized a longitudinal design to trace changes in student attitudes throughout the course of medical training. The most provocative work was done by Leonard Eron (1955, 1958), who, using paper-and-pencil tests, noted an increase in cynicism and a decrease in humanitarianism when contrasting freshmen with seniors. Yet he found no such trends when he compared nursing and law students.

The advantages of the first approach are that its design is simple and that it yields quantitative information regarding attitudinal changes over a period of time. The disadvantage is that it deals with a narrow range of variables, the data from which rarely generate interpretative insights; that is, the investigator must look elsewhere for explanation. For instance, Eron postulated that the observed increase in cynicism and decline in humanitarianism are due to the neurotic anxieties allegedly typical of medical students.

The question of whether medical school does, in fact, foster cynicism while weakening or destroying idealism and humanitarianism has been the subject of an interesting series of studies and essays stimulated by Eron's work. The findings of some studies seem to substantiate his conclusions (Gordon and Mensh, 1962; deBrabander and Leon, 1968); but those of others contradict them (Miller and Erwin, 1959).[25] None, however, has disputed his claim that medical students lose much of their initial idealism. "That some form of disenchantment occurs," Bloom (1963, p. 87) notes, "is too universally reported to ignore." Still remaining, however, are such debatable questions as the following: What changes, if any, occur in replacing the initial idealism? And what events and processes account for such changes?

The second research approach is exemplified by *Boys in White: Student Culture in Medical School* (Becker et al., 1961), which is a detailed case study of a single institution. In studying the sociocultural milieu at the University of Kansas Medical School, these investigators utilized participant observation and discussion with medical students. The complexities of student subculture were investigated through intensive fieldwork rather than by a "test and run" strategy, to trace specific attitudinal traits. The researchers' focus was on the interactions among students and their social environment; they analyzed the collective understanding, perspectives, and working agreements that develop informally among student communities in adapting and finding solutions to their common problems.

The richness of the Becker data easily generates plausible explanations. The apparent increase in cynicism, for instance, is explained as being a situational adjustment rather than a permanently fixed personality trait carried into medical practice (Becker and Geer, 1958; Becker, 1964). Student cynicism, they say, is due to disillusioned reactions to the unexpected academic realities of medical school. For, instead of assuming responsibility for patients as they had imagined they would do, idealistic students find an academic dilemma of major proportion. However:

> As school comes to an end, the cynicism specific to the school situation also comes to an end, and their original and more generalized idealism about medicine comes to the fore again, though within a framework of more realistic alternatives. Their idealism is now more informed although less selfless (Becker and Geer, 1958, p. 55).

Subsequent research (Gray, Moody, and Newman, 1965) tends to support the view that medical school graduates have less cynicism and more humanitarianism than they had as medical students.

The intensive fieldwork of the Kansas study, performed over a period of six months, has added significantly to the understanding of the problematic issues involved in socializing medical students and has illuminated the following matters with which students must deal during the course of their school experience: the existence of ambiguity and uncertainty in a profession that prides itself on its rationality and competence; the fact that the students' technical knowledge cannot be as detailed and extensive as the faculty requires; the formation of a student subculture for purposes of mutual protection and assistance; and the problems of choosing a specialty, with all its personal and career implications (Levinson, 1967, p. 262).

The Kansas study, however, tells more about student adaptation to medical school than it does about their professional development, and more about situational adjustment than about the enduring changes that students undergo in various socializing conditions. Levinson notes,

> The authors' primary interest is in the young man's effort to become a medical student and to manage the demands and stresses confronting those who have the status of student in this organization. The longer-term career consequences are of less immediacy both for the student and for the investigator. Or, put another way, their focus is not primarily upon the students as budding physicians but rather upon students collectively as low-status workers trying actively to adapt and "make out" within a strongly hierarchical organization (Levinson, 1967, p. 259).

Present Study

My intent in this study has been to incorporate the strengths of the aforementioned studies and of other pioneering efforts. Without neglecting minority views, I have tried to capture the collective conscience (or student culture) that emerges from and is altered by the various experiences that confront students. In doing so I endeavored to ascertain basic changes in attitudes and values that affect subsequent medical careers. Because it is not restricted to an elaborate analysis of only a few variables,[26] the study deals in a broad way with the interplay of environmental contexts and the emerging personality outlook of the physician-to-be.

As mentioned in the preface, the theoretical scheme utilized is compatible with the work of Levinson (1967), and I seek to explore in the present study each dimension of this conceptual framework. Examined first are the medical recruits (or socializees) who constitute the study population—their backgrounds, their reasons for selecting medical careers, the process by which they gained admittance to medical school, and their methods of financing their medical education (Chapter 2). Then attention is turned to the primary socializing agents (Chapter 3) and the classmates who, as a collective body, alternately adapt and react to the established system (Chapter 4).

The analysis then deals with the socializing mechanisms and processes that shape medical recruits into doctors—the curriculum that represents the faculty's formalized blueprint for "building" doctors (Chapter 5), and the challenging trials and adversities inherent in the medical school experience that necessitate adaptive learning and change (Chapter 6).

The final section analyzes the emerging outcome of medical socialization by tracing the attitudinal changes that become incorporated into the personality fabric of young men and women soon to "pop out" as physicians. First, their evolving attitudes about patients are examined (Chapter 7), and then changing views about doctors and their profession are explored (Chapter 8), as well as the various medical specialties (Chapter 9). Finally, the analysis deals with the students' emerging self-attitudes (Chapter 10) and their personal attributes and values (Chapter 11). The final chapter (Chapter 12) provides a summary and interpretation of findings.

Throughout this conceptual analysis is woven the intensely human experiences of very real medical students—men and women who, as this book is read, have already blossomed into full-fledged professionals trained to meet the complex health needs of a dynamic mass society. Here, then, is the story of an entire class of medical students—a group destined to have an important impact upon the health and well-being of many.

NOTES

1. See Chapter 5 for a discussion of the medical school curriculum.
2. For the information of the nonmedical reader, a straight internship requires training for an entire 12-month period in only one medical specialty (e.g., internal medicine, surgery, or pediatrics); a mixed internship involves training in more than one specialty (e.g., 6 months in surgery and 6 months in internal medicine).
3. Such an attitude seems to be partly a defense against the damage done to

the egos of first-year medical students by the pronounced drop from the high status they enjoyed as premed students, and partly a reaction to an intense disillusionment that occurs in the first weeks of school when they discover themselves to be held in low esteem by faculty and hospital staff alike.

4. Blumer's comments concerning the subjective approach to studying social processes are apropos:

> To catch the process, the student [investigator] must take the role of the acting unit whose behavior he is studying. Since the interpretation is being made by the acting unit in terms of objects designated and appraised, meanings acquired, and decisions made, the process has to be seen from the standpoint of the acting unit. It is the recognition of this fact that makes the research work of such scholars as R. E. Park and W. I. Thomas so notable. To try to catch the interpretative process by remaining aloof as a so-called "objective" observer and refusing to take the role of the acting unit is to risk the worst kind of subjectivism—the objective observer is likely to fill in the process of interpretation with his own surmises in place of catching the process as it occurs in the experience of the acting unit which uses it. (Blumer, 1962, p. 188)

5. As a panel analysis, the research technique consisted of collecting and analyzing data through repeated interviews with a sample of individuals in a natural rather than a laboratory setting (Levenson, 1968). For discussions of this approach, see Christie and Merton (1958); and Rosenberg, Thielens, and Lazarsfeld (1961). Wall and Williams (1907) is a good source of information about such longitudinal studies. For a longitudinal field work of nursing students, see Olesen and Whittaker (1968). Also see Lesser (1974) for a unique longitudinal study of medical students presented through more than 300 artistic renderings.

6. For a longitudinal analysis of individual medical students, see Milton J. Horowitz (1964).

7. Durkheim's phrase, "collective conscience," or "collective consciousness," while not popular among some sociologists, is used to refer to the "social climate" of the class. By using this concept (Durkheim, 1938), however, I wish neither to reify it nor imply that this collective product is merely the sum of its parts. Instead I mean that the group thinking, feeling, and acting may be different from the individuals who compose it.

8. The first scale, the *Medical College Environment Index*, was developed by Edwin B. Hutchins and produced by the Association of American Medical Colleges, Evanston, Illinois. For further information on the two tests developed by Leonard D. Eron, see Eron (1955).

9. For an essay concerning how interviewers condition medical students to elicit certain attitudinal responses, see Howard S. Becker (1956).

10. That the study of Becker et al. (*Boys in White*, 1961) appears to lack insight about the affective aspects of medical socialization, as Levinson (1967) has charged, is probably due to the short-term segmental relationships the researchers had with the subjects.

11. Some of the insights resulting from this analysis are given in Chapter 6 and in Coombs and Goldman (1973).

12. Since Louis Stein was in the class that began a year earlier than my study population, his observations also allowed me to compare two classes with regard to certain attitudes. No pronounced differences were noted. Some of his observations are incorporated into Chapter 4; see also Coombs and Stein (1971).

13. Before the data processing was complete, materials involving some 365 items of information completely filled four legal-size filing cabinets. Svalastoga (1970) observes that sequential research is definitely not a one-man job but rather a task for research teams. Because of the problems and the length of time involved, he says, "Sequential research demands a continuously high level of motivation. If in doubt, that is, whether or not to engage in sequential research, the answer ought to be obvious: Do not do it."

14. See Chapter 9 for a discussion of changing student views about the surgeon.

15. Blake P. Boyle, who served as my research assistant at the time of the study, was coding supervisor throughout the entire project. His services were invaluable.

16. Although during the internship year the study population became scattered over the entire country, I kept in touch by mail and do have data on the internships and residencies entered into and the final specialty choices of my cohort. (See Chapter 9 on specialties.) Understanding of the later stages of career development was also enhanced through interviews with 13 physicians who had practiced for an average of 12 years.

17. Concerning women in medical school, see *Why Would a Girl Go Into Medicine?* (Campbell, 1974) and pertinent journal articles: Winner (1975); Nadelson and Notman (1974); Howell (1974); Gross and Crovitz (1975); Cohen and Korper (1976); Hilberman et al. (1975); Howell and Hiatt (1975); Letter (1974); Ris (1974); and Spiro (1975). On ethnic/racial minorities in medical school, see McCarthy (1975); Evans and Jackson (1976); Dresden, Collins, and Roessler (1975); Smith (1976); Macy Foundation (1975); Johnson, Smith, and Tarnoff (1975); and Gaines (1975).

18. For instance, Rothman (1972) provides evidence to support the view that "the assumption of relative stability of characteristics of medical students across classes cannot be considered as axiomatic." At Harvard, for example, Funkenstein (1968) reports that three types of students can be differentiated on the basis of career interest and aptitude: the scientist, the psychiatrist, and the clinician. In my study, however, most students were of the last type; very few showed inclination for scientific or psychiatric careers.

19. For more detailed information, see *New York Times* (1966) and Kerr (1972).

20. The similarity of problems and administrative concerns at the various schools was apparent among participants at my institute on "Psychosocial Aspects of Medical Training," as is the case each year at annual conferences of the Association of American Medical Colleges and at meetings of student groups.

21. To aid in identifying idiosyncratic features of this particular class and medi-

cal school, I have had two medical students—one from a different class in the study institution and the other from another medical school—critically read the entire manuscript and, based upon their own experiences, point out such features to me.

22. For good reviews of this subject, see Merton, Reader, and Kendall (1957); Clausen (1968); and Goslin (1969).

23. This section has benefited greatly from the essays of Brim and Wheeler (1966).

24. See, for example, Kennedy and Kerber (1972).

25. For a review of the literature on this subject, see Reeves (1964) and Gray and Newman (1961).

26. No doubt a large variety of theoretically and practically important inter-relationships exist among the hundreds of measures treated here as dependent variables. But limitations of space and time forbid such elaborate analysis here. Since these analyses are of secondary importance to my design, they must be set aside for future study.

2. Medical Recruits: A Portrait of the Study Population

We are a bunch of people who are as different as we can possibly be: Our ways of life, our schooling, and our families are all different. Our only basic similarity is our effort and desire to become doctors. (A freshman)

MY STUDY CLASS entered medical school in the fall of 1967 and graduated in the summer of 1971. There were 62 medical recruits and 58 graduates. Fifty-four of the graduates were original students and four were additions to the class. Of the original eight who did not remain with the class until graduation, two graduated at another time or another place. As Table 2-1 shows, the fluctuation in the number of students over the four years also caused a fluctuation in the number of participants in this study. The unfolding drama of adaptation and self-change among these participants was extracted from 229 interviews completed over a four-year period.

BACKGROUND CHARACTERISTICS

As the freshman suggested in the lead-in quote, recruits, being strangers, tend to view one another as entirely different. Yet when their backgrounds are examined, many similarities become apparent.

Personal and Demographic Characteristics

The 62 first-year medical students in this study were selected from some 1,600 applicants; thus each filled a position sought by 25.8 others.[1]

At the beginning of the freshman year, most students were in their early twenties. The modal age was 22. Only two students were over 25; one

23

TABLE 2-1. Four-Year Fluctuation of Study Participants.

Year of Study	Students at Beginning of Year	Changes in Student Numbers Over Year			Students Unavailable for Interview	Resulting Participants	
		Dropped [a]	Added [b]	Remaining		Number	Percent
FR 1967–68	62	3	0	59	0	59	100.0
SO 1968–69	59	1	1	59	2	57	96.6
JR 1969–70	59	3	3	59	1	58	98.3
SR 1970–71	59	1	0	58	3	55	94.8

[a] Withdrew, repeated, or transferred from school.
[b] Transferred from another school or held back from previous year.

was 26, the other 29. (Persons over 25 were not encouraged to apply as freshmen.)

All but one were Caucasian, and only 4 percent of the class were women.[2] Seventy-eight percent were Protestant, 12 percent were Jewish, and 7 percent were Catholic; those of the Mormon and Moslem faiths constituted the remainder.

One-fourth of the entering freshmen were married; but the number had increased to 41 percent by the beginning of the next school year. In the junior year, married students numbered half the class, and by graduation six out of ten students were married. During the four years, 3 percent of the class became separated or divorced from their spouses.

Slightly more than three-fourths of the entering class had been reared in the eastern part of the United States and another 15 percent hailed from the western states, principally California. The remainder came from the Midwest (5.0 percent) or a foreign country (2 percent). All but 8 percent (who came from very small towns) were reared in urban areas;[3] among these urbanites 14 percent were reared in a megalopolis. The largest number, however, came from middle-size cities having populations of 50,000 to 250,000.

Family Background

Most students considered themselves to be of middle-class origin; only one indicated an upper-class family background and two others working-class backgrounds.* Fathers' incomes were estimated by more than half the class as being $10,000 or more per year,† and by one-fifth as exceeding $20,000 annually.‡

More than half the fathers and slightly less than half the mothers had attended college. Four out of ten fathers were college graduates; 30 percent had gone on to graduate or professional school.[4] One-fourth of the mothers were college graduates; 7 percent had gone on to graduate school. Only 15 percent of the fathers and 12 percent of the mothers had not graduated from high school.

Occupations of the fathers were interestingly varied. One out of seven

---

* Students were shown a card listing various socioeconomic statuses and asked to specify which was most descriptive of their own family. Results are as follows: upper class, 1.7 percent; upper middle class, 28.9 percent; middle class, 44.1 percent; lower middle class, 20.3 percent; working class, 3.4 percent; lower class, none; and unknown, 1.7 percent.

† This figure may be compared to 37 percent of families in the United States earning less than $10,000 in 1968, reported by Smith and Crocker (1971).

‡ Actual breakdown by class: $20,000 or more, 22.0 percent; $16,000–19,999, 6.8 percent; $12,000–15,999, 18.6 percent; $8,000–11,999, 20.4 percent; $4,000–7,999, 18.6 percent; below $3,999, none; and unknown, 13.6 percent.

was a physician, and an additional 4 percent were in medically related fields. Twelve percent were in food-related businesses, and 10 percent were in the insurance field; an additional 5 percent were in each of the following: the armed services, church ministry, construction business, and education. The remainder represented such careers as furniture dealer, funeral director, steel mill inspector, farmer, and pilot, and varied from a rural mail carrier to an executive vice president of a large corporation.

Seven out of ten students represented families with fewer than four children. The typical student was either the first-born (44 percent) or an only child (14 percent);[5] two were from sets of twins whose other twin was attending another medical school. The others were mostly second-born (28 percent) or third oldest (7 percent).

Typically, the students' parents were married, living together, and getting along quite well with one another. Ten percent of the mothers were widows; another 5 percent were deceased. Only one student came from a home where both parents were deceased, and 4 percent were from families where the parents were either separated or divorced.

In contrast to the student who had lost both parents and felt his growing up thereafter was "an emotional struggle," more than half the class recalled their childhood environments as being warm and affectionate; another third had moderately happy memories. Only a few (7 percent) had unhappy memories of long duration, recalling major interpersonal conflicts with their parents.

Academic Background

Entering freshmen received their undergraduate training at a variety of American colleges and universities (see Dubé, 1974b). In all, 39 institutions of higher learning contributed to their premedical training. Only three universities contributed three or more students to the class; 13 students had attended the parent institution of the medical school. State universities were well represented, as were private universities and colleges.

Prior to medical school enrollment, all but 8 percent of the class had graduated with a B.A., B.S., or A.B. degree.[6] One out of ten had achieved the Master's degree, and 2 percent had the Ph.D. In terms of academic scholarship, 8 percent had either a perfect record (a grade-point average of 4.0 throughout all four years of undergraduate work) or were within 0.2 of a point of a perfect college record. Grade averages of one-fifth of the class exceeded 3.5 (of a possible 4.0); one-third ranged from 3.0 to 3.49; and 37 percent averaged 2.5 to 2.99.* With regard to achievement on the Medical College Admission Test (MCAT), 12 percent ranked in the 90th

---

* Five percent had grade averages of 2.5 or less.

percentile, 14 percent in the 80th percentile, 19 percent in the 70th percentile, 25 percent in the 60th percentile, and 12 percent in the 50th percentile; 18 percent fell below the 50th percentile.[7]

DECIDING ON A MEDICAL CAREER

Clearly, medical recruits have much in common. But as the freshman
earlier quoted indicates, their greatest similarity is in the desire to become
physicians. This becomes evident through exploration of such questions as:
At what point in life do recruits decide to become doctors? What factors
and events affect their decisions? What influences do their parents have
upon them? And what careers might they have chosen if medicine had not
been accessible to them? [8]

Time of Decision

The decision to become a doctor comes early in the lives of most
students. Even before entering college, three out of every five had made
that decision. Of this number, 29 percent decided during high school, and
14 percent during junior high; 21 percent recalled only that they had
"always" wanted to become doctors. One of the latter declared that he
was simply "born to be a doctor." But the desire to study medicine did not
come into sharp focus for one-third of the class until they were in college*
and not for 3 percent until they were in postgraduate training.

Influencing Factors and Events

The most influential factors attracting students into medicine were
interest in science; contact with influential physicians; favorable concept
of the doctor's status and role; comparison of a medical career with other
careers; and prior medical employment.[9]

Interest in biological sciences led more than half of the class in the
direction of a medical career.† Students found, however, that these courses,
no matter how enjoyable, did not satisfy their need for interpersonal involvement. "Being stuck away in a laboratory for pure science's sake was
not an appealing prospect," is the way one student expressed it.

---

* Seven percent decided in the freshman year, 15.2 percent in the sophomore year, 8.5
  percent in the junior year, and 1.7 percent in the senior year.
† Biological sciences are mentioned by 52.5 percent of the class; these courses are, of
  course, prerequisites for admission to medical school.

The impact of personal contact with influential physicians was especially strong when these physicians were relatives. As previously mentioned, one of seven students had a father who was a physician (the mother of one of these was a physician also), and 7 percent had grandparents who were doctors. Moreover, 3 percent of the class had either a brother or sister in the medical profession; 17 percent had at least one uncle engaged in medicine; and 12 percent had a cousin working in the medical field. These students indicate that such close acquaintance with medicine was largely responsible for their interest in the field.

A favorable concept of the doctor's status and role was inbred early in most students. One need not be a doctor's son to note the deference and respect physicians enjoy. And their activities are obviously exciting. Witnessing doctors at work in an emergency room of a hospital, for example, sold one student on a medical career. "I was there with my brother who had been hurt," he recalled. "I watched them wheel in a little boy; they pulled back the curtain and it really caught my imagination watching them work." Medical dramas on television reinforce such feelings by projecting an exciting professional life full of challenge and stimulation. They also portray the doctor as an independent person, an individual who has achieved the enviable position of setting one's own timeclock and being one's own boss. Having contact with interesting people and enjoying high status and financial rewards are also the physician's happy circumstance. It is not surprising, then, that students are encouraged to aspire to such a career.

Summer jobs in medical settings stimulated some candidates to pursue careers as doctors. Three out of 10 students attributed much of their zeal for becoming doctors to previous work in hospitals as orderlies, X-ray technicians, surgical assistants, or volunteers. Two others attributed their ambition to having worked in rehabilitation centers, and one even felt that his work in a mortuary had contributed to his desire to study medicine.

Interestingly, a few seemed to come to medicine through an emphasis on the negative aspects of other careers; that is, they ended up choosing medicine by eliminating other fields. For them, teaching was too repetitious, chemistry too lacking in social contact, engineering too ordinary, etc.

Parental Encouragement

Not one student voluntarily expressed parental influence as a motivating factor, and comments related to parents were usually evoked only by explicit questioning. Apparently, students were very sensitive to being regarded as less than adult and therefore avoided giving the impression of being under parental influence.

Upon probing, I learned that few parents were outwardly negative about a medical career for their children. The widowed mother of one was worried about the financial burden of medical school and others were concerned about the demands a medical career might have upon emotional or physical health, as well as home life. Such parents were not opposed but only anxious for their sons or daughters to be happy in their chosen careers. The physician father of one student "tried to talk me out of it," the student said, "but he was really only making sure that I knew what it entailed."

Half the class portrayed their parents as providing encouragement without pressure. Once the decision to become a doctor had been established parents typically became excited at the prospect. For instance, a Jewish student described this moment as the "fulfillment of a Jewish mother's dream. Once you get accepted into medical school," he said, "your stud points go way up! All your mother's friends who have daughters become interested. Their feeling is that being a doctor is almost as good as being a rabbi. And no one has more prestige than a rabbi!"

Alternative Careers

Generally speaking, few medical students give serious consideration to any career other than medicine. Only 24 percent could think of an alternative career when asked what field they would have gone into had medical school been inaccessible. (Nine percent had selected government service, and 5 percent each had selected dentistry, law, and business.) The others had no recollection of having considered anything else. If forced to make a second choice, however, almost half the class would have attended graduate school in a scientific discipline in order to train for a medically related career. And even this alternative was regarded as a waiting station for productive study while reapplying to medical school. Although a few had taken the Graduate Record Examination as an extra form of insurance, these students could not really visualize themselves as becoming anything other than doctors.

GAINING ADMITTANCE TO MEDICAL SCHOOLS

The process of gaining admission to medical schools occurs in three stages: (a) The applicants select the schools they wish to attend, (b) the schools then identify acceptable applicants, and (c) the schools select the first-year classes. It becomes increasingly difficult to select the most qualified from the vast number who apply each year as more qualified applicants seek admittance than the freshman classes can absorb. As an example, total first-year enrollment in the United States expanded from 9,479 students in 94 medical schools in 1967 (Jarecky, Johnson, and Mattson, 1968) to 12,361 students in 108 medical schools in 1971, and then jumped to 15,613 students in the 116 medical schools in operation in the 1976–77 school year ("Datagram," 1977).[10]

The medical school that was the locale for my research attracts many students from the national applicant pool, and its Admissions Committee uses the same evaluation techniques as other medical schools. As previously noted, these criteria include grade-point averages, MCAT results,[11] the quality of premedical education, professorial letters of recommendation, and impressions of applicants from the admissions interviews.

Some critics are questioning the merits of this more or less standardized application process on the ground that it may be dysfunctional for the medical system. That is, they observe that "the very qualities which are so often negated in the medical application process may be those that are the most striking characteristics of the effective doctor." [12] For example, Jason (1972) maintains that selection procedures are often directed at finding individuals who can survive the first year of medical school, when nearly all the attrition occurs but when few of the characteristics of the effective physician are required.

Application Process and Applicants

At the time my study group applied for medical school, there were 18,724 competitive applicants who submitted a total of 93,332 applications for first-year classes in U.S. medical schools, an average of 5.0 applications each (Stritter, Hutton, and Dubé, 1970). Most of the study subjects adhered to this pattern by applying to six or seven medical schools. However, 15 percent applied to more than 10 schools, and 5 percent restricted their applications to only one, the study institution. The median number for the entire class was five, which matches the national average for applicants at that time.

The average student attended application interviews at three medical schools, and almost one-fourth of the class were interviewed by five or more schools. Others cancelled additional interview appointments because they had already been accepted by the subject school. Of the 41 percent who received offers from only one school, 5 percent had applied only to the study institution. Thirty-six percent had offers from at least two schools, 16 percent had at least three offers, and 7 percent received four or more offers.*

---

* Since many students terminated applications elsewhere once they had committed themselves, these figures should not be construed as truly accurate. Had the students not terminated further applications, other offers might have been made.

Application Interview

As previously mentioned, the value of conventional techniques for selecting medical students is increasingly coming under attack. For instance, Gough (1971, pp. 13–15) points out that ratings by interviewers in the admissions interview [13] generally define a clear pattern of preference despite the fact there is little evidence that these preferences forecast superior performance. Generally, the sensible, well-organized, and tactful applicant is preferred to the individualistic, outspoken, and seemingly difficult applicant.

Some two-thirds of the class believe that faculty interviewers rate intelligence and academic ability as the most desired qualities. In this view, the ideal applicant is "studious, hard-working, and bright," but he or she must also be "well-rounded." The "bookworm" type who limits himself exclusively to scholastic pursuits does not make a strong impression.

Since intelligence and academic ability have already been demonstrated, the interview is, students feel, a final check to screen out "weirdos" and to determine if the student is "a fairly decent guy or gal." It is a "testing situation" designed to see how well candidates can handle anxiety and pressure. For example, one candidate was handed a sheet of paper and asked to identify the 50 famous people whose names were listed so the interviewer could observe his emotional reaction under pressure. Another prospect was heavily quizzed about his religion and his views about birth control, abortion, and other controversial topics. Still another was put on the defensive when a psychiatrist walked into the room, shook hands and promptly announced, "You are nervous, aren't you?" Such experiences convince students that the most highly valued personality trait is the ability to "keep one's cool," to maintain a confident, poised manner under pressure; as one freshman observed, "It is not so much what you answer that counts but how you answer."

A good deal of role-playing and bluffing is used by some applicants during the interviews. They try to impress the interviewer with ready-made answers for anticipated questions. This approach is justified by the fact that they simply cannot afford a wrong answer since it might jeopardize what they have struggled so long to attain. For this reason applicants try to project whatever image the interviewer seems to be seeking. Usually this means trying to appear alert, friendly, dedicated, concerned, service-oriented, and self-confident; so they give a good handshake and try to make a favorable appearance in all possible ways. "You put on a facade and hand out all the big words you can," a freshman explained; "and when you're asked what you do in your spare time, you emphasize that you go to museums instead of movies."

An equal number, however, see role-playing as violating their feelings of personal integrity. In their view, being honest is more important than being liked. Moreover, it is to one's advantage, they say, to play it straight; and so they do. Among these students—and there are only a few—are those who are so confident of being accepted that they feel no necessity for bluffing; for such students it is simply a matter of which school to select. In rare cases the highly confident may even give jarring responses to the interviewers. For instance, when asked why he wished to become a doctor, one student, who had tired of such "motive mongering," replied, "I want to become a god, save the world, and earn over $100,000 a year."

Role-playing is encouraged in big and impersonal schools, students say, by the manner in which the faculty members question and drill the applicant. But in smaller schools, where the atmosphere is more informal, applicants feel more at ease and have less need to put on a facade. The hospitality at such schools also seems to help students reveal their true attitudes and feelings.[14]

School Selection

The principal factors that influenced students to select the study institution rather than another school were geographical location, reputation, and anticipated friendliness. For a few, necessity was the deciding factor.* The school's location, either near their homes or else far enough away to be of contrast, was important to many. Those who had completed their undergraduate work at the parent institution were given a chance to continue a successful and pleasant affiliation. For many candidates, the school's reputation for academic and clinical excellence cloaked it with prestige. But overriding all these advantages was its reputation for friendliness. Discouraged by projections of cutthroat competition and huge classes at larger schools, students were favorably impressed by the smaller student-body size and more favorable student/faculty ratio and by the enthusiasm exhibited by those who escorted them on campus during their application interviews.

FINANCING MEDICAL EDUCATION

Admittedly, financial support is of great concern to medical students during their prolonged professional education. Of utmost importance is information regarding the average annual expenses of medical students and also the manner in which most medical students finance their education. Yet, given today's uncertain economy, statistics like these become obsolete

---

* Scholarships offered 15 percent of the class complete financial support, while 5 percent of the students had no other offers.

almost as fast as they are printed. The costs of medical education have shot up so sharply within the last two or three decades,[15] and means of meeting these costs are undergoing such massive upheavals, primarily because of uncertain policies in government funding of medical education,[16] that reports of actual expenditures and sources serve only as comparative data. With this background in mind, then, the financial assistance that was generally available to medical students at the time of this study is examined and compared with the manner in which my population obtained financial aid for medical school training.

According to a U.S. Department of Health, Education, and Welfare survey conducted in 1968, the year my study began, medical students reported average annual expenses of $4,394, an increase of $817 (23 percent) in four years' time; the average annual expenses for single students were $3,421 * and for married students, $5,727 (Smith and Crocker, 1970, p. 22). (Students at private schools averaged about $850 more than students at public schools, the difference being due to higher tuition costs in private schools.)

In addition to receiving some financial help from their families, most medical students tap a variety of other sources of financing to complete their medical education. Married students tend to rely heavily on their spouses for income; single students as a rule depend more on their families, their own earnings, outside loans, grants, and monetary aid from other sources such as military reserve pay (Ceithaml, 1965). According to Smith and Crocker (1971), more than three-fourths of the income reported by medical students during the year this study began was derived from their earnings, their spouses' earnings, or family loans.[17] The average amount of income reported from their earnings and savings was $1,606 for married students and $1,238 for single students. Both the number who received help from their families and the average amount of help they received were larger in private than in public schools. Of the two-out-of-five students who borrowed money, 32 percent borrowed from the Health Professions Educational Assistance Act (HPEAA) funds, averaging $1,178 per loan. Thirty-two percent of all medical students also held a scholarship or non-refundable grant, the average amount being $1,057. In addition, 23 percent reported that they worked during the beginning school term (Smith and Crocker, 1970, p. 30).

Financial assistance at the school where I conducted my study is available from a variety of sources, and each student who accepts a place in the entering class is considered a candidate for scholarship aid. Most scholarships are awarded according to financial need, and loans are available solely on that basis. When a student is accepted, he receives a school Finan-

---

* In 1974 the average annual expenses for single students were $5,280, an increase of about 54 percent in seven years' time, according to the 1974–75 bulletin of the subject medical school.

cial Aid Application Form and a Student Financial Statement. After the forms are processed, an estimate of the amount of financial aid available for a particular student is made, and he is notified regarding a tentative award. This award does not represent a commitment on the school's part, however, since considerable amounts of aid are dependent on government funding.

Of the several sources of financial assistance open to students,[18] two or more often combine to provide adequate support. Methods and attitudes concerning the handling of funds remain fairly constant throughout the four years.

Financial arrangements with parents vary from no help whatsoever to token gift amounts, partial support after scholarships and loans, and complete support. Those students who receive no help at all say they neither expected nor wanted such help. The majority who accepted parental aid dislike the idea even though they are grateful for it, and some express their guilt feelings openly. "It bothers me," one said. "I hate to tap somebody on the shoulder and say, 'Could you spare $20,000?'"

The reactions of those paying for their education through loans differ. Some are confident that they will have no difficulty in repaying the loans later. Most, however, borrow only as a necessary evil and suffer anxiety over being in debt so long. Money from odd jobs or summer employment is rarely sufficient for their needs. A few obtain financial support by committing themselves to medical service in the military.

Married students have a somewhat different story. Most of them rely heavily on their spouses' incomes for the largest part of their living expenses and on loans to cover tuition and the actual training expenses. Many married students rationalize that their companions like the idea of their becoming doctors and are more than willing to shoulder the responsibility, although a few students dislike feeling dependent on their mates. Another few, however, feel satisfaction that their spouses can be part of a "team effort." After four years, a senior summed up his feelings this way:

> I feel great. I don't owe anybody anything for my education. I was afraid I would have to borrow from my father when they cut back the loans and I didn't get one. But we were able to save $2,000 each year ourselves for the tuition; and it really feels good to know that my medical education, my M.D. degree, is mine and my wife's, and nobody else's. No one else helped us do it. It's a very proud feeling.

SUMMING UP

Students in an entering class of medical recruits, hailing as they do from all parts of the country, may appear to be, as the freshman quoted earlier said, "as different as we can possibly be." In reality, however, important similarities exist; most students are unmarried white Protestant firstborn or only children between 21 and 23 years of age from stable middle-class homes.[19] Moreover, all have been to college and, for the most part, have taken similar courses in the biological sciences. And, having been reared in a mass society (watching the same television shows, reading the same syndicated news releases, etc.), they have shared a great number of common experiences.

But, as the quoted freshman correctly observed, the greatest similarity among recruits is their common desire to become physicians. Background information reveals a striking picture of medical recruits as persons having an extraordinary degree of personal commitment to this career. Rather than floundering in search of a meaningful direction, like so many of their youthful peers, these students decided on a medical career at an early age; most have not even entertained the possibility of any other career. Moreover, all have overcome formidable obstacles in gaining admission to medical school, such as competing successfully for the best grades and politicking effectively to impress premedical advisors and medical school admissions committees. And, equally impressive is their demonstrated willingness to shoulder heavy financial burdens and in other ways sacrifice personal pleasures in order to achieve their goals. Such commonality makes clear that career socialization is well underway before a recruit even gains admission to medical school.

Since recruits come to medical school so highly motivated, the potential of effective socialization is greatly enhanced. But as we shall presently see, their initial commitment and enthusiasm are not always grounded in reality. And because of this, severe adjustment problems can result as students begin the long and strenuous climb up the career ladder to physicianhood.

NOTES

1. Each year since 1967 the number of students applying for admission has increased markedly. For example, 6,007 persons applied for the entering class in 1973, or 67.5 students for each of the 89 places in the first-year class. In 1975, the number of places for entering students rose to 101. This increase is partially explained by the nationwide increase in the number of students interested in pursuing careers in medicine (Dubé, 1974a). But since most students apply at several medical schools (8.65 each in 1975), these odds are not quite so overwhelming as they appear to be. Figures reported for 1975–76 indicate that the acceptance rate was 36.3 or about three applicants for every medical school seat in the country (Gordon, 1977).

2. At the time of this study, the national norm for entering female medical students was between 8 and 9 percent of all medical students (Bowers, 1968); since then it has risen to 24.7 percent ("Datagram," 1977). In the years 1968–69, total entries of U.S. minorities in medical school were 4.2 percent ("Datagram," 1972); eight years later they totaled 12.1 percent ("Datagram," 1977).

3. I have used the Census Bureau definition of "urban"—a place with 2,500 or more inhabitants.

4. National data at the time the study was initiated show that medical students were from the upper end of the educational scale; 35 percent of them reported that their fathers had graduate or professional training beyond college in comparison to only 5 percent of all males 25 years of age and over in the United States having this amount of education (Smith and Crocker, 1970).

5. Current literature is heavily documented with discussions that relate order of birth to achievement. Many studies (Cobb and French, 1966) show an unusual frequency of oldest sons among male medical students. Schachter (1963), however, contends that the repeated findings of firstborns among eminent scholars are not related to birth order but merely reflect that scholars "derive from a college population in which firstborns are in marked surplus." For further discussion of the relationship between birth order and academic achievement among medical students, see Shaver, French, and Cobb (1970).

6. See Sedlacek (1967) for national figures concerning the types of degrees earned prior to medical school entry at the time of this study.

7. Since 1961, approximately 97 percent of all medical school applicants and 99 percent of the accepted applicants have taken the MCAT, which, as has been noted, is used by admissions committees of medical schools in conjunction with undergraduate grades, interviews, and recommendations in making admissions decisions (Nelson, 1972).

8. Some prospective medical students, of course, abandon their plans. For studies on this, see Funkenstein (1961) and Levine, Weisman, and Seidel (1975).

9. See McDermott et al. (1973), for a discussion of changes in the 1970s with regard to student motivations.

10. See Culver's (1963) discussion on the premedical education and selection of medical students. For a thorough study of applicants to medical schools from 1964 to 1973, see the following series of articles: Johnson (1965), covering the years 1964–65; Mattson, Johnson, and Sedlacek (1968), covering 1966–67; Jarecky, Johnson, and Mattson (1968), covering 1967–68; Stritter, Hutton, and Dubé (1970 and 1971), covering 1968–69 and 1969–70, respectively; Dubé (1975) for the period of 1970 through 1975; Dubé and Johnson (1976) for the 1974–75 school year; "Datagram" (1976a,b) for figures on applicants and total enrollment for 1975–76; and "Datagram" (1977) for information covering the 1976–77 school year. For other figures, see also Crowley (1975b).

11. Erdmann, Mattson, Hutton, and Wallace (1971), in "The Medical College

Admission Test: Past, Present, and Future," summarize the history of the test, its operation and how it is scored, and its problems and potentialities. Many of the problems have finally been resolved as students began taking for the first time in the spring of 1977 the New MCAT (American Association of Medical Colleges, 1977).

12. See Seegal (1964). See also Levitt and Rubenstein (1967).

13. For a descriptive study of those who typically comprise Medical School Admissions Committees, see Oetgen and Pepper (1972).

14. See Hubbard and Howard (1967) for a comparative analysis of the advantages and disadvantages of large versus small medical schools.

15. Whereas total resource costs for a senior medical student at, for example, Duke University in 1943 were estimated at $1,950 (Davison, 1952), yearly costs at this school at the time of this writing ran as high as $25,000, according to William G. Anlyan, Duke's vice president for health affairs (*Medical World News*, 1974). This figure represents a 1,182-percent increase in 30 years.

Actual tuition rates paid at the same school in 1943 were $450 (one-quarter of the total medical-school resource cost of $1,951), whereas the amount paid in tuition in 1974 was up 600 percent to $2,700 (just a little over one-tenth of the institution's estimated total resource cost of $25,000).

Although these figures may seem high, they fall within the framework recently reported by the Association of American Medical Colleges (1974a). Estimated annual costs of undergraduate medical education programs surveyed at 12 medical schools ranged from $16,000 to $26,000 per student in total resource cost—a prorated amount of all expenses involved in operating a medical college and teaching hospital.

Total resource costs of medical education are now coming under increasingly closer scrutiny, particularly through studies such as those conducted by AAMC (1974a) and the Institute of Medicine (1974), to bring out the *actual* cost of educating an undergraduate medical student (including instruction, program administration, research, and clinical activity).

16. Although tuition rates have risen sharply over the past three decades, tuition has diminished greatly in significance as a source of support for the total medical education structure and services ("Datagram," 1971). Further, it has been tacitly understood that federal and state governments contribute substantially in supporting the undergraduate medical education process, a policy that has been endorsed and accepted as standard, as indicated in reports issued by the Association of American Medical Colleges (1974a) and the Institute of Medicine (1974).

Although the general trend is for increasing government support of medical-school training, research, and operations (Crowley, 1975b, pp. 1344–1351), there have been some reports that funding may be reduced so that "only the rich will be able to attend medical school" (*Medical World News*, 1974). Such shifts in education financing patterns could appreciably affect the more recent trend of broadening medical school populations to include more students from minorities and a wider range of socioeconomic backgrounds.

17. Smith and Crocker (1970, p. 24) itemize the sources and percentages of

income of all medical students for 1967–68 as follows: own earnings and savings, 24 percent; spouse's earnings, 29 percent; gifts or loans from family, 25 percent; loans from Health Professions Educational Assistance Act, 8 percent; loans from medical school, 1 percent; other loans, 3 percent; nonrefundable grants from Health Professions Educational Associate Act, 2 percent; nonrefundable grants from state governments, 1 percent; all other sources, 6 percent. (Loans guaranteed by the American Medical Association were less than 0.5 percent.)

18. For general financial information and specific scholarship and loan sources, see *Medical School Admission Requirements, 1976–77, U.S.A. and Canada,* 26th Edition (Association of American Medical Colleges, 1975), Chapter 4. One such loan source is funded by physicians in practice who are members of the AMA (Crowley, 1975a).

19. Concerted efforts have been expended over recent years to alter this traditional pattern by recruiting medical students from minority groups (Blacks, Indians, Chicanos, etc.) and, of course, from among women. So, although the study population is typical of the classical medical-school pattern, today's classes tend to be represented by a larger number of minority students. Yet, by working their way through college and in other ways participating in mass society, minority students who apply to medical school have in many ways internalized traditional middle-class values and aspirations. In any case, the study population is probably representative of the masses of students who have preceded them through medical school and now are practicing physicians.

PART II

THE SOCIALIZING NETWORK

3.   Faculty and Hospital Staff

There's a caste system here, a rigid hierarchy, but you have to be around a while to figure out how it works. (A junior)

A GREAT MANY INDIVIDUALS comprise the faculty and staff of a medical school and teaching hospital. A bewildering mass of personnel—some in white, gray, tan, or blue uniforms or "lab coats," some in the green garb of the operating room, and others in ordinary street clothes—busily circulate among the rooms and corridors of the medical center complex. At noon, the hospital cafeteria is a focal point where many paths cross. It is indeed a colorful blend of sight and sound as hospital personnel gather to share refreshment and conversation.

Although beginning medical students may be bewildered by the large variety of employees, they soon learn to differentiate among them and to peg them in their proper places in the hierarchy.[1] But, because of the rapid vertical mobility among prospective doctors, their own positions in the ranking system are not always clear to them.

In the student's eyes, professional status within the teaching hospital is generally divided into two major categories. The first consists of those who have achieved an M.D. or Ph.D. degree or are aspiring to obtain one or the other.[2] The second includes everyone else in the hospital structure, from nursing supervisors and registered medical technologists to orderlies and cooks in the kitchen.

Three classes of people comprise the first category. First and highest ranking is the faculty, whose primary responsibility is to teach students. Faculty members have their own levels of status, from instructors and assistant professors to associate professors, professors, and department heads. Below the faculty on the status ladder are "Fellows," who have completed specialty training and are subspecializing in a second residency (e.g., pediatric cardiology), and "house officers" or "house staff," who are taking their internship or residency training in the hospital and instructing medical students at the same time. Their standings in the hierarchy, depending on their specialties, range from interns through first- and second-year residents up to chief residents. And below the house staff is the student body itself, comprised of freshmen, sophomores, juniors, and seniors.

Ranking highest in the second major category—those not on the M.D. or Ph.D. path—are the nurses, followed by medical technologists and other allied health workers who have completed their formal training. Also in this group are those who have graduate working status but have not yet entirely completed their training, such as student nurses, other full-time students, and hospital support personnel. Much can be learned from all these staff members, by example if not by precept.

Entering medical students, of course, are only dimly aware of all these divisions and subdivisions. They learn fast, however, especially if a registered medical technologist (who usually has a B.S. degree) is mistaken for an X-ray technician (usually with minimal training beyond high school), or a senior nursing student for a beginner.

FACULTY: BASIC SCIENTISTS VERSUS CLINICIANS

At the time of this study, the full-time faculty consisted of nearly 400 persons, almost all of whom had doctoral degrees.* The most obvious distinction among them, then as now, is that one segment comprises academic specialists in disciplines basic to medicine (anatomy, biochemistry, microbiology, physiology, pharmacology, etc.), while another group consists primarily of clinicians. The first group, referred to in medical school as basic scientists, is composed largely of Ph.D.s. They deliver didactic lectures and supervise laboratory exercises, then spend their remaining time in research and related activities. Clinicians, by contrast, are generally less concerned with basic research and "pure" academic issues. Although they may also give lectures and conduct research, much of their time is spent in patient-related activities. Their teaching is usually done at the bedside in the hospital and in the outpatient clinics.

Basic Scientists and Clinicians as Viewed by Students

Both faculty groups, of course, are charged with the responsibility of preparing medical students for their future roles as physicians, but their approaches to this task are often seen in sharp contrast, and students are

* Eighty-two percent had the M.D. degree, 12 percent were Ph.D.s, and 2 percent had both of these degrees. Most of the remainder were doctors of dental surgery, veterinary medicine, or theology. There were a few whose highest degree was the master's and one or two who had only a bachelor's degree.

quick to make comparisons.* "They are as different as night and day," said one junior. "It's like comparing apples and oranges."

Academic Versus Clinical Orientation

Basic scientists, being more oriented toward a theoretical or "pure science" approach than the more pragmatic clinicians, believe that knowledge need not be practically useful to be valuable. Hence, their respective disciplines are generally presented in as much detail as possible, with little discernible concern for practical significance.

This academic preoccupation provokes much criticism from students, most of whom have a strong clinical bent. Such professors, students complain, are not in touch with the larger clinical picture. "They get all hung up in their own little speciality area," said one senior. "They're not aware of what is happening right next door in the hospital."

In the students' view, basic-science instructors regard them not as medical students aspiring to become physicians but as graduate students specializing in their own disciplines. Their courses are said to include too much needless academic detail. "They're wasting our time making us learn all this insignificant baloney," students complain. "They've just been cooped up in their labs too long," a senior said. "They ought to be taken out on the hospital wards and shown where all of these molecules and chemicals really fit in. They'll find them in human beings, not in test tubes."

Clinical faculty members, on the other hand, generally ignore the academic distinctions—the detailed minutiae and esoteric theory—and emphasize instead the larger patterns relating to clinical situations. "They don't specialize in trivia," one student puts it. Yet they must know enough of the details to diagnose and treat illnesses. The choice of therapy, clinicians maintain, should depend not on academic theory, but on its record of effectiveness. Their stance proclaims, "Who can argue with results?"

Teaching Versus Research Interest

Generally speaking, clinicians are seen as being more interested in teaching than their basic-science colleagues, who are often preoccupied with their own research projects and regard teaching as an interfering chore. They often appear in the lecture room, present a series of facts in rapid

* This information was obtained by asking each year, "How do faculty members in the basic sciences seem to compare with the clinical faculty?" I realize that "clinicians" and "basic scientists" as described in this chapter are ideal types. But as far as student stereotypes are concerned, these ideal types are realities. There is evidence, however, that after graduation medical personnel view medical school physicians, as compared to community-based practitioners, as being more academic than clinical. For example, see Kendall (1965) and Houser (1965) for discussions dealing with medical educators versus community practitioners.

succession, then quickly retreat to their laboratories. As one student observed, "They throw out the material with the attitude, 'Catch it if you can; if you can't, tough luck.' " Then on "judgment day" students must "regurgitate" all that has been "thrown at" them.

Moreover, research-oriented professors seem reluctant to engage students in discussion, answer their questions, or in other ways spend time with them. When these professors are also viewed as dogmatic and authoritarian, as some of them are, students feel repressed. "They spoon-feed us and don't give us credit for being able to reason or think for ourselves," students grumble.

So it is not surprising that clinicians are regarded as better teachers than the basic-science professors. Rather than requiring students to memorize innumerable detailed facts, clinicians seem more concerned about their ability to apply what has been learned. This quotation is illustrative:

> The doctor will present a patient and then pick our brains, asking, "What did you observe?" He writes the responses on the board and then says, "All right, now, what do these facts suggest?" Ideas pop up from everywhere, and he doesn't give any put-downs. He never says, "Of course it couldn't be that," or implies, "That's stupid." After he writes all of our ideas on the board he says, "All right, let's evaluate these alternatives. Mr. So-and-So, what did you think of this interpretation? Give me the pros and cons." He makes us call forth academic material and apply it.

A natural selection process may account for some of the differences between the basic-science and clinical faculties. Since teaching positions as a rule offer less money than a physician could earn in private practice, the clinical faculty is made up largely of physicians who enjoy medical trainees and the opportunity to teach them.

By contrast, Ph.D.s attracted to medical school are often of the opposite type—those whose interest in teaching is secondary to research. Those interested primarily in teaching stay in colleges and universities where teaching opportunities abound and where students who specialize in their disciplines are more appreciative of what they have to offer. Whereas college professors ordinarily teach two or more courses, a Ph.D. in medical school generally gives only a few scattered lectures or else supervises laboratory work. Obviously, this is a desirable arrangement for one who does not enjoy teaching.

In recruiting Ph.D. faculty, medical schools tend to emphasize the opportunity for research rather than the responsibilities for teaching. When I was offered a faculty position at the medical school, for example, it was made clear that more than half my time would be free for independent research. Other advantages include good research facilities and increased chances of getting research grants, as well as a better salary than most colleges can offer.

Aloofness Versus Empathy

As compared to clinicians, Ph.D.s seem distant and aloof; generally speaking, little camaraderie exists between them and their students. "We're just tolerated," a freshman observed. But students often feel a sense of kinship or brotherhood toward many members of the clinical faculty. Several factors contribute to this relationship.

First, clinicians have more face-to-face contact with students. Whereas basic-science professors typically deal with students en masse during class lectures or laboratory sessions, clinicians usually work with groups of only three or four at a time. This situation allows participants to learn one another's names and in other ways to become personally acquainted.

Because they are constantly meeting and working with people as individuals, clinicians usually develop a social *savoir faire* that may enhance their relationships with students. As one third-year student put it, "I can communicate better with the clinical faculty members because they're used to talking with people rather than mice."

Another factor is that the clinicians have themselves been through medical school and therefore have more empathy with students. "They know what we're going through and are sympathetic to our plight," a freshman explained. Because they are of the same "species," it is natural for prospective doctors to identify with the clinical faculty and emulate its example. Clearly, clinicians serve as role models, and students identifying with them learn much through imitation. This informal process accounts for the lion's share of the transformation of students into physicians.

Although members of the basic-science faculty play an important role in teaching medical students, they rarely serve as role models, and they display few of the paternal or fraternal attitudes toward medical students that clinicians often do. The social distance between students and basic-science professors led one sophomore to say, "I have the feeling that they don't even like us."

Basic Scientists and Clinicians as Viewed by Each Other

Because members of the faculty are so highly trained and well qualified in their specialties, it is natural for them to respect one another, regardless of whether they are clinical or academic specialists. More than a fourth of the class note that M.D.s and Ph.D.s have a high regard for one another and appreciate the others' contributions. "Both types are needed," a senior said. "Clinicians can't help the patients without new knowledge coming from basic research; and this information is of little value unless someone applies it on behalf of the patient." Yet, at the same time, the relationship between basic-science and clinical professors seems to be characterized by mutual condescension and strained tolerance. Students note that each group has a professional pride that causes it to feel superior to the other.*

In the clinicians' scheme of values, clinical perspicacity is of primary importance. Although a Ph.D. professor may be a recognized authority in his field, much of what he teaches is irrelevant from the clinical viewpoint. This attitude comes through to students during the early stages of their clinical training, when clinicians sometimes denigrate basic scientists by saying that much of what they teach is either impractical or erroneous. This quotation from a third-year student is illustrative:

> Dr. —— walked in the first day and said, "I'm going to find out what you know." Then he presented a hypothetical case and asked students what they should do. When nobody gave the answer he wanted, he told us to forget what we had learned, because if we tried to do things the way we had been taught we'd probably kill the patient.

Clinicians often tend to feel that their Ph.D. colleagues are too pre-occupied with their academic specialties to be concerned with the purely human aspect of medicine. While ignorance of clinical techniques and their specific applications is understandable, Ph.D.s are not easily excused for losing sight of the patient as the ultimate focus of both clinical and academic medicine. After a Ph.D. professor had lectured to a class of third-year students, the physician in charge of the course remarked: "Boy, you sure can tell that fellow doesn't have to work with people for a living!"

But the Ph.D. does not accept the inferior posture to which clinicians would assign him; far from it. Instead he typically displays a condescending attitude toward clinicians, whom he regards as mere technicians whose understanding of the principles they apply is limited and superficial. Said one senior, "I heard a Ph.D. remark that the M.D. is no more than a TV repairman—a technician who 'tunes up' the human mechanism."

Ph.D.s feel superior to physicians because of their specialized training in research and the scientific method. Even when M.D.s engage in research, basic scientists tend to look down their noses at them. Having devoted an entire career to one specific area of science, the Ph.D. sees the M.D. researcher as poorly trained, lacking the knowledge to set up good studies with proper controls. "Some of the stuff they publish," one Ph.D. said, "is really shallow."

It is galling to the Ph.D. when the news media credit the clinician for new advances in medical technology derived from basic research. "Clinicians get all the glory for new advances," a junior said, "when much of the

---

* When third-year students were asked, "How do the Ph.D.s seem to view M.D.s?" 12.1 percent replied that Ph.D.s had favorable impressions of M.D.s while 44.8 percent thought that they had unfavorable feelings; the remainder were uncertain. When the question was reversed, 34.5 percent indicated that M.D.s held favorable views of Ph.D.s, while 51.7 percent felt they had unfavorable attitudes.

legwork has been done by the researcher; the public doesn't understand that most medical research is done by Ph.D.s rather than M.D.s."

With such reasons to feel superior, basic-science professors can easily become envious and resentful of physicians who make more money and have higher community status.[3] "The Ph.D. feels he has worked as long and hard to achieve his doctoral degree, but is not recognized like the M.D.," a senior said; "The latter is always in the limelight." This feeling may account for the student-perceived tendency of the Ph.D. to resent medical trainees, whom he regards, to quote a freshman, as "stupid boobs who will soon be making more money than I am even though they know much less."

Faculty members seldom disparage each other openly, but most students are aware of the behind-the-scenes politics, the continual jockeying for honor and recognition in the social network of the medical school. The obvious differences between the Ph.D. and the M.D. faculty present a ready arena for status one-upmanship.

PERCEIVED FACULTY ATTITUDES TOWARD STUDENTS

Faculty members, of course, are charged with the primary responsibility of training medical students and preparing them for their future role as physicians. How they regard students and interact with them has a major impact on student adjustment and career development.

Views of Students at Progressive Stages of Training

Freshmen

Initially, the relationship between students and faculty is not a happy one. Only one in ten freshmen perceives the typical faculty member as having a favorable view of students.* Little camaraderie or sense of emotional closeness exists between first-year students and their mentors. During this year most teaching occurs in the lecture room or laboratory; there are few intimate teaching situations. Moreover, several instructors are in-

---

* Conversely, almost half the freshmen (45.8 percent) felt that the faculty viewed them unfavorably, a figure which steadily dropped to an almost imperceptible 5.5 percent in the senior year. These views were expressed in response to the question asked each year, "How does the typical faculty member look upon medical students this year?" During the freshman year, one-third of the class responded "some favorably, some unfavorably," but this number, too, rapidly diminished to 5.5 percent in the senior year.

volved in freshman courses, and this does little to enhance interpersonal rapport. Few go out of their way to become personally acquainted with students or even to learn their names. "It's almost like a machine," one student commented. "The faculty pushes the button and we do the work. Everything is programmed and our feelings are not considered; it's very impersonal."

Some professors, usually those with strong research orientation, make it clear that teaching is a bothersome interruption of their work. "They just put up with us," a freshman complained. "They have to teach in order to stay on the faculty, so they just go through the motions. Some of them act like they don't care whether you drop out or not."

Even more irritating are instructors who display condescending attitudes. With striking frequency, freshmen complain about being treated like "high school kids," "children," or "infants." They feel this way when required to attend lectures and labs or when given unsolicited recommendations about how they should study or budget their time. After excelling academically in college, freshmen find it a bitter pill to swallow to be regarded as unmotivated and incompetent. "They don't seem to understand that we're 23 or 24 years old, with intelligence obviously above average," a freshman charged. "We ought to be treated more like adults now than when we were in college."

Having been conditioned in college to think independently, to budget their time, and to express personal views openly, freshmen react strongly to the authoritarian climate of the medical school. This is how one course was presented:

> The professor introduced himself, very straight-faced and sober, and stated, "This is not liberal arts. Is that clear? Clear? Clear?" He went around the room saying "Clear?" as though he were threatening us and setting himself up as an enemy of some sort. It was a "them against us" type of situation.

Student dignity is insulted by the laboratory manual that says, "Students will *study* . . .," with the word "study" underlined. Such tactics reduce the freshman's self-concept from that of an intelligent and mature person possessing impressive credentials and high aspirations to that of an untried "greenie" who must prove himself or herself anew. "They regard us as complete dummies," one observed. "They view their job as drilling knowledge into stone."

Sophomores

Fortunately, by the second year, most students feel that the faculty attitude has improved considerably. Nearly half of the sophomore class comment favorably on their mentors' view of students. "We're one notch up on the ladder," a sophomore explained, "and we're treated accordingly."

Although basic-science instructors are still resented for their teaching style, they are believed to display a less condescending attitude. Surviving the rigors of the freshman year is proof enough, students feel, that they are both able and dedicated. "After all we've been through in making it this far," a sophomore declared, "they've got to respect us." Such feelings of accomplishment no doubt color student views of the faculty.

A common feeling among sophomores is that their professors are now beginning to see them as future professionals—more as physicians-in-training than as immature children. Sophomores feel that the faculty, although by no means regarding them as equals, at least gives students credit for having the potential for becoming such.

The realization that sophomores are on the threshold of clinical work motivates the faculty to give them more of the necessary "meat." "They act like it's their last chance to teach us some basic facts before we go out and descend on the poor patients," a sophomore commented. Being better informed than freshmen, sophomores are more stimulating to teach, and faculty members are more likely to listen to their views. "Last year it was all memorization and regurgitation," a sophomore pointed out, "but this year we get more chance to express opinions. They respect us for having survived to this stage, and they don't talk down to us."

Juniors

More than two-thirds of the junior class perceive the faculty as having a favorable view of students. Nearly all of the third-year instructors are M.D.s rather than Ph.D.s, and students feel that they are now looked upon as future colleagues. Happily, students are impressed with the tolerance and patience shown them by the clinical faculty. "None of them makes fun of us," one said. "And if we come up with an idiotic diagnosis, most of them will try to explain where we're wrong."

As in previous years, however, faculty members make it clear that students must remember their place. Although not treated as inferior, they are expected to maintain the proper student-teacher relationship.

Seniors

Feeling accepted by the faculty is a typical experience among fourth-year students; only a handful perceive any unfavorable faculty sentiment. Realizing how hard students have had to work to arrive at this stage, the faculty seems willing to grant them a greater degree of status and clinical responsibility. Although still not considered equals by any means, seniors are treated "almost the same as younger colleagues, part of the clinical team." Accordingly, faculty members are more likely to go out of their way in helping them learn. "It's really a now-or-never situation," said one senior, "and they feel a responsibility to produce good doctors."

During the senior year it becomes clear to students that their professors regard them as their finished product, and naturally they want their own product to be good. "They have a genuine interest in fourth-year students," said one, "because these are the people who are going to represent their school. When meeting a physician from another medical center they want to hear, 'We've got Sally ____ from your school and she sends her regards,' or 'Bill ____ is with us—he's really doing a great job.' "

During this year members of the clinical faculty begin to show considerable personal interest in the students, asking about future plans with "almost a parental concern." Some students, however, see an ulterior motive in this—"They look at us as potential candidates to fill the interns' places here," one senior said; "they try to entice good students into their programs." But, whatever the motive, this personal attention is happily received.

Faculty Definition of Student Success

A dramatic change in the faculty's criteria for judging success occurs at the end of the second year when students are, in effect, handed over from one faculty group to another. According to most freshmen and sophomores, the faculty's criterion of student success is academic achievement. Operationally defined, a good student is simply one who excels on tests.*

The natural tendency of academicians to evaluate students by scholastic standards is reinforced by the necessity of evaluating them en masse. As previously mentioned, few professors become personally acquainted with students during the basic-science years; consequently, they resort to traditional techniques of testing and grading in order to measure student interest, initiative, and ability.

While recognizing the importance of academic achievement, the clinical faculty evaluates students to a large extent on qualities other than book-learning. According to juniors and seniors, they are judged not only by how basic medical knowledge is grasped, but also by the way it is applied to clinical work and performance of assigned duties.† At this stage successful students are those who can take a good history, conduct a proper physical exam, and then develop a reasonable diagnosis on the basis of the informa-

---

* This information was obtained by asking students each year, "From the faculty's point of view this year, what is a successful student?" While high academic achievement is considered most important by 50.0 percent in the freshman year and 52.6 percent in the sophomore year, it drops precipitously in the clinical years—to a mere 1.8 percent in the senior year.

† Clinical competence and concern for patients are not even mentioned in the freshman and sophomore years as faculty criteria for student success; but in the final two years clinical competence is mentioned by 43.1 percent of the juniors and 45.5 percent of the seniors; and concern for patients by 17.2 percent of the juniors and 14.5 percent of the seniors.

tion obtained. They keep neat charts and remain in close touch with their patients' progress.

A good student also feels a responsibility for the welfare of the patients and spends enough time with them to develop rapport. They are regarded as "total persons" rather than pieces of unfeeling protoplasm.

Only one criterion of success remains significant throughout all four years: the display of interest and initiative.* Two comments—the first by a freshman and the latter by a senior typify this view:

> A teacher gets a bigger kick out of someone who is really interested and uses himself to the maximum than out of the smart guy who knows it all at the start and gets the highest grades.

> The most disastrous thing you can possibly do is to show a lack of interest.

Expected Student Role with Faculty

It is generally understood by students at all stages of training that they are expected to observe certain behavioral standards when with the faculty. Initially, more than one out of three students feel that they can act normally when with the faculty; but the number who feel this way declines: 36 percent during the freshman year, 30 percent in the sophomore year, and 17 percent in the junior and senior years. Through increasing exposure to the faculty, students come to know more and more clearly what their mentors expect of them.

Interest and Enthusiasm

As previously mentioned, students are expected, first and foremost, to show an active and sincere interest in medicine and in their own medical training. They display this interest by being punctual at classes and at their assigned duties, listening attentively, and participating actively while on the job.

The importance of fulfilling faculty expectations in this regard was made dramatically clear when a four-year student was dropped from school, reportedly because of a "bad attitude." (Remotivated and humbled by the experience, this student was soon readmitted.)

Respect

While most professors want a student to be inquisitive and show a desire to learn, it is abundantly clear that they also expect to be approached

---

* The response "shows interest and initiative" was given by 34.5 percent of the freshmen, 29.8 percent of the sophomores, 41.4 percent of the juniors, and 54.5 percent of the seniors.

CARNEGIE LIBRARY
LIVINGSTONE COLLEGE
SALISBURY, N. C. 28144

with courtesy and deference. "Invariably, respect must be shown," a junior commented. "This they demand."

Some students regard this deference as nothing more than is due an older and more experienced person. One such student, a junior, stated, "Whenever I see a third- or fourth-year student talking to a staff man with even a hint of sarcasm I just cringe; somebody ought to really put that person down. The faculty deserves respect."

The majority of students, however, feel that "this respect bit" is carried too far; that the expected degree of deference extends considerably beyond the normal requirements of social grace. While generally going along with the faculty expectation, these students feel inhibited by a hierarchical view of the student–instructor relationship. They feel stifled when required to act subserviently, to "be seen but not heard," and to regard every word that falls from their mentors' lips as gospel. So they secretly deride instructors who convey the impression, "I am wonderful; I speak, and you listen." And these same students express disgust with obsequious classmates who "act like the local lackey, parroting 'Yes, sir' or 'No, sir' to everything the faculty says."

Professional Behavior

Faculty members expect students to act professionally, to behave in a manner befitting their status as future doctors: Although faculty members may recognize the students' needs to have some fun, they make clear that such diversions must not interfere with the learning process. Giggling, being indolent, or playing pranks are taboo. As one freshman put it, "They expect us to be mature and not go around slapping people on the butt; no horseplay."

But students complain about mentors who "almost seem afraid to smile." One student said, "They want us to act like our mothers just died. With them it's strictly business all the time." Fortunately, most mentors are not so rigid, and they encourage students to relax and be more open and natural. With such instructors students feel freer to express opinions, ask questions, and even argue a point of view—in a respectful manner, of course—for even these faculty members like to be treated courteously.

HOSTILITIES BETWEEN STUDENTS AND FACULTY

During the first two years of medical school, hostility toward the faculty is often like the volcano that steams and rumbles but somehow fails to erupt. Seven out of ten underclassmen confess to feelings of resentment toward their instructors. However, only one in ten upperclassmen feels much animosity in that direction.

Even when resentments run high, during the first two years, open expressions of belligerence toward faculty members are rare. Freshmen are especially insecure. Few of them will openly assail their mentors. "I'm scared to take them on," one commented. "I'd be slitting my own throat." There is not much freshmen or unmarried underclassmen can do except get together in gripe sessions and "let off steam by bitching and talking about quitting. We blow out the instructors we're annoyed with, but only behind their backs." It is reassuring to students to hear classmates express the same complaints and to know that they are not the only ones who feel frustrated and hostile. "It just feels really good to be able to cut loose sometimes," a freshman said. Married students, of course, often complain to their spouses to relieve their tensions.

This early antagonism is usually blamed on such grievances as "busy-work" activities that needlessly waste time; lack of clinical orientation in lecture and laboratory work; dull, uninspired teaching; thoughtless scheduling of exams and activities that create avoidable pressures; and trick examination questions and other unfair testing methods. Vexations that are mentioned less frequently include faculty members' ignoring student opinions and suggestions for improving the curriculum; demeaning or embarrassing responses to students, such as laughing at their questions; underestimating students' motivation and maturity by assuming that they have to be forced to work; and general antagonistic attitudes that make students feel that faculty members feel punitive toward them.

These complaints diminish markedly when students become upperclassmen. Those resentments that persist usually are focused on irritating personality traits of mentors, unwillingness to give students clinical responsibility, assignment of students to repetitive chores that have little instructional value, and conceited attitudes about themselves or their specialties accompanied by disparagement of other clinical services. But these irritants rarely have much energy behind them. "It's nothing at all like the first two years," a junior commented, "just little things usually due to fatigue or misunderstanding." When personality conflicts exist between a student and a faculty member, the student merely keeps his distance when possible and finds solace in the fact that rotation to the next service is not far off.

Thus, as students gain confidence and feel more secure, their peer group is utilized less and less often for ventilation and emotional support. The proportion who rely on classmates for these purposes declines from 83 percent in the freshman year to 54 percent in the sophomore year, 33 percent among juniors, and only 9 percent among seniors.* The lower

* Open expression of hostility takes an interesting turn: a modest 20.3 percent during the freshman year jumps, as pressures build, to 50.9 percent in the sophomore year. Then as students begin their clinical apprenticeships there is a dramatic drop to 8.6

statistics during these last two years reflect not only the greater proportion of married students in the class but also the fact that upperclassmen actually feel much less hostility. When occasional irritation does surface among advanced students, they usually avoid direct confrontation. "Most of us just shut up and sail along."

Direct Confrontation

As always, there are exceptions to the norm. Some students will occasionally challenge a faculty member directly. Although one out of five freshmen and half the sophomores prefer an open manifestation of antagonism, only a few are willing to risk their tenuous status by being too visible in such attacks. Admiring classmates point to one brave soul who dared to tell an unpopular professor, "I've been talking with some of the upperclassmen and they tell me this course isn't worth a damn." Such directness, though, is rare. Usually militant students try to avoid being conspicuous when giving the faculty a bad time. Passive–aggressive techniques are more typical—such as inattention or indifference during a lecture or half-hearted participation during a question-and-answer period. "We just sit back and don't take notes," a freshman said. "When a ridiculously easy question is asked, nobody will raise a hand to answer it; that frustrates the instructor."

More overt techniques such as laughing, grumbling, or jeering during a lecture are also used, but those who use them avoid identification. Another technique is the use of loaded questions designed to embarrass professors: "If we can get away with it, we will try nailing the instructor on a question, backing him into a corner and then watching him squirm." Such actions, of course, only antagonize the professors and reinforce their perceptions of students as immature, thus escalating interpersonal hostilities.

Hostility peaked during the second year, when a formal request by a class representative was totally ignored by the instructor. This request was for the elimination of required discussion groups, unanimously judged by classmates to be "busywork." Frustrated by this "gross waste of time" and angered by the instructor's unresponsiveness, the class voted to boycott the activity. Upon learning of this plan, the instructor was reportedly "purple with rage." Because of their vulnerability, students backed down from their

---

percent in the junior year and zero during the senior year. Group action as a means of expressing hostilities also rises sharply between the freshman (1.7 percent) and sophomore years (19.3 percent), but levels to 6.9 and 9.1 percent, respectively, in the remaining two years. Most interesting of all was the response that "expressing hostility isn't necessary," which rises from zero during the sophomore year to 81.8 percent in the senior year. The actual question posed was: "How do students vent their hostilities toward unliked faculty members?" The responses show clearly that hostility is primarily a phenomenon of the basic-science years.

planned boycott; but their hostilities continued to run high. "If the term doesn't end soon," said one, "it's going to boil over into something fierce."

The only other group uprising occurred during the senior year when, as previously mentioned, a student was asked to withdraw from school even though he was in the top half of the class academically. When the promotions committee offered no specific explanation for his dismissal, the class as a whole demanded the student's reinstatement. The possibility of being forced to leave school after four years of hard work and an enormous financial investment was very upsetting to all, and the incident provoked considerable suspicion and ill will among the student body. "We really raised a stink," one said. "If this can happen to one of us for no apparent reason, then it could happen to the rest of us, too—and we don't like that idea at all!" (As previously mentioned, this student was later readmitted; but how much influence classmates had in the decision is a matter of speculation.)

Explanation of Faculty Hostilities

Whenever a Ph.D. seems antagonistic, students have a handy explanation: He is simply taking out his ill humor on students because he is a "frustrated physician"—a person who wishes, either overtly or subconsciously, that he had gone through medical school himself. More than a third of the class express the belief that these mentors were dropped from medical school or were unsuccessful in gaining admittance in the first place.* A sophomore said:

> We had a conference with Dr. ——, and everybody knew he was out to get us and that we were out to get him, too. He asked questions we couldn't answer, and we returned the favor. He was trying to embarrass us and vice versa. I've heard that he started med school but dropped out because he couldn't make it.

Students supported this view by pointing to Ph.D.s who openly acknowledged having quit medical school. Why would such a person seek employment at a medical center, students reason, unless the old flame is still burning?

Those who see their Ph.D. mentors as medical school rejects theorize that these individuals harbor a generalized hostility for the medical profession. "It's a defense mechanism for coping with their own failure," a senior declared. "They give terrible lectures and then get out as fast as they can;

---

* During the freshman year interviews, many students spontaneously commented that Ph.D. faculty members were medical school rejects. So, in the second year I asked the entire class, "Do you think that the Ph.D. staff members would, if they had their wish, prefer to be physicians?" There were 36.8 percent who categorically agreed "yes" and 12.3 percent who thought that some would but most would not.

they just don't give a damn, because they've probably been rejected from medical school."

Since a medical career clearly has more appeal to medical students than a career in basic science, students tend to project these values onto others. For instance, a sophomore said, "Dr. _____ is so interested in anatomy he must have wanted to be a surgeon; I can't understand why he didn't go on and become an M.D." And, referring to an admired professor who is "smart as a whip," another sophomore said, "With a mind like his, why would he be satisfied with physiology?"

Students are quick to point out, however, that this view of the Ph.D. faculty as frustrated M.D.s is not universally applicable. Some of the basic scientists are obviously dedicated and satisfied with their careers. Commenting about such instructors, a sophomore said, "They are so wrapped up in their own work and enjoy it so much, I figure that must be what they wanted to do."

A few students recognize that the view of Ph.D.s as frustrated doctors is, to some degree, an ego defense on the part of their classmates. "During the first two years we're made to feel like we don't know anything, and we don't. So, as a defense mechanism, we look down on the Ph.D. professors." On this theme, a sophomore said:

> There is a great deal of snobbery on the part of medical students toward the Ph.D. Believe it or not, Ph.D.s are considered second-class citizens. It's amazing that anyone could look down on a Ph.D., but in this strange little world it happens.

The sophomore then added, "The honest medical student will admit to having an enormous ego, as big as a stomach. The need to find some way to be on top results in putting down the Ph.D. instructor." When each group tries to put down the other, a vicious cycle is established. Although pride is temporarily bolstered by such means, a high price is paid in anxiety and discontent.

OTHER MENTORS AND ROLE MODELS

Teaching medical students, of course, is primarily the responsibility of the faculty, but other hospital personnel also play an important role in preparing them for their future. One learns to be a doctor not only through formal tutoring (classes, laboratory sessions, conferences, and so forth) but also via informal processes such as imitation and role-playing. And in these more subtle ways, medical personnel other than the faculty can play an important role. The techniques of patient management, for example, may be learned from observing a variety of hospital personnel in action.

Interns and Residents

Except in second-year pathology and radiology courses, underclassmen have very little contact with the interns and residents who make up the house staff. But in their junior year, when assigned to work on the hospital wards with "service patients" (those who cannot afford a private physician), students deal regularly with the house staff.* Speaking of the latter, a junior said, "It's the main source of teaching. If the house staff is good, you learn a lot; if it's not, you don't learn much." [4]

During the senior year, students work mostly with private patients and thus have closer contact with the attending physicians who make up the clinical faculty. But contact with the house staff still remains an important source of learning.

Although interns and residents are primarily interested in developing their own clinical proficiency while completing their training, they also act as mentors for medical students who accompany and assist them as they go about their hospital duties. Such physicians teach as they work, both by example and by precept.

In the teaching role, some house officers, of course, are more competent than others. Good teachers act as role models and also take time to explain principles and procedures and to answer students' questions. They keep students alert to potential learning situations and provide opportunities to perform clinical procedures.

Most members of the house staff are rated as at least adequate in the teaching role, although a few are viewed as incompetent. Preoccupied with their own training, the latter seemingly make no effort to teach, either because they are too busy or simply not interested in teaching.

House officers who regard teaching as a burden ignore students or assign them menial chores. Concerning the first approach, a junior complained,

> They'll just go about their business, not making any effort to include us in what they're doing; on rounds they'll put their heads together, muttering words that we can't hear. And since we know nothing about the patient, who looks perfectly okay, we wonder what's going on. It's like sitting back and watching a movie without sound.

Even more irritating, though, are house staff who use students only as assistants to complete routine and distasteful chores such as organizing charts, writing progress notes, and running errands—whatever the house officer wants to avoid doing. "Some of the house staff people act like you're

---

* I learned about student attitudes concerning the house staff by asking these questions: (a) "How have residents treated you this year?" (b) "How have interns treated you this year?" and (c) "What does the house staff do that is most irritating?"

their coolie," a senior complained. "They say, 'Go do that'; 'Find this for me'—and they think that's the extent of what they should teach." *

Nonetheless, students are, generally speaking, quite tolerant of house officers, pointing out that they have a heavy work load and many pressures. ("It's really not their fault; they're often so busy they don't have time to stop and answer what seems to them to be a silly question.") Others sympathize with the residents' desires to further their own training. ("The big problem is that they're still trying to learn, too, so they want to do everything they can themselves. In their position, I'd probably be doing the same thing.")

Clearly, students identify with house officers, and this makes it easier to overlook their shortcomings. After all, just a short time ago they were medical students, too. And since interns are so close to their own status level, career identification is accentuated. But this is not to say that house officers are immune to criticism. Residents, for example, are occasionally portrayed as aloof, uninterested, and condescending in their attitudes toward students: "Sometimes they treat you like you're not a full member of the human race."

Interns, however, are rarely described in this manner. In fact, one student maintains, "I've never had a bad intern." The latter are consistently portrayed as being friendly and willing to go the extra mile in helping students gain clinical experience. "They're pretty nice because we're both in the same boat," a senior remarked. In fact, some interns are personal acquaintances who graduated in the previous class. So, as one senior noted, "When they're so close to us, it's uncomfortable for them to lord it over us."

Nurses

The nurse's role as mentor is complicated by an ambiguous status relationship with medical students.† They realize that, once they earn the M.D. degree, nurses must follow their medical orders. Yet when just beginning clinical work, they are in fact subordinate to the nursing staff in experience and in practical knowledge.[5]

As they begin work on the hospital floors, prospective doctors must depend on nurses for such essential information as the location of equipment and drugs; and they also learn from them much about the practical techniques of patient management and the basics of hospital routine. Most

* Nearly half the senior class (43.6 percent), compared to only 6.9 percent of the juniors, expressed resentment toward the house staff for imposing menial tasks. The difference is probably due to the eagerness of fourth-year students to take on greater clinical responsibility. In the junior year, any chores can seem new and challenging.

† Data on nurses were obtained by asking (a) "How have the nurses treated you?" and (b) "What have they done that is most irritating?"

third-year students, therefore, admit that, regardless of their future relationship, nurses deservedly have higher status. "They know much more about what's going on and have greater facility with the practical aspects of medicine than I do," a junior acknowledged. "They know more about drugs and things that are learned only by practical experience—like making sure the oxygen is turned off before doing a blood count." This recognition is occasionally reinforced by house officers, who instruct students to "be nice to the nurses. Most of them know more than you do."

It is especially easy for students to respect nurses who have specialty training or are in charge of hospital wards. For example, much can be learned from nurses who have worked for years in an intensive care unit or with emergency resuscitation. As one student expressed it,

> In an emergency code-red situation some nurses are trained to assume the responsibility for getting things going even before the doctor arrives. They'll make sure that the anesthesiology department is called and will have the proper equipment there even before the doctor orders it. Just watching them is a learning experience.

Most students realize, too, that as far as the daily operation of the hospital is concerned nurses are far more important than students. "When we go on vacation for two weeks," a senior observed, "everything goes on just the same without us. But when a nurse goes on vacation, they have to find a replacement. They're absolutely necessary."

But as students gain more competence and begin to assert themselves, their status relationships with nurses change and become confused. Interpersonal problems can occur when students begin to resent their subordinate status and try to compensate. "We've been subordinate to everyone for too long," a junior complained. "I really hate being subordinate to nurses, too; some of them act uppity and try to call all the shots." As students achieve more independence, realizing that they are well along the road to becoming interns, they find it more difficult to accept a status inferior to that of nurses.* As one explained, "It's just kind of an awkward position to be in. You know you will soon be directing them; yet at the present time you're not performing any vital function."

Most nurses are pleasant and cooperative, and when students are not too aggressive, nurses find satisfaction in contributing to their education. But students can also be troublesome. "Nurses resent us for the time it takes to run around and look after us," one remarked. "We distract them from their work. Most of them are nice, but sometimes I get the feeling they don't want to mess with us, like they'd love to stomp on us."

---

* At the peak of their status strivings, 60.3 percent of the junior class expressed complaints about nurses as uncooperative, resentful, hard to get along with (crabby, bitchy, hostile), condescending, and questioning of students' authority. By the end of the fourth year, after seniors had established greater authority, the percentage of students who criticize nurses in this way dropped to 16.7 percent.

Because nurses have so much informal authority on the hospital floors, it is easy for them to deflate the ego of an overaggressive student. They can simply ask a technical question, "knowing damn well," as one student put it, "that we don't know the answer." Or they can confront a student with the fact of his or her student status, saying (by implication), "You're only a student; what do you know?" Such an approach can really rouse the student's ire: "When they treat me like I'm still a medical student," one said, "it burns the hell out of me."

When a student gives a medical order to a nurse, the latter may reply with a challenge or—worse yet—adopt the mentor role, telling the student that the task (completing a certain form, for example) is not a nursing staff responsibility. "You tell nurses to do something and it may not get done," a junior complained. "They'll look at your name tag, and if there's an M.D. on it they'll do it; if not, they'll tell you to go take a powder."

Despite such problems, however, slightly more than half of the juniors say that nurses are generally helpful, cooperative, and understanding of medical students. And things improve even more during the senior year when students have greater clinical experience and work more closely with the attending physicians who serve private patients. This exposure confers higher status upon them. Consequently, nurses generally show greater respect. "They treat us more like doctors now," a senior observed. "When they call us 'doctor,' there is less sarcasm in their tone."

Because of this status transition it is not surprising that students increasingly see their position as superior to that of nurses. Whereas one-fourth of the freshmen regard themselves as having higher status, 52 percent of the seniors share this view. After being "low person on the totem pole" for so long, seniors find much satisfaction in the realization that, as one expressed it, "The nurse has reached a status plateau. Her career potential is realized, but ours is only beginning; so things are much better for us."

Allied Health Workers

Other potential mentors are the various medical technologists and other allied health workers who have had specialized training in particular aspects of medicine (inhalation therapy, for example). The benefits can be reduced, however, when students regard themselves as having superior status.

In the first year of school, the students' contact with allied health personnel is minimal. It comes as a jolt when they find that these specialists do not always look up to them. "I learned this summer," a sophomore exclaimed, "that paramedics rate themselves above us; they look down on medical students as having silver spoons in their mouths and as having aggressive, know-it-all attitudes."

In second-year laboratory courses like hematology, technologists sometimes serve as instructors. "This is their big moment of glory," a sophomore said, "and they can't help having a holier-than-thou attitude." It is ego-deflating when the medical technologist projects a superior attitude, saying in effect, "You dummy, can't you even stick a needle in a vein?"

Technicians enjoy greatest respect from medical students during the third year, when the students are groping about trying to learn new procedures and find their way around the hospital floors. At this time, as a junior indicated, the technician's specialized training is most highly valued: "We may know a lot more about test tubes, calorimeters, and things like that; but we don't know beans when it comes to helping sick people. The paramedical staff is much more competent in clinical work."

By the end of the junior year, however, students typically feel that the status situation is reversed; more than half of the class feel that they have outdistanced the medical technologists and other allied health workers. At this time it is particularly aggravating when the latter act as if they know more than students. "It really gets on your nerves," a junior said.

Toward the end of the senior year little doubt exists—at least in students' minds—about who has the upper hand. The student's newly acquired sense of authority is illustrated by one senior's comment: "A lot of the time paramedics can deal quite effectively with things, and you must realize that they are part of the clinical team. But if I need a syringe, I'll say, 'Would you get me a syringe?' I say it politely, but I mean for that order to be carried out."

Status relationships notwithstanding, these allied health workers, like nurses and house staff, can play a helpful role in the socialization of the emerging physician.

SUMMING UP

Learning to be a doctor is profoundly affected by the complex social structure that exists at the medical center. During their sojourn in medical school, students must learn to deal with a wide variety of personnel, all of whom have a specialized role in the ongoing operation of the medical complex. Acquiring the ability to function effectively in this bureaucratic maze of technical human interrelationships is no small achievement.

The principal participants at the medical center involved in the training of rising medical practitioners are (a) the faculty, (b) the house staff, and (c) nurses, technicians, and other health workers. Although the faculty is formally charged with the main pedagogical responsibility, all who are involved help in one way or another in preparing students to be doctors. In word and deed, they serve as socializing agents.

Students' receptiveness to such influences, however, is affected by their status relationships with these potential mentors. Those with greatest socialization impact upon medical students are those whose status the students covet. Because they naturally identify with those who have already traveled the same career path, doctors' words are especially valued and their actions and attitudes imitated. Clearly, such persons are mentors in every sense of the word.

Although much can also be learned from nurses and other allied health practitioners, the students' anticipated status—the realization that, as physicians-to-be, they will soon be giving medical orders to such personnel—can reduce the potential socialization impact of these clinicians. Status conflicts can also lessen the benefits of basic-science instruction, even though the Ph.D.s hold faculty status. Although these professors can play an important role in indoctrinating students with the background knowledge necessary to clinical practice, students are usually less than appreciative. Rarely, if ever, are the basic-science mentors regarded as role models, no matter how personally charming they may be. Clinically oriented students are not interested in devoting their professional lives to obtaining and promoting specialized knowledge about one particular facet of science, such as the biochemistry or physiology of the body. Rather, clinicians are interested in the body per se in all its ramifications pertaining to health and sickness. In short, their orientation is practical and substantive rather than theoretical and formal.

Because medical students expect their mentors to display the former rather than the latter orientation, their disillusionment is great, especially during their exposure to the basic sciences. I believe that this social–structural feature of the training institution underlies many of the adjustment problems that confront medical recruits en route to physicianhood.

NOTES

1. For an analysis of the medical center as a social system, see Bloom (1971). See also Bloom (1973).
2. In 1961, undergraduate medical students in the United States comprised almost half the student population taught by medical school faculty. By 1972, however, medical students accounted for only two out of five students. The others consisted of interns, residents, and pre- and postdoctoral students in the basic and clinical sciences and full-time equivalent students in the other health professions (Association of American Medical Colleges, 1974c).
3. For a discussion of academic advancement procedures for Ph.D.s as compared to physicians, see Marshall et al. (1973).
4. For further discussion of the house officer's teaching role, see Brown (1970).
5. See Rockoff (1973) for an excellent essay on the interaction between nurses and medical students.

4. Classmates

The class is close, but I wouldn't say that it's one cohesive unit. It all depends on whether we get in a jam. When we're threatened, we congregate in a group and come out ahead together. But basically we're independent people. (A sophomore)

MEDICAL SCHOOL is sometimes compared with a submarine that submerges with its crew of students and, over the next four years, makes only occasional contact with the outside world.[1] Since students are completely engrossed in their studies or spend most of their waking hours confined either to the medical school or to the hospital, they feel "totally immersed in the sea of medicine," * even to the point of "drowning." One student expressed it this way:

> You just feel submerged and have to fight to learn what's going on in the rest of the world. You spend so much time around the hospital that you feel you're going to die from inhaling hospital air.

A natural consequence of relative isolation from the social world outside their medical community is that students become very well acquainted. "When you go through so much together," one said, "you get to know these people real well; I guess it's kind of a closed system."

What happens interpersonally when classmates spend so much time together in a closed system? Answers unfold through examining the developing patterns of friendship, by dissecting some of the interesting features and, finally, through looking at the social processes related to class diversity and/or cohesion.

---

* Seeking to learn how universal this feeling might be, I asked students each year, "How close to reality is the statement, 'Medical school becomes almost as closed an environment for its students as a submarine does for its crew'?" Since only 10.5 percent of the freshmen disagreed with this statement as compared to 14.3 percent of the sophomores, 49.2 percent of the juniors, and 54.6 percent of the seniors, apparently the submarine analogy becomes less applicable to the situation as the would-be physicians proceed through school.

INTERPERSONAL ATTRACTION

Since students are initially anxious to find others of their own kind with whom they can communicate easily, entering classes soon form into small groups. As a rule, there are only a few who prefer to go their own way independent of their classmates. For the most part, students are quite dependent upon their classmates for emotional sustenance and academic well-being. They expect one another to be friendly and to extend help, compassion, and understanding when needed.

In order to gain some understanding of the nature of interpersonal attraction, I asked students each year to identify their best friends, as well as the persons with whom they spent the most time. Freshmen usually gave the same names in answer to both questions.

Propinquity

During the first semester, many friendships are formed around the dissection table in gross anatomy. Because classmates are assigned alphabetically in groups of four to study the same cadaver, their friends often have names beginning with the same letter as their own or a letter close to it in the alphabet. "Naturally, if you spend 16 weeks with three other people at the same table," one said, "you get to know them well." And this friendship pattern is reinforced when students are alphabetically assigned to partners in other laboratory courses as well.

Antagonisms, of course, occasionally develop among laboratory partners in such close working relationships. More often, however, the stressful first-year conditions of medical school cement friendships. In a backward glance, a senior compares these work groups to "military squads behind enemy lines where success and safety depend upon mutual cooperation and good will."

One might ask, then, "How enduring are friendships formed in this manner? Do they carry over and, if so, for how long?" One sophomore's view is fairly representative of what happens: "It varies from semester to semester and year to year. As the lab groups change around, you find yourself hanging around with the people who are in your present group."

Students who room together or live in the same neighborhood also tend to form friendships and to spend leisure time together. But the number of students who continue to live together after the sophomore year decreases,* since an ever-increasing number marry as they proceed through school.[2] And when married, students tend to spend time with their spouses

---

* The number of single students who live together rises slightly from 15.5 percent in the freshman year to 19.3 percent in the sophomore year, but drops to 8.8 percent in the junior year and to 10.9 percent in the senior year.

and with other married students. "I don't see too much of my last year's friends any more," one remarked. "Now that I'm married, I do a lot more with married students, especially my last year's dissecting partner, who is married, too. Married couples are included in my circle of friendships now."

The most noticeable change in friendship patterns occurs between the sophomore and the junior years. Not only are more students married, but also they are no longer together in large classroom settings as they were the year before. Instead, they find themselves rotating 'in small groups through the various clinical services of the hospital. In the last two years the class is divided alphabetically into three broad groupings, or sections. The students in each section then rotate as a group through each of the three major specialty divisions—internal medicine, surgery, and OB/GYN–pediatrics.[3] In this manner, each group spends one-third of the year in each of these three divisions.

Within each section there are further subspecialties and programs into which students are subdivided; consequently, only a handful of students actually have much interpersonal contact with each other during the day. Accordingly, as one junior explained, "The persons we work with are chosen for us. We're divided into groups of four and then paired off." This work arrangement can, of course, contribute to the development of close friendships, yet there is also an increasing tendency toward individualization, as is illustrated by the fact that more and more students find themselves spending time with no one person in particular. As one points out, "Emphasis is now definitely off the class and onto what you are personally learning on the floor."

Common Backgrounds

Although students who work or live in close proximity often form friendships, previous research makes it clear that interpersonal attraction is also influenced by common background.[4] In this respect, medical students, like most other people, are most comfortable with those who share a similar way of thinking as a result of a common background. A few, however, claim to thrive best on challenging contact with students of different backgrounds. But no matter how important background factors are during the first year, they become lost to students as they proceed through medical school. Freshmen and sophomores, for example, are very much aware of each other's backgrounds: "There are a lot of Northerners in the class," a Southern student said, "and it's a shock to be around them." But these features lose visibility and importance to juniors and seniors who no longer evaluate one another in terms of such identifying traits. In this regard, four years of medical-school processing acts as a "melting pot," wherein such distinguishing background traits become dissolved. A senior observed, "It's not like the first two years when the Southerners sat with the Southerners and the Northerners with the Northerners; now, everyone has become 'equalized.' " In reply to my question, "With whom do you spend most of your time, and why?" slightly more than one-fourth of the freshmen mentioned that they spend their time with those of similar background. But in subsequent years almost no one referred to social origin. Similar results are found in reply to the question, "Whom do you prefer as an intimate friend, and why?"*

From the standpoint of socialization theory, this is significant. An old campus cartoon illustrates this point. The first frame of a series of pictures shows a variety of people being pledged to a college fraternity. As the frames move along, the distinguishing traits of these people are gradually extinguished until they all appear in the last frame to have the same hairstyle and to be smoking pipes (at that time, the sophisticated thing to do). Perhaps medical school is much the same, with easily identifiable traits being the criteria by which students respond to one another during the early years. But as they proceed through medical school, their distinguishing traits become blurred, and a commonality emerges. Having shared the intense experiences of basic-science training, upperclassmen have much more in common than not; their shared status of prospective doctor overrides all identifying status symbols. Consequently, they become increasingly unaware of background traits and less likely to stereotype one another by such traits. This tendency does not escape the attention of observant students. Said one:

> Medical school is comparable to an assembly line where distinguishing background traits are lopped off and different parts and materials are added to make a final product. The peculiar habits and practices of freshmen are pretty well done away with, so that by the time they become seniors they have been molded into a sort of uniform image.

Common Interests, Attitudes, and Values

As students' ranges of acquaintances increase, new friendships are formed. Social and extracurricular activities often become a basis for acquiring new friends. Double-dating is one such activity. Some classmates also form friendships through playing tennis or sharing similar activities. But only a few actually form friendships with those having totally different attitudes and values. One such student, a maverick, described his

---

* Less than 5 percent of the students in the sophomore, junior, or senior year mention similar backgrounds as a reason for spending time with persons. Likewise, whereas about 15 percent of the freshmen and sophomores mention similar backgrounds as being important in a friendship, only two students in the junior and senior year do so.

liking for such a relationship: "There are so many things that we don't share as far as attitudes and views go that it almost makes it interesting just to say 'hello' to him."

Common interests, compatibility, and similar attitudes and values, unlike background factors, remain important in the clinical years. This "value homophily" (sharing of similar values) among close friends is not greatly affected by the year of medical training but is a fairly constant factor in interpersonal attraction.*

Students' relationships, however, seem to be rather fluid in nature. For example, only a third of the sophomores cited as their best friend the same person they had named the previous year. Also, an increasing number replied "no one in particular" when asked to name their most intimate friend. This indicates that classmates tend to become more independent and to rely less heavily upon each other for emotional rewards as they move through school.

INFORMAL CONDUCT NORMS AND SANCTIONS

Along with the early friendships that develop among students, informal conduct norms and sanctions also emerge. As a group entering medical school, students are aware of only the most obvious behavioral standards. At the same time, their insecurity as newcomers creates a desire to conform and to be accepted. The question is, "Conform to what?"

With such competitive students as these, norms develop quickly around study habits and students' perceptions of their scholastic ability. In addition, how they behave in the classroom and on the hospital floors and how they relate to their peers and to the faculty become issues of importance. These dimensions of student culture were explored by asking such questions as (a) What do your classmates do that is most irritating? (b) What do you do to discourage this? (c) What do your classmates do that wins the greatest approval? and (d) How do you encourage these acts? Results show that during the first two years classmates are much more critical of each other than they are thereafter. For example, whereas only a few freshmen and sophomores could respond to the first question by stating that

* The results of this study indicate that 24.1 percent of the freshmen, 33.3 percent of the sophomores, 14.0 percent of the juniors, and 27.3 percent of the seniors were aware of spending the most time with "friends having common interests." (This was learned when I asked, "With whom do you spend the most time, and why?") Similarly, 37.9 percent of the freshmen, 45.6 percent of the sophomores, 21.1 percent of the juniors, and 30.9 percent of the seniors mentioned that similar attitudes and values were significant in intimate friendships. For a review of literature on interpersonal attraction, see Coombs (1966); and for a related study, see Coombs (1969).

nothing irritated them, more than a third of the juniors and half the seniors gave this response.*

Study Behavior

Initially, beginning students try to learn all the material assigned to them. Although they soon realize that this is an impossible goal, they do not readily overcome a fear of falling behind their competitive classmates whom they imagine as being hard at work all the time. Consequently, even when their books are set aside, they find it difficult to relax. It is not surprising, then, that moderation in studying emerges as a behavioral standard permitting classmates to disapprove of those whose study behavior differs from the norm in either direction. Anyone who goes too far one way or the other—studying more than others or not studying hard enough ("those who don't really give a flip about the work")—falls into disfavor.

Underclassmen who "don't do anything but study, who know it all, and who are on top of everything" are generally frowned upon. And although a classmate who stays an extra hour in the laboratory or library may be "a nice person," such students make others uncomfortable. To bring these study behaviors in line, classmates use disapproving facial gestures and derogatory terms such as "hot dog," "gunner," and "grade hog." Only those who are well-rounded and achieve high grades through their own natural abilities without becoming bookish "boxed-off intellectuals" earn the respect of classmates.

By the senior year, though, student views change; not one senior offers any criticism that another is working too hard. This is probably because there is less competition among classmates and more emphasis on personal learning, so that students are less threatened by the activities of overzealous classmates. At this stage, it is accepted that "everyone is working and learning as much as possible."

Classroom Behavior

Another type of student who is heartily disliked by classmates is the one who uses unfair tactics to make a favorable impression. Such students, labeled "pseudo-intellects" by their peers, pretend to know more than they really do and ask "brown-nose" questions of the instructor only to make an impression, not to learn. "This type tries to impress you by talking

---

* In response to the question, "What do your classmates do that is most irritating?" only 5.1 percent of the freshmen and 8.8 of the sophomores indicated that nothing irritated them, whereas this response was given by 37.9 of the juniors and 50.9 percent of the seniors.

about research done the preceding summer," one complained, "and always comes up with a question to ask in class; you know damn well that the answer to the question was known before it was asked."

In the preclinical years, when students are under a good deal of pressure and spend most of their time in the classroom, the motivation, timing, and appropriateness of questions are acutely important; students are easily annoyed by classmates who repeatedly ask too many questions in the classroom, especially when the answers are of no benefit to the class as a whole or may cause them to remain during such discussion when it is time for the class to break.* Consequently, classmates pressure those who violate this norm:

> We come right out and let the jerk know. For instance, several of us got mad when —— asked questions all the time. So we made derogatory comments whenever the dope raised a hand. We must have gotten the message across because he stopped.

Other techniques of social control are also used, such as hissing, booing, grumbling, and laughing out loud at the offender. In one instance, a student brought a hotel desk bell into class and "dinged" it every time a "stupid question" was asked. Sometimes these techniques are also used during lectures to harass unpopular professors, but there are mixed reactions to such harassment. Some students, generally those who sit near the heckler, offer support; but others, who are embarrassed or distressed by such behavior, say,

> It's gotten to be almost cruel; you can always hear these comments coming from the back of the class. Some people laugh openly at the teacher in class; they always seem to be ridiculing someone. When the professor happens to hear them, the rest of the class seems embarrassed.

The class reacts differently, however, when such treatment is given to a professor who has treated them unfairly or has damaged their self-esteem. In these instances, students feel that "any time a student can wheel a professor around by proving an error or making a point that hasn't been brought out in the lecture, the whole class is upgraded."

Whereas one in ten freshmen and one-third of the sophomores voice irritation about classmates who are rude to professors, only one student in the final two years even brings up the topic. Two things probably contribute to this change of attitude. First, fewer classroom situations exist, so such issues are less likely to occur. And, second, the vast majority of the professors in the last two years are clinicians rather than basic-science professors. As previously mentioned, this results in greater identification with and respect from the students.

---

* "The waste of time that is brought about by excessive questioning" is named as a source of irritation by 16.9 percent of the freshmen and 29.8 percent of the sophomores, but by only 6.9 percent of the juniors and 1.8 percent of the seniors.

Clinical Behavior

The techniques used by freshmen and sophomores to bring disapproved behavior into line generally disappear as students move into the clinical years; only a very few upperclassmen refer to "gunners" and "hot dogs." Occasionally a clinical student mentions "putting down a hot dog" by singing or whistling "I wish I were an Oscar Mayer wiener." But the old booing, hissing, laughing, or cutting others down with verbal labels are increasingly replaced by straightforward statements of disapproval to the offender. Generally speaking, though, clinical students apparently feel little need to express disapproval.* The most common complaint among clinical students is "work dodgers who leave someone else holding the bag to do their scut work." For example, one made his disapproval apparent to a shirking classmate by the statement: "Last night I started four I.V.s for you when you were on call. I guess they couldn't reach you down at the brewery." Such complaints, though, are uncommon among clinical students.

Student Cooperation

Although not averse to criticizing their classmates, especially during the competitive basic-science years, students expect considerable cooperation from one another. Because of heavy pressure, they view medical school as a give-and-take proposition. This is never more apparent, for example, than in the freshman year when classmates study together and lend lecture notes to those who miss or fall behind. Despite pressures created by competitive course grading, there is a "tremendous amount of teaching among the students." As one noted,

> We really hash this stuff around. Plenty of answers that I've put down on tests were not completely the result of my own thinking but might have come from a phone call to another student the night before.

Clearly, the most approved attitudes and behaviors are helpfulness and cooperation.† In this atmosphere, one who is conceited or in other ways shows exaggerated self-concern quickly becomes unpopular. "The person who knows the answer to your question and won't give it to you" quickly earns a bad reputation for "not giving a damn for anyone else." But the

---

* As many as 41.4 percent of the juniors and 63.6 percent of the seniors fail to name even one irritating thing about their classmates, whereas virtually everyone has a list of complaints during the first two years.

† This response is given by 23.7 percent of the freshmen, 15.8 percent of the sophomores, 26.2 percent of the juniors, and 30.9 percent of the seniors in answer to the question, "Which attitudes and behaviors bring the most approval?"

most disliked student of all is the "phony who is friendly with you in order to get something out of you."

Students also expect cooperation and consideration from one another in the clinical years, even though they see each other less. For instance, they may cover for a classmate who is burdened with too many cases by "working up" a patient. Or they may share information or teach newly acquired skills to each other:

> One of us may say, "Hey, Phil, I've got a good murmur; come on over and see what you think." Or, I'll go up to Suzanne, who's interested in internal medicine, and ask her about the electrocardiogram because she's studied it more. But by the same token, when she asks me what the normal baby is supposed to weigh at six months, I can help her.

For these reasons clinical students sometimes conclude, "We're teaching each other just about as much as the house staff is teaching us."

DIVERSIFYING FACTORS

Initially students tend to classify their classmates as follows: those who are more oriented to work or to play; those who are single or married; those who are Northerners or Southerners; and those who are activists or passivists in relating to the faculty.* But these perceived distinctions become increasingly blurred as students move into the clinical years. Only two freshmen are unable to identify any social categories in contrast to more than a third of the seniors.†

Orientation to Work or Play

Because incoming students are very competitive and have their social antennae out for gauging appropriate behavior, they are quick to note which classmates are oriented more to work or to play. Accompanying their awareness of the enormous amount of material to be learned is a desire to maintain some balance in their lives. So it does not take long to note which students are "gunners" or "hot dogs," which are "regular guys and gals," and which are "hell raisers." As they advance through school, however, students become more confident in their own abilities and less aware of these differences. In fact, only one senior makes any mention of this work–play difference.‡

* Some individuals, of course, fit easily into several categories.
† To 10.5 percent of the sophomores, 15.5 percent of the juniors, and 36.4 percent of the seniors, these distinctive characteristics are no longer identifiable.
‡ Comparisons between "gunners" and "regular guys/gals" are mentioned by 49.2 percent of the freshmen, 26.3 percent of the sophomores, and 29.3 percent of the

72   THE SOCIALIZING NETWORK

"Gunners"

Those dubbed as "gunners," "bookers," "hot dogs," or "grade hogs" have earned their names as the result of their seemingly complete preoccupation with achieving high grades. Rarely seen outside the library, these students hardly finish one quiz before they begin studying for the next one. Preoccupied with academic detail, they strive to know every fact and to amass an enormous amount of information. As previously mentioned, however, their grades are achieved at the expense of their social lives. Their severest critics, the "hell-raisers," view them as socially inhibited and as "weirdos, the ones who are always in the corners of the library studying by themselves." Said one,

> You see some people who are always in the library reading—seem to be booking. How much they know, I'm not sure. Most of us do our work and go home; but after putting in a full day these people don't feel right without picking up a book just to be reading.

"Regular Guys/Gals"

Generally speaking, about 80 percent of the class are viewed as "all-around nice people" who work hard, because there is no other way, but who do not much care for constant study and would often prefer to be doing other things. Being more practical and less oriented to the printed page than the extremely studious, these students are more selective in what they study and how they study. Although they join the "gunners" in the library just before examinations, they tend to relax when the pressure is off. In this way, most of these students find they can adapt to the vicissitudes of medical training, although they, too, sometimes feel a necessity for "getting out and being free—escaping." Pet irritations of these students are the "rote learning of the basic-science years" and the fear that they might become "warped" in this closed environment. "I've almost forgotten how to carry on a normal conversation," one of them lamented. "Everything that pops into my mind is medically related." Because these students are usually extraverted, sociable types, they find joy in the prospect of going on the hospital floors and having variety in their work.

"Hell-Raisers"

The "fun-seekers," "social studs," "swingers," and "goof-offs" earn their reputation by a manifest desire to "get out and have as much fun as

---

juniors. No seniors make any mention of "gunners." Likewise, 47.5 percent of the freshmen, 29.8 percent of the sophomores, 8.6 percent of the juniors, and only 1.8 percent of the seniors make mention of "hell-raisers"—fraternity or sorority types who like to appear "cool" and sharp.

possible" through continual dating, drinking, frivolity, and telling tall tales. Whereas most students try to live it up a little after examinations and on free weekends, the "hell-raisers" cannot wait; they have a "really big blow-out after *every* quiz." Their capability for hard work does not deter them from interrupting their studies for pool or a game of cards. The "gunners," their worst critics, view these classmates as "wasting a lot of time to-gether—they sit around and gab, play bridge, and just wander around wasting time, instead of doing anything constructive." Although the "regular guys/gals" do not feel comfortable around the "hell-raisers" as a group, they do enjoy their company as individuals and seem to be more sympathetic toward them than are the "gunners." "This is just their way," one said. "They'll probably do as well as anyone else and they are good people relaters."

Marital Status

Whether a classmate is married or single is much more significant in the freshman year than at any time thereafter.* In this year, single students rely heavily upon one another for relaxation and social life. (As mentioned, only one-fourth of the freshmen in my study population were married.) The unmarried students eat together in the hospital cafeteria and congregate in the library during the week; they date, drink, and attend theater and athletic events together on weekends.

Married students as a group appear more serious-minded, stable, and mature than single ones. Some classmates also consider them to be less friendly. One obvious reason for this is that married students tend to group together because of friendships formed by their spouses, and this automatically excludes them from some of the social life they might have enjoyed with their unmarried classmates. Even so, the amount of time that medical students have available to spend with their wives or husbands is not great. From a spouse's point of view, a mate's inaccessibility is the greatest problem.[5]

Single students complain that married classmates are noticeably unenthusiastic about chipping in for expenses for such things as class parties. Consequently, single students tend to label them as "do nothings."

The distinction between the single and the married, however, becomes less noticeable during the clinical years as an increasing number marry. As one senior notes,

> Most students are married now. There's less tendency to form cliques. Where the single and the married tended to separate in the first two years, now the tendency is to mix more.

* The difference in marital status among classmates is noted by 57.6 percent of the freshmen, 26.3 percent of the sophomores, 10.3 percent of the juniors, and 10.9 percent of the seniors.

Geographic Origin and Student Activism

The tendency to identify social categories most strongly during the freshman year is also seen by the way Southerners and Northerners perceive each other. Initially Southerners consider classmates from the North and the West Coast to be "Yankees," and look upon them as loud, obnoxious, arrogant, aggressive, and conceited. They describe the Yankee students this way: "If they want to say something, you damn well better let them say it because you're not going to get anything said if you don't."

In like fashion, the so-called Yankees tend to look upon their Southern classmates as naive, passive, extremely one-sided about political and racial problems, and always anxious to preserve the status quo. In their view, Southerners are still "yearning for the good old days, and are so passive that they act hospitable to any and every individual, regardless of whether it's someone they like or not."

Initially, students who fit either of these stereotypes tend to stick together, especially when they have more in common than just geographic origin. For example, Jewish students from Northern states tend to congregate. On the first day of school, a freshman observed, "You could almost divide the room right down the middle aisle into Northerners and Southerners." And this division carries over outside the classroom. As one student said, "Southerners have their own parties to go to; Northerners and Westerners go somewhere else."

The apparent difference between the Southerners' and the Northerners' temperaments is best illustrated by an incident that occurred in the sophomore year. At one point, when students became greatly upset over the treatment they had received in a particular class, some wanted to boycott the class; others did not. Those in favor of boycotting were seen as being from the North and the West Coast, while those who wanted to keep the status quo and not offend the professor were seen as being from the South. But instead of being labeled "Northerners" and "Southerners," those from the North were called "liberal radicals" and those from the South, "passive conservatives." The conservatives' view was this:

> The liberals want to boycott the whole thing—to tell the department chairman how pointless the assignments are, what a waste of time they are, and, if he doesn't agree, then boycott! The conservatives just want to tell him and then let him decide. I don't think the liberals have the right to speak for the class by telling the faculty what we want done.

But the liberal activists had a different view:

> My parents always said, "Southerners are so darn slow they're frustrating." I'm finding this to be true. Southerners are resigned to accepting anything the faculty has to offer regardless of whether or not it seems worthwhile. They're very passive and almost apathetic.

Such stereotypes wane, however, by the senior year, when comments about geographic origin become minimal.*

Other Groups and Aggregates

At the outset of medical training a few other special-interest groups are also recognized. These groups include (a) athletes who play ball together on weekends; (b) various religious groups, particularly the Jewish students; (c) "loners," who appear only when they have no choice but to work with others; and (d) a few "philosophers," who circulate from group to group, depending upon which seems most interesting to them at the time.

These perceived differences, like others previously mentioned, diminish in visibility as graduation approaches. "I can't define distinct groups any more," a senior admitted. "Some friendship groups remain, but each year they become a little less definite than they were before." In short, students come to be more individualistic and preoccupied with a common career focus as they move through school. And, since they have more and more acquaintances, the earlier interpersonal liaisons no longer assume the same importance they once did. Graduating seniors become more self-sufficient socially as well as intellectually.

STUDENT COHESIVENESS

As previously mentioned, most students, especially in the early years, are dependent in great measure upon their interpersonal liaisons with one another for academic and emotional well-being. These liaisons lend support and strengthen them in the face of stress and uncertainty and make student life tolerable. Thus the class is characterized by an underlying unity of "in-it-togetherness."

Classmates as Supportive Colleagues

When they need help with an emotional problem, most beginning students turn to a classmate since he or she is "in the same boat."† Since

---

* Each year the number who mention the North–South dichotomy (that is, Yankees versus Rebels) drops. This dichotomy is mentioned by 23.7 percent of the freshmen, 17.5 percent of the sophomores, 6.9 percent of the juniors, and only 3.6 percent of the seniors. Only one student in the junior year and no seniors made any mention of student activism.

† During all four years, the students indicated that the ones they would seek out for help with emotional problems would be their classmates. This response is given by

peers are more accessible and less threatening, a student rarely pours out real troubles to a faculty member. Concerned with establishing and maintaining a good image, such students generally try to hide their anxieties from those in authority. "You don't want the faculty to think you are any more screwy than they already do," a freshman points out. So when faculty members are sought out, students usually select someone who is "out of the mainstream" of the course work and "who won't judge but will help to find out what is best for you." As most first-year students agree, though, "A student who is in your situation and beating it is the one to talk to."

In the sophomore year, reliance on classmates reaches its peak, probably because of the great stress occasioned by academic pressures during this time. And although students rely less on their classmates for support after this year, more than a third of the seniors still indicate that classmates are their "principal source of emotional support."

During the clinical years, however, some students rely on faculty members and house staff, those with whom they have rapport.* Also, as there are more married students in these years, an increasing number mention their marital companions as the persons most apt to provide them with help.† A male student, for example, stated,

> I'll go home and talk with my wife about a lot of things that I won't talk with anybody else about; she understands and listens.

One of the women students gave her husband credit for always finding time to listen and sympathize, even though he had a demanding job in addition to the constant strain of coming up with money for her school expenses. It is indeed fortunate that many spouses feel it their duty to patch up their mates emotionally and send them back into the arena.

"Beating the System"

Notwithstanding the competition for grades, medical school nurtures a certain camaraderie among those struggling to get through; classmates soon develop a strong sense of cooperation in working together to "beat the system"; i.e., streamlining course requirements that seem difficult, meaningless, or unreasonably burdensome.‡ The methods by which classmates

---

47.5 percent of the freshmen, 59.9 percent of the sophomores, 46.6 percent of the juniors, and 34.5 percent of the seniors.

* Reliance on staff is mentioned by 22.4 percent of the juniors and 27.3 percent of the seniors.

† The spouse is named by 13.6 percent of the freshmen, 19.3 percent of the sophomores, 31.0 percent of the juniors, and 36.4 percent of the seniors as the one most often turned to for help with emotional problems. This increase, of course, reflects the fact that each year more students are married.

‡ As to whether or not it is possible to "beat the system," 59.3 percent of the freshmen, 22.8 percent of the sophomores, 12.1 percent of the juniors, and 18.2 percent of the

cooperate in this regard are many. One that involves an important group effort is the informal communication network established by classmates to deal successfully with the faculty. This network is used to learn mistakes made by previous classes as well as the trials and errors of their own group. Upperclassmen are sought after for old examinations, lecture notes, laboratory reports, and advice about professors and their courses. These aids then spread among the class as photocopied advice and hand-me-down materials, making it generally known "what you have to do and what you don't need to do."

Working together like this, students are better able to predict if a professor is going to be easy or tough, fair-minded or tricky—"twisting words around so that you interpret the question wrong." And they also determine what they are expected to learn, based upon what they believe the professors view as important.

Another method of "beating the system" is in cooperative efforts to save time by cutting corners in assignments and exercises that seem unrelated to the students' professional development. Especially in freshman laboratory courses, students cooperate by dividing up the work among a larger group so that each person does only a specialized part of the experiment; sometimes one group will average its results with those obtained by another group. This technique saves time and does not seriously curtail the learning experience; for as students say, "If things don't come out the way they are supposed to, you can always look up last year's book or find somebody's data." They rationalize it this way:

> We don't do our lab assignments together just to get out of work but because we want to learn more while we are doing something else; the amount of time required is not proportional to the amount learned.

Instead of feeling that they are shirking responsibility, students regard themselves as handling an undesirable situation intelligently by minimizing the time spent on irrelevant tasks. They claim, as one student put it, "If there is something there for us to learn, we will really work at it; but it is ridiculous to spend a lot of time on some trivial point." So, while there are those who consistently attempt to "play it straight," readily admitting there *is* a system to beat, students who are ingenious at cutting corners are often rewarded by having more time for independent study and even getting better grades. A freshman experience illustrates this point. Laboratory instructors in a particular course, bothered by seeing a majority of the students leaving early, sought to penalize them by calling for laboratory reports before the assigned date. The only ones penalized, however, were those who had conscientiously done the assignment, since they had not yet

---

seniors indicate that it is. But as they proceed through school, students increasingly deny that it is necessary or desirable to "beat the system." That is, more and more they tend to identify with the system and become an established part of it.

had time to complete the write-ups. Those who had pooled their efforts had already completed their reports and had gone on to study other materials.

As students move into the clinical years, they more often do as they are supposed to do, primarily because the material seems more practical and related to their goals. A typical reply to my inquiry about ways to "beat the system" is: "I don't think this question applies any more." That is, students now identify with the goals and methods of the established system; and because the system is personally relevant, they emulate their instructors, feeling that to attempt to "beat the system" is to foolishly short-change themselves. This view is in marked contrast to the basic-science years.*

Even so, some upperclassmen note that it is easy to short-cut the system if one is so inclined. One merely appears at strategic times and sloughs off at other times. "As long as you show up and make your presence known," they claim, "you can still pass." One student elaborates,

> You can persuade someone to look at your patient for you, copy the resident's work-up, make yourself scarce when you think you are wanted to do someone else's scut work, put in fewer hours than are expected, and come late and leave early, because there is no effective supervision or check on your performance. You can even ignore the fact that you are on call and probably get by.

According to one senior, "Anyone who goes through the first two years and then keeps his mouth shut and shows up for rounds can get through and beat the system." But clinical students feel that the demands made upon them are not unreasonable, and consequently they have no motivation for not meeting these expectations. "It's not a system that you want to beat," a senior said. "You're *part* of it!"

Competition and Conflict

In addition to having high personal standards and being competitively oriented, entering medical students are aware that class standing influences their chances for good internship appointments. They are, however, hopeful that class competition will be minimized, because most of them are fatigued from the competitive struggles that were necessary for gaining entrance to medical school. Consequently, a prevailing attitude is, "I'm not trying to compete with anybody except myself." Said one student,

> Most of the class are pretty decent about the whole thing. For example, if I find something significant on a histology test, I try to set up the one behind me by leaving the pointer right on it.

* In contrast to only 8.5 percent of the freshmen and 7.0 percent of the sophomores, 58.6 percent of the juniors and 41.8 percent of the seniors claim they have no desire whatsoever to "beat the system."

Despite this general outlook and the efforts of medical school administrators and some professors to minimize student competition, some
"grade hogs" find it important to beat everyone else by continually "shoot-
ing for higher grades than others get." These individuals defend their
fierce competitiveness by saying, "We've been competitive all our lives to
get into med school, and it's just natural that we will continue to be
competitive here." Some even complain to their professors for a few extra
test points just so they can score higher than others. One such student, a
a most unpopular fellow, always investigated to see if anyone had gotten
a higher grade; if his was not best, he felt bad and the next time studied
even harder. And when such students ask others about their test scores,
competitive spirits are aroused. A student commented,

> One guy who used to sit next to the one I worked with would say, "Don't
> you think it's immature for two people to compete for grades?" My friend
> was rubbed the wrong way by this and has been trying to outdo him on the
> quizzes ever since.

A certain amount of competition is to be expected, of course, among
those who are high achievers. Thus it is not surprising that my question,
"Have you noticed any competition or hostility between classmates this
year?" evoked affirmative answers. Although it is well known that "some
people just plain don't like each other," interpersonal conflict is usually at
a minimum; and students rarely display their feelings openly. To my knowledge, suppressed hostilities became apparent only once. This was at a
freshman Christmas party after students had been drinking, and "the
things that came out were amazing." As one freshman said, "Certain
people had been bugging others all along and I never realized it. We almost
had three fights right there."

Considering the fact that classmates spend long hours together during
times of high tension, surprisingly little conflict is shown. As described by
one student, "doing tedious lab work with the same students, sometimes
from ten in the morning till three in the afternoon, can make you frustrated and irritable; and you may come out with a few biting words."
Other than admitting to becoming "a little tight and edgy" at examination
times, however, students usually affirm that they "get along very well." "It
is more amazing," one student stated, "that there are no open hostilities in
a class this size."

During the clinical years the principal sources of competition among
students stem from (a) desires to make good impressions on the clinical
instructors, and (b) personality clashes. Juniors report that those who
used to compete for grades resort to more subtle means, such as demonstrating their knowledge to clinical instructors in front of their peers. For
example:

> If there is a brown-noser in a group, he or she will ask the resident lots of
> questions or go to the other extreme and answer every question the resident

asks. These people learn as much as they can on one thing and then manipulate so they can ask questions on it. During a conference or lecture this type always waits until the end and then asks a question when the answer is already known; everybody just sort of says, "Well, there goes the meathead again."

Seniors, however, generally feel that competition has dissipated * and any hostility flare-ups are likely to stem from simple personality differences. They agree that at this stage they are concentrating on becoming good doctors with little thoughts of cutthroat competition. Competition is also discouraged by the fact that grades are de-emphasized and exams are infrequent in the clinical years. Even then examinations are often oral, and the results are usually not returned. Also, when assigned to different clinical services, students have little contact with most of the class and there is no basis for comparison with the work of others.

Class Unity

Because new recruits soon become entrenched in fairly strong interpersonal relationships amid small groups, one does not expect to find any substantial unity among the class as a whole. But friendships do not remain static; group memberships are open and overlap. There are few well-formed cliques, and not many students perceive a social hierarchy of any kind, although a vague pecking order exists based upon class standing. There is no outward show of social superiority.

Considering that class members are individualistically oriented and come from a variety of backgrounds, the degree of class unity is striking. Nevertheless, the class is not a single homogeneous unit, for there are many viewpoints on every issue. But because they share common goals and experience stressful situations together, they do develop a certain camaraderie. One freshman phrased it this way: "We're all in the same kettle, so we might as well jell."

Although preclinical students often mention "being in it together," they make no such comments when they become juniors and seniors. No longer do they have contact with the larger class as a unit because of their rotations into different clinical specialties. Each student is more on his or her own and follows a schedule that is different from that of classmates except for the fairly rare occasions when class meetings or lectures are held. "You can go for months without seeing somebody," a junior remarked. "Unity is almost nonexistent; you're all spread out—here, there,

---

* To the question, "Have you noticed any competition or hostilities between classmates this year?" an affirmative response was obtained from 69.5 percent of the freshmen, 71.9 percent of the sophomores, 37.5 percent of the juniors, and 27.3 percent of the seniors.

and yon. You just never get to see old friends." Thus clinical students acknowledge that much less unity exists for them than in former years.

SUMMING UP

The comparison made at the beginning of this chapter between medical students and a submarine crew leaving for a long journey is appropriate. Participants are relatively out of touch with the world as they knew it and must, of necessity, depend primarily upon each other for comfort, support, and companionship. Both crew and student body are submerged in depths they could only imagine—one in a tangible ocean, the other in a swirling sea of knowledge.

But at the journey's end, the submarine joins the larger fleet and its crew scatters among the other vessels. "Now it's more like we've traded the submarine for an aircraft carrier," a senior remarked. "We're still on water and can't set foot on land, but we can move around more." Clearly, things are better; not only is the feeling of confinement less pronounced, but participants have higher status, more knowledge, and considerable practical experience. One might say they have obtained their "sea legs."

Until the journey's end, medical recruits occupy a subordinate position in the formalized system, thereby remaining vulnerable to the will of the staff. However, the informal system that spontaneously forms among recruits—sometimes called "student culture"—provides collective protection and relief from stressful experiences and personal anxieties. This salient principle is noted by the sophomore quoted at the beginning of the chapter: "When we're threatened, we congregate in a group and come out ahead together."

The collective nature of professional socialization in medical school has other important ramifications as well. One is that classmates learn much from each other. Another is that the group processes tend to round off idiosyncracies among individuals in the class. When an individual tries to succeed in a threatening environment, security is enhanced by being like everyone else or, conversely, having everyone be like oneself. So, during the initial period of stress and insecurity, conduct norms quickly develop; and classmates exert considerable pressure upon one another to stay in line with these expectations so that a few do not make others feel guilty or look noticeably bad. This homogenizing process has the effect of blurring distinctive individuality.

Upon entering medical school, recruits are acutely aware of the individual differences existing among classmates. But as the collective process grinds away, the various statuses that once gave identity to individuals (Northerner, Jew, and the like) become obscured and give way to a single uniform status shared by all students—physician-to-be. Increasingly, as they proceed through school, classmates are only dimly aware of identifying stereotypes that were once so visible. "Everyone is more alike now than in the past," a junior observed.

As graduation approaches, attention shifts to how well classmates play the role pertaining to their common status, as defined by student culture. And these criteria of interpersonal success provide the social looking glass whereby professional self-identities are formed.[6]

NOTES

1. Material in this chapter relating to the first two years of medical school is taken from Coombs and Stein (1971).
2. However, the opposite also occurs; that is, some get divorced. To understand the dynamics of marriage as related to medical training, I interviewed approximately 200 spouses of medical students, interns, and residents affiliated with the teaching hospital where I conducted this study. An analysis of these data will be presented in a future volume.
3. See Chapter 5 for a description of this teaching arrangement.
4. For a review of the literature on the effect of social background on interpersonal attraction, see Coombs (1966, p. 166).
5. For a discussion of the medical marriage, see Coombs (1971b).
6. Perhaps relevant here is Goffman's (1961) discussion of "total institutions" that tend to strip the self of its old features and then rebuild it along new dimensions.

PART III
SOCIALIZING MECHANISMS
AND ADVERSITIES

5. Medical School Curriculum

We've done academic work for an awfully long time. So when we finally
reached the clinical years I felt like shouting, "This is it; come on troops!
Boy, now I can try my wings!" (A junior)

FOR MORE THAN HALF A CENTURY little change has occurred in the basic organization and form of medical curricula in the United States. The classical pattern has comprised two years of required course work in the basic sciences followed by a clinical apprenticeship. But since the 1960s, gusty winds of change have swept over the fields of medical academia. Stimulated by large financial incentives from the federal government aimed at reducing the doctor shortage,[1] many institutions have moved toward three-year schools and abbreviated basic-science curricula.[2] The premise is that our nation's health care problems can be effectively reduced by (a) increasing enrollment, (b) building more medical schools, (c) shortening the training period, and (d) improving training effectiveness.[3]

Externally induced incentives such as these, reinforced with internal pressures due to student unrest, have created among medical educators a climate for change, and have resulted in an anxious ferment to improve the established system of medical training. Seeking beneficial changes, more and more medical schools have embarked on reorganization and revision of their curricula and schedules.[4]

The main organizational objective at most schools has been to reduce problems resulting from the rigid territorial lines that have developed between academic departments, described in medical circles as a "hardening of the categories." Attempting to utilize an interdisciplinary and coordinated teaching approach, many schools have developed courses organized around the individual organ systems of the body, such as the cardiovascular system, for example. Rather than offer separate courses in biochemistry, pathology, physiology, and so forth, taught by instructors who have little idea of what is taught in other departments—the traditional approach—such schools schedule interdisciplinary lecturers to cover materials that pertain to particular organ systems—the new approach. By integrating the basic sciences, the administrators of these medical schools seek to eliminate duplications between departmental offerings and reduce the basic-science material nonessential for clinical work.

Complementing these less formal curricular changes has been the elimination of grades and class standing, the traditional techniques of evaluation, which are being replaced with a pass/fail system wherein students are evaluated and ranked, not with a grade (A, B, C, D, or F), but simply with a "satisfactory" or "unsatisfactory" rating. This evaluation system is intended to have a wholesome effect by decreasing anxiety and student competitiveness while enhancing creative study and self-motivation.[5]

Other popular departures from traditional pedagogical techniques have included the addition of social and behavioral sciences to the curriculum, clinical experiences and patient contact from the opening day of school, and opportunities for active student inputs into the planning of course content and elective selection.

Yet after only a few years' experimentation with these departures from the established way of doing things, the pendulum has swung back toward the traditional system. At some schools, such as Harvard and Yale, for example, there has been a strong trend toward retrenchment and reinstatement of the traditional approach, wherein students take several departmental courses during a semester, study the material, and then are tested on it.[6]

Critics of the new system accuse curriculum committees of lowering academic standards, making course material too superficial, and taking away much autonomy from preclinical departments. And they also oppose the pass/fail grading system, which seems to have become inextricably linked to the new curriculum, as being a step backward, not forward. Grades are beneficial, they say, because they help students assess their own performance, motivate them to work harder, and thereby enhance competition in the national marketplace for the most prestigious internships. And when students studying under the new system do poorly on the national board examinations, fuel is added to the fire of these critics.

While students generally prefer the self-learning emphasis of the new approach rather than the faculty-directed techniques of the old, or traditional system, it is often a mixed blessing. For although students are relieved from competitive pressures, the new system places a heavy burden on them to overcome inertia, fatigue, and procrastination.[7]

Despite these trends and countertrends, one can only speculate about the future direction of curricular revision in this country; whether the pendulum will take large or small swings in one direction or the other remains to be seen. But whatever form and organization future curricula may take, of this point we may be sure: The curriculum represents the faculty's best thinking and efforts regarding the proper training of medical recruits. The curriculum is its formalized blueprint designed to shape medical students into doctors.

TRADITIONAL CURRICULUM

The vast majority of medical school graduates in this country have experienced a traditional system similar in broad outline to the one that existed at the medical school where I conducted this study. Organizational details of this classical design have varied from school to school, of course, but the overall structure and form are remarkably similar, consisting of approximately two years of basic-science course work followed by a two-year clinical apprenticeship.[8]

The purpose of the curriculum is, as the school catalog from the study institution indicates, "to provide a solid foundation for the student to enable him or her to develop continuously as a physician during internship, residency, and practice." To this end, the school attempts to give students the knowledge, skills, and attitudes basic to all fields of medicine. Specific objectives established for the curriculum are to provide a knowledge of

a. normal human beings and the common disorders of structure and function that result from disease, injury, or birth defect;
b. the way in which physical, chemical, biologic, psychological, social, and genetic factors affect people in health and disease;
c. the skills and resources within the profession and community that relate to the prevention or cure of disease; the limitation of disease, and the promotion of health;
d. the social, ethical, and historical settings and traditions associated with medical education and practice.

In addition, the curriculum is intended to help each student

a. understand himself or herself so that patients and their problems can be better understood;
b. establish habits of continuing self-education;
c. become thorough and accurate in all observations, recording, and interpretations.

Through opportunities for practical clinical experience, students are advised that physicians can "cure sometimes, relieve often, prevent frequently, and comfort always."

First Year

During the first year, students at the study institution concentrate on normal structure and function. The courses in anatomy (including gross anatomy, histology, and neuroanatomy), biochemistry, and microbiology are supplemented with a course entitled "Perspectives in Medicine" (a two-year interdisciplinary course dealing with the historical and sociologic

FIGURE 5-1. First-Year Schedule

First Semester
(First Unit — 5 Weeks; Second Unit — 11 Weeks)

Time	Monday	Tuesday	Wednesday	Thursday	Friday	Saturday
8:00-8:50	Gross Anatomy	Gross Anatomy	Perspectives in Medicine	Perspectives in Medicine	Psychobiology	
9:00-9:50	Gross Anatomy	Histology[a] or Neuroanatomy[a]	Histology	Histology[a] or Neuroanatomy[a]	Histology	Gross Anatomy
10:00-10:50						
11:00-11:50						
1:00-1:50	Preparation Time	Gross Anatomy	Preparation Time	Gross Anatomy	Preparation Time	
2:00-2:50						
3:00-3:50						
4:00-4:50						

[a] Histology is taught during this period for the first five-week unit in place of neuroanatomy; for the remainder of the semester (the second, eleven-week unit), neuroanatomy is taught at this time in place of histology.

Second Semester
(16 Weeks)

Time	Monday	Tuesday	Wednesday	Thursday	Friday	Saturday
8:00-8:50	Biochemistry	Microbiology	Biochemistry	Microbiology	Biochemistry Perspectives in Medicine	Microbiology
9:00-9:50						
10:00-10:50						
11:00-11:50						
1:00-1:50	Biochemistry	Preparation Time	Biochemistry	Preparation Time	Preparation Time	
2:00-2:50						
3:00-3:50						
4:00-4:50						

concepts of medicine, the scientific method, biostatistics, and medical genetics) and occasional lectures in psychobiology (an introduction to psychiatry and the behavioral sciences). Figure 5–1 is the daily calendar of hours that students follow during each semester of the freshman year. Figure 5–2 indicates the number of hours spent in each course during the first year.

Second Year

In the second year, disease is the main focus of study. An understanding in biologic abnormalities in structure and function is gained through correlated courses in pathology, pharmacology, and physiology. As Figs. 5–3 and 5–4 indicate, these courses consume a lion's share of the sophomore's time. A few lectures in psychopathology and a continuation of "Perspectives in Medicine" round out the offering. The course in psychopathology deals with normal and abnormal mental mechanisms, personality deviations, and the more common mental disorders.

To prepare students for future clinical assignments, eight weeks are set aside at the end of the sophomore year for teaching them the principles of clinical practice. In an interdisciplinary course entitled "Introduction to Clinical Medicine," students are instructed in the basic skills of taking medical histories, conducting physical examinations and laboratory tests, and interpreting the findings obtained. This course comprises a series of lectures, demonstrations, and case presentations. Toward the end of the course, students are given opportunities to examine patients in the hospital wards and to discuss their findings with the instructors.

During this eight-week period, students are also introduced to the

FIGURE 5-2. Summary of Hours—First Year

	FIRST SEMESTER (FIRST UNIT—5 WEEKS; SECOND UNIT—11 WEEKS)	SECOND SEMESTER (16 WEEKS)	TOTAL HOURS
Anatomy			
Gross	85	183	—	268
Histology	60	63	—	123
Neuroanatomy	—	66	—	66
Biochemistry	—	—	288	288
Microbiology	—	—	192	192
Perspectives in Medicine	10	21	32	63
Preparation Time	60	132	192	384
Psychobiology	5	11	—	16
	220	476	704	1400

FIGURE 5-3. Second-Year Schedule

First Semester and Second Semester (First Unit — 24 Weeks)

Time	Monday	Tuesday	Wednesday	Thursday	Friday	Saturday
8:00–8:50	Physiology or Pharmacology	Physiology or Pharmacology	Physiology or Pharmacology	Physiology or Pharmacology	Physiology or Pharmacology	Physiology or Pharmacology
9:00–9:50	Pathology		Pathology		Pathology	Pathology
10:00–10:50	Pathology		Pathology		Pathology	Pathology
11:00–11:50	Pathology		Pathology		Pathology	Pathology
1:00–1:50	Psycho-pathology	Physiology or Pharmacology		Physiology or Pharmacology		
2:00–2:50	Preparation Time	Physiology or Pharmacology	Preparation Time	Physiology or Pharmacology	Preparation Time	
3:00–3:50	Preparation Time					
4:00–4:50	Preparation Time					

Second Semester (Second Unit — 8 Weeks)

Time	Monday	Tuesday	Wednesday	Thursday	Friday	Saturday
8:00–8:50	Surgery Lecture	Human Reproduction	Surgery Lecture	Human Reproduction	Surgery Lecture	Human Reproduction
9:00–9:50	Preventive Medicine	Preventive Medicine	Surgery Lab	Preventive Medicine	Surgery Lab	Physical Diagnosis, Clinical Lab Methods, Intro. to Medicine
10:00–10:50	Preventive Medicine	Radiology	Surgery Lab	Radiology		Physical Diagnosis, Clinical Lab Methods, Intro. to Medicine
11:00–11:50	Perspectives in Medicine	Physical Diagnosis, Clinical Lab Methods, Intro. to Medicine	Perspectives in Medicine	Physical Diagnosis, Clinical Lab Methods, Intro. to Medicine	Preventive Medicine	Physical Diagnosis, Clinical Lab Methods, Intro. to Medicine
1:00–1:50	Preparation Time	Physical Diagnosis, Clinical Lab Methods, Intro.	Preparation Time	Physical Diagnosis, Clinical Lab Methods, Intro.	Physical Diagnosis, Clinical Lab Methods, Intro.	
2:00–2:50	Preparation Time		Preparation Time			
3:00–3:50	Preparation Time					

	FIRST SEMESTER	SECOND SEMESTER		TOTAL HOURS
	First Unit		*Second Unit*	
	16 WEEKS	8 WEEKS	8 WEEKS	
Human Reproduction ...	—	—	24	24
Introduction to Clinical Medicine	—	—	136	136
Pathology	192	96	—	288
Perspectives in Medicine .	—	—	16	16
Pharmacology	68	81	—	149
Physiology	244	79	—	323
Preparation Time	176	88	48	312
Preventive Medicine	—	—	48	48
Psychopathology	16	8	—	24
Radiology	—	—	16	16
Surgery	—	—	48	48
	696	352	336	1384

FIGURE 5-4. Summary of Hours—Second Year

fundamentals of surgery and radiology. Lectures on human reproduction, marriage and family health, preventive medicine, perspectives in medicine, and the history of medicine complete the curriculum.

Third and Fourth Years

In the third and fourth years, students spend most of their time in small groups on the hospital floors in various clinical assignments. Third-year students rotate their schedules so that during each quarter (fall, winter, and spring) they serve a clerkship in one of the three major clinical services, as indicated in Fig. 5–5: a surgery clerkship, a medicine clerkship, and a clerkship in OB/GYN and pediatrics. By the end of the junior year, each student will have had experience in each of these clinical areas. In the senior year, a fourth (summer) quarter is added (Fig. 5–5), and the curriculum is divided into four sections: The first three are the major clinical services, while the added quarter is devoted to a supervised elective that holds particular interest for the student.

Each class section is further divided into small groups that rotate through the various subdivisions of each clinical service. During the surgery clerkship, for example, students may rotate through general surgery, thoracic surgery, ophthalmology, urology, neurosurgery, orthopedics, and plastic surgery. The medicine clerkship includes general medicine, cardiology, dermatology, hematology, metabolism, and gastroenterology. Neurology is included in both medicine and pediatrics.

FIGURE 5-5. Clinical Assignments—Third and Fourth Years

Third Year

Quarter	Section I	Section II	Section III
Fall	Medicine	Surgery	Ob-Gyn/Pediatrics
Winter	Ob-Gyn/Pediatrics	Medicine	Surgery
Spring	Surgery	Ob-Gyn/Pediatrics	Medicine

Fourth Year

Quarter	Section A	Section B	Section C	Section D
Summer	Medicine	Elective	Ob-Gyn/Pediatrics [a]	Surgery
Fall	Surgery	Ob-Gyn/Pediatrics[a]	Elective	Medicine
Winter	Ob-Gyn/Pediatrics [a]	Surgery	Medicine	Elective
Spring	Elective	Medicine	Surgery	Ob-Gyn/Pediatrics [a]

[a] Divided as follows: Half quarter—Obstetrics and Gynecology; Half quarter—Pediatrics

During clinical rotations, groups of three or four students are assigned to a member of the house staff who conducts daily teaching exercises. Members of the staff also lead daily teaching rounds with groups of about six students. The usual format of conducting rounds in a teaching hospital is as follows: One of the house staff gives an abbreviated diagnosis to the students in a conference area, which may or may not be followed with short lectures by the attending physician. The entire group then visits the bedside of the patient, the attending physician checks the validity of the findings, and students are allowed to participate to some degree in observing, touching, and checking. The group then retires to a quiet area to discuss the case and its possible management. The next case is then introduced.[9]

The purpose of the clinical clerkship is, of course, to provide students an opportunity to work closely with patients and to observe disease processes firsthand. Bedside teaching helps students gain applied knowledge and practical experience in the basic clinical procedures.

During the third year, students work with "service patients" in the hospital wards, those receiving free physician care because of their inability to pay a private physician. Here they learn methods of history taking and physical examinations and diagnosis, correlation of laboratory studies, and general therapeutic principles through ward rounds and ward classes. In addition to taking medical histories and performing physical examinations, they attend operations on their assigned patients and participate in daily ward conferences with the staff. They are also expected to spend as much time as possible reading about the various disorders under consideration.

A variety of short courses presented during this third year (Fig. 5–6) offers capsule overviews of numerous clinical areas: anesthesiology, applied medical genetics, dermatology, neurology, neurosurgery, obstetrical and gynecological pathology, obstetrics, ophthalmology, orthopedics, otolaryngology, radiology, surgery, and urology. These courses usually consist of didactic lectures as well as clinical demonstrations. Other courses offered to juniors include a continuation of the behavioral science course in marriage and family health and two special offerings: "Medical Jurisprudence" (in the Department of Preventive Medicine and Genetics) and an interdepartmental course entitled "Medical Education for National Defense" (MEND).

Also included in the third- and fourth-year programs are teaching clinics, which are offered through the medical, pediatrics, psychiatry, and surgery departments. In these clinics, actual cases are discussed, then illustrated by patients from the wards. In surgery, the history, physical examination, diagnostic techniques, and treatment of a case are discussed after presentation by a student. In the third-year weekly psychiatry clinics, various fields of present-day psychiatry, mental hygiene, and psychiatric social work are covered, and the taking of psychiatric histories is demonstrated and practiced; senior students spend one-half day per week for two quarters assigned to the psychiatry service.

Aside from these teaching clinics, almost all of the fourth year is spent in clinical clerkships (Fig. 5–7). Here seniors are expected to apply their improving skills to a more detailed study of disease mechanisms and therapy. In addition to dealing with ward "service patients" as they did in the third year, they are exposed to private patients in the hospital. They also gain experience in the outpatient department and in the emergency room, and make daily hospital rounds with the attending physician and house staff. Emphasis is placed on the development of clinical judgment, and students are expected to formulate their own ideas of the best diagnostic and therapeutic approach in each case.

One requirement for graduation at this school is a senior dissertation— a paper that is most often a critical discussion of some area of medicine.

FIGURE 5-6. Third-Year Schedule

Time	Monday	Tuesday	Wednesday	Thursday	Friday	Saturday
8:00-8:50 (F) (W) (S)	Otolaryngology	Anesthesiology Dermatology Dermatology	Neurology Neurosurgery Ophthalmology	Radiology Radiology Urology	Med. Genetics Orthopedics M E N D	
9:00-10:50		Clinical	Clerkship			
11:00-11:50	Pediatrics Clinic	Medicine Clinic	Surgery Clinic	Prev. Med. (W) Psychiatry (F and S)	Ob-Gyn Clinic	
1:00-3:50		Clinical	Clerkship			

F—Fall Quarter; W—Winter Quarter; S—Spring Quarter.
Clerkship time is arranged by services with the equivalent of one afternoon per week unscheduled.

FIGURE 5-7. Fourth-Year Schedule

Time	Monday	Tuesday	Wednesday	Thursday	Friday	Saturday
8:00-10:50		Clinical		Clerkship		
11:00-11:50		Medicine Clinic	Surgery Clinic			
1:00-4:00		Clinical			Clerkship	

Clerkship time is arranged by services, with the equivalent of one afternoon per week unscheduled.

The topic for this dissertation must be selected and approved in the third year.

HOW STUDENTS ARE EVALUATED

The M.D. degree is conferred upon those who have successfully completed four years of specified study in the medical sciences. In order to graduate, each student must also pass Parts I and II of the examinations given by the National Board of Medical Examiners. Part I is usually taken at the end of the sophomore year, and Part II at the end of the senior year.

Performance in Basic-Science Courses

In the basic-science courses, the grading system is similar to that employed by most undergraduate schools; grades are given on the basis of frequent examinations. The final grade in each course is reported to the Dean's office, where the information is used to rank students from high to low in class standing.

If a student's performance falls short of school standards, he or she is called to meet with the Promotions Committee, a faculty body that reviews the progress of each student at the end of each grading period. Some students may be required to repeat a particular course, or even an entire year. In rare instances, a student may be required to withdraw when it is evident that he or she is not qualified to continue.

By contrast, high achievers are honored for outstanding performance, usually at an annual gathering such as an honors convocation. At that time, several certificates and awards are given by the faculty and financed in part by pharmaceutical houses, in recognition of exceptional achievement. A gift is usually given the individual with the highest class standing.

Performance in Clinical Work

The performance of students during the clinical clerkship is rated by the clinical faculty on the basis of twelve factors listed on a "Student Evaluation Form." [10] These factors are: (1) Information Gathering; (2) Utilization of Laboratory; (3) Problem Solving and Clinical Judgment; (4) Implementation of Management Plan and Understanding of Impediments to Optimal Patient Care; (5) Relationship to Patients; (6) Relationship to Colleagues; (7) Relationships to Paramedical Personnel and Community Facilities; (8) Professional Satisfactions; (9) Conceptualizations About Disease; (10) Work Record; (11) Emotional Stability; and (12) Overall Competence.

Each of the first nine factors and Factor 12 on the "Student Evaluation Form" are rated on a twelve-point scale, as follows:

1–3—Poor

4–6—Marginal

7–9—Good

10–12—Excellent

To insure uniform interpretations of these performance factors, descriptions of the "effective" and the "ineffective" student are given on the Evaluation Form for each of the first nine categories.

Factors 10 and 11 (Work Record and Emotional Stability) are scored differently, with *yes* or *no* responses to specific questions. The student's rating on Factor 12 (overall competence) is based on the judgments recorded for Factors 1–11.

The descriptions of all twelve factors, which are given below with the basis for rating each, are paraphrased from the "Student Evaluation Form."

Performance Evaluation Categories

1. INFORMATION GATHERING. Concern here is with the student's skill in obtaining and organizing diagnostic information from the patient. An *effective* student elicits an accurate, perceptive, and appropriate history; avoids general stereotyped expressions; correlates the facts from all facets of the history into a meaningful conception of the patient's circumstances; conducts an accurate and appropriate physical examination; records information in a systematic fashion and writes careful progress notes; and uses available time effectively to reach a reasonable end point with each patient. By contrast, the *ineffective* student takes a ritualistic history that exhibits little concern for the individual patient's problem; ignores or fails to explore leads; writes a history full of cliches and unsubstantiated summations; focuses the physical examination on preconceived notions of what should be found and makes it uneven in depth; takes notes that are disorganized and inadequate for guiding subsequent decisions about management of the patient; and makes inefficient use of time with no clear goal in mind.

2. UTILIZATION OF LABORATORY. This pertains to the student's ability to use laboratory facilities and to interpret laboratory results. The *effective* student is discriminating in the use of laboratory facilities; uses knowledge of basic sciences in justifying requested tests; and interprets results in the light of the case at hand, integrating and evaluating them with other data

about the patient. The *ineffective* student is indiscriminate in the use of the laboratory; does not have a clear rationale for his or her laboratory orders; is interested only in the laboratory result itself and whether it is normal or abnormal; and usually accepts the laboratory report as the final arbiter of action, failing to integrate it with other findings or to evaluate it in light of the total picture.

3. PROBLEM SOLVING AND CLINICAL JUDGMENT.   This concerns the student's ability to use the information gained to arrive at a diagnosis and to develop a sound plan of management. The *effective* student is responsive to unexpected findings and seeks to determine their implications; takes all the data into account before reaching a decision and regularly tests alternative hypotheses; approaches the diagnosis objectively and avoids prejudgment; has a sound rationale for therapeutic decisions, and makes provisions to monitor the patient's progress and to modify therapy as required. The *ineffective* student is unable to interpret unexpected results and often ignores them; works at random, without perceptible hypotheses, and leaves loose ends; approaches therapy with cookbook style; makes little effort to monitor the patient's progress; and switches tactics often, paying little attention to basic therapeutics.

4. IMPLEMENTATION OF MANAGEMENT PLAN AND UNDERSTANDING OF IMPEDIMENTS TO OPTIMAL PATIENT CARE.   These are concerned with the student's understanding and ability to consider various social, economic, personal, and familial obstacles to optimal patient care. The *effective* student seeks to treat more than the immediate health problem when other factors in the situation affect the general well-being of the patient; is aware of the specific social, economic, personal, and familial conditions that affect the management of each patient and compromise the patient's compliance; takes realistic account of these factors in outlining a plan of management with each patient; and adapts the treatment to meet specific needs. The *ineffective* student focuses only on the immediate health problems; tends to treat the patient in a rigid, stereotyped manner, as another case of diabetes, hypertension, and so forth, without adapting personal management to the specific circumstances of each patient; tends to blame vague social forces and the individual patient for any lack of compliance; practices shortsighted management; and adapts poorly to special situations.

5. RELATIONSHIP TO PATIENTS.   This pertains to the student's willingness and ability to establish an effective relationship with patients. The *effective* student establishes and maintains a comfortable professional rapport with patients; tends to overcome communication problems; protects the confidence of the patient and provides appropriate explanations to the patient and family; encourages the patient to express personal ideas, attitudes, concerns, and anxieties; conducts own contacts with the patient in a way that reflects kindness, respect, and honesty; and practices a ma-

ture, gentle, and accepting approach without overinvolvement. The *in-effective* student gives no evidence of interest in the patient as a person; presents a stereotyped approach and cold manner, making no attempt to overcome problems of communication; fails to provide adequate guidance to the patient and family, or is tactless and indiscreet in discussions with them and discourages the patient from expressing private thoughts and anxieties; is harsh and inconsiderate and may exhibit overt disapproval of the patient; or may, on occasion, become overinvolved.

6. RELATIONSHIP TO COLLEAGUES. This deals with the student's skill in establishing appropriate professional relationships with classmates and attending staff. The *effective* student seeks professional contact with staff and peers; is straightforward in approaching them and raising constructive questions about the concepts they present; is available to assist as required and offers advice in a tactful and discreet manner; recognizes personal limitations and exercises initiative within those limits; and seeks advice and consultation when needed and makes good use of the contributions of others. The *ineffective* student may be quiet, insecure, and uncommunicative; may attempt to minimize professional contact with staff and peers; may be alternately defensive, tactless, inconsiderate, or overcritical toward them; and displays rigidity in habits, and is unwilling or unable to give or take advice gracefully or request required assistance.

7. RELATIONSHIPS TO PARAMEDICAL PERSONNEL AND COMMUNITY FACILITIES. Of concern here are the student's willingness and ability to make effective use of paramedical personnel and community resources in planning the total care of the patient. The *effective* student recognizes the skill of other members of the health team and is discerning in the use of paramedical and public health facilities and personnel; is aware of their specific contributions and will make an effort to establish contact with them and to seek their assistance when appropriate; and deals with them as professional colleagues, effectively integrating their contribution into the total care of patients. The *ineffective* student fails to recognize the professional skills of other members of the team; has only vague notions of the role of paramedical and public health personnel and facilities; makes little effort to establish professional contact for the purpose of mutual understanding; rarely utilizes such resources; and deals with them as subordinates rather than as professional colleagues and does not integrate their efforts into the total care of the patient.

8. PROFESSIONAL SATISFACTIONS. These pertain to the student's attitudes toward various aspects of professional responsibilities and opportunities in dealing with the patient. The *effective* student is willing and able to accept responsibility for the care of assigned patients; can tolerate the inevitable disappointments and obtain satisfactions from work with patients for whom no quick successes are possible; handles frustrations

through constructive thought and modifications in approach; is open to the ideas of others; and continues to develop individual knowledge and skills. The *ineffective* student is easily frustrated in the absence of quick success or, if faced with alternatives from which to choose, has developed a rigid system of behavior and expectation and is intolerant of change; derives little satisfaction from work except in the most rigid setting; and demonstrates little interest in utilizing professional experience to develop knowledge and skills.

9. CONCEPTUALIZATIONS ABOUT DISEASE. These relate to the student's ability to take a variety of approaches in analyzing problems of disease. The *effective* student can think validly about a situation in abstract terms; can separate a disease process from its effect on the patient as a biologic organism, can utilize various systems of categories (anatomic, physiological, psychosomatic, etc.) in analyzing the disease process; and is willing to use abstractions arrived at in this way in thinking about disease. The *ineffective* student is always pragmatic; avoids realities beyond the situation at hand; limits own ability to think about disease and restricts personal scope to a single approach; and is too amenable to suggestions, has little independent thought, and values few ideas for their own sake, whether right or wrong.

10. WORK RECORD. This deals with rating the student's work performance. Rather than utilizing the usual 12-point scale, the faculty member simply checks one of three responses ("yes," "no," or "insufficient information to judge") to the following questions:

a. Did you find the student ambitious? (Would the necessary clinical tasks be undertaken without repeated requests?)
b. Was he or she available when needed?

11. EMOTIONAL STABILITY. This has to do with how the student reacts under various stressful circumstances. The student is rated by "yes" and "no" responses to the following questions:

a. Adaptability (Do hostile, critically ill, physically attractive or unattractive, or otherwise unusual patients exert unfavorable influence?)
b. Flexibility (Do sudden changes in patient condition or in attitudes of others cause undue disturbance to the student?)
c. Physical appearance (Is grooming, personal hygiene, or apparel at any time bizarre or inappropriate?)
d. Intellectual honesty (Does he or she copy house officer's work-up or quote unread references, etc.?)
e. Professional demeanor (Is behavior at any time unprofessional, offensive, bizarre, unethical, or unusual in any way?)

12. OVERALL COMPETENCE. This category is for judging the student's overall performance in the clerkship and is rated on the basis of scores on the previous eleven factors.

Faculty Rating Procedures, Known and Unknown

Staff members are encouraged to offer comments about the student's performance on any or all of the twelve factors on the rating form and about anything else that is considered relevant in evaluating the student's overall competence. To insure the greatest possible fairness of evaluation, raters are asked to consider the performance of students in each category before moving to the next category; and whenever an unsatisfactory rating is given, the rater must specify the exact circumstances that led him or her to this conclusion.

Despite the formal, highly structured method of evaluating student performance just described, the rating procedure is generally not formally made known to the students themselves.[11] The semisecrecy with which grading occurs in medical school could perhaps be likened to the way physicians typically handle laboratory results. Patients are seldom allowed to obtain their own laboratory results, even though their own bodies were tested and they paid for the service; instead, the results seem to become the personal property of the physician in charge. Students, like patients, apparently must accept this paternalistic posture on the grounds that their physician mentors are *the* authorities and know what is best.

However, even though students did not at the time of the study have access to information pertaining to their own performance evaluations, their concepts of appropriate clinical behavior generally seemed to correspond with the standards described on the rating form. This commonality reinforces the idea that most learning for the clinical role occurs informally through modeling, rather than through didactic instruction.

HOW STUDENTS EVALUATE THE CURRICULUM

The criteria by which students evaluate courses and clinical rotations remain fairly constant throughout all years of school. When asked why certain courses or clerkship experiences are considered better than others, students say that good ones have the following characteristics: interesting subject matter; effective presentation of material; clinical relevance (topics and experiences that will be useful in future medical practice); and well-organized components (to maximize amount learned per unit of time).

Interest in Subject Matter

One-fifth of the class base their choice of a best course or service primarily on personal interest. When one is vitally interested in the topic, the work is a joy rather than an effort; lectures and reading assignments are hungrily devoured. Concerning one course, a sophomore said, "I just ate it up; I must have read two or three unassigned books on the subject." Yet, a classmate had this reaction to the same course: "I found it completely boring and unenlightening; the work was a drudgery, and I had to force myself to do it."

The relationship between interest and work enjoyment holds true for clinical services as well. Pediatrics rotation, for example, can be either enjoyable or not, depending on how well one relates to children. Such basic interests unquestionably influence the choice of a medical specialty. (Refer to Chapter 9.)

Presentation of Subject Matter

In each year of medical school, the quality of instruction remains important in winning the approval of students. The courses and rotations judged best are those taught by dedicated instructors who demonstrate a genuine interest in helping students learn. They prepare the material well and present it in a clear, concise, and interesting manner. Even those offerings that otherwise hold little appeal are enjoyable when well presented.

Courses taught by poorly prepared professors frustrate students. This is because their lectures are disorganized and they compensate for inadequate preparation by "speeding up and hurrying through those areas where they are fuzzy."

Students also take a dim view of lecturers who use them as a captive audience for discussing their latest research. These professors seem to regard teaching as a chore, a necessary evil that detracts from their primary interest. So when given teaching assignments, they may simply drone on about their research activities.

Students comment frequently on how much they prefer the one-to-one learning experiences in the clinical setting. But clinicians, like their basic-science colleagues, vary in tutorial interests and talents. In some services, staff members make themselves accessible and take time to explain procedures and answer questions. Describing one such service as "the most outstanding" in his experience, a junior remarked, "Those on the staff make sure that we participate in every way possible, doing as many procedures as we can. They let us write orders and challenge us intellectually. And they don't limit their teaching to their own specialty, either; they'll sit down and talk about the patient's social as well as his medical problems."

But, unfortunately, some clinical mentors seldom make themselves available to students, and their teaching is limited to instructing them on the performance of routine chores. "They don't read our write-ups and sometimes not even our progress reports," a junior complained. "So there is no way of knowing whether we're doing a good or bad job." Rounds on one service are described like this:

> We'll sit there for an hour going over the patients' charts. The resident doesn't discuss them with us, but may say to the intern, "Mr. So-and-So spiked a fever; what shall we do?" But we are never included in the conversation, and our opinions are never asked. After flipping through the charts, the resident will walk into a room and just make immaterial conversation with the patient—like "How are you today?" or "You should eat your food." Nothing is pointed out to us that we should notice; we are just ignored.

Whatever learning takes place on such rotations depends primarily on one's own initiative and ability to find answers to questions in the library. It is understandable that students feel cheated.

Clinical Relevance of Subject

At all stages of training, students strongly favor courses and services that have obvious clinical relevance—those that clearly pertain to the role of the practicing physician.

Basic Sciences

Students have a hard time seeing the clinical relevance of some material presented during the first two years. "We take dictation, cram it all into our heads, and then regurgitate it for exams," a freshman grumbled. "Then two weeks later it is all forgotten." Students fail to see how the rote memorization of "myriad trivia" prepares them to be physicians. "I feel cheated," a freshman lamented. "I'm not learning enough of the right things; a lot of what I'm studying, I'll never use again."

Even basic-science courses, however, have their bright spots. Although anatomy requires a great deal of memorization, it is the most highly praised freshman course, since it clearly relates to clinical medicine. "It's the real nitty-gritty, the stuff we've just got to know," a freshman observed. "It gets us started on what medicine is really about."

Anatomy instructors are praised for taking the trouble to make the course clinically relevant. In this course, very few lectures are given. Instead, students read up on an aspect of anatomical structure and then use the cadaver as a visual aid to observe what they have read. By asking frequent questions as to how the information is medically useful, the instructor helps students perceive clinical applications. "He really made me feel like I was doing something worthwhile," said one freshman. "It wasn't just learning for learning's sake but something we will be able to use as doctors. He was the best teacher we had because he got *us* to do it."

In other popular basic-science courses, patients are brought in to illustrate particular points. During the second year, nearly half the class find these clinical presentations the most worthwhile activities of all, for actual patients help bring course materials to life. Pharmacology, for example, is a favorite sophomore course because patients (either live or on videotape) are used to illustrate the treatment of particular diseases such as "diabetes mellitus," and the subject is then discussed from a variety of angles. "Actual problem solving in clinics makes it easier to learn than when we just memorize notes," a sophomore explained; "I remember much better when I see patients than when I simply memorize a long list of drugs from a sheet."

Other praiseworthy activities include autopsy case reports in pathology, visits to patients' homes with a public health nurse, and a preceptor program that allows underclassmen to accompany clinical students as they go about their hospital activities.

Clerkship Experience

Department services vary considerably in their ability to meet student needs. Those judged as worst provide students only minimal responsibilities for patient care; instead of doing, they merely observe. Speaking of such a rotation, a junior lamented, "I feel more like a spectator than a doctor; they act like every procedure is open-heart surgery. I feel as useless as a fifth wheel."

By contrast, the "best" services encourage students to feel responsibility for patient care, allowing them to do as much as they feel competent to handle. For example, a house officer, without revealing his or her own diagnosis, may ask students what orders they would write for treating a patient; then the merits and shortcomings of their views are discussed. When students must think for themselves in this manner, morale is improved and the learning process is enhanced.

Students naturally prefer rotations that permit them to participate in clinical procedures. One such service, described as "a tremendous opportunity," allows students to become actively involved in surgical procedures. "Often the surgeon would map out what was to be done, the resident would do it, and we would assist," an enthusiastic junior exclaimed. "We scrubbed in every day!" Such mentors adapt a philosophy that, in order to learn something fully, one must "see one, do one, and then teach one." "You can read or observe all day," a senior said, "but unless you actually get immersed in the work by doing things yourself, it's impossible to get a real grasp on the subject."

In the various outpatient clinics, students see the most patients and are given the most responsibility. "That's where you see it all," a senior commented. The outpatient clinic often resembles an office practice, where a majority of the patients have ordinary illnesses—a situation quite different from that encountered on the ward of a teaching hospital. And to make things even better, students have a good chance to see patients before the attending doctor or resident does. Obviously, being the first to perform a work-up on the patient provides a much better learning situation than being third or fourth in line and knowing the previous work done by the senior physicians.

The hospital emergency room also provides an excellent clinical experience. Comparatively large numbers of patients with a wide variety of medical problems are seen here, and students are given considerable responsibility. As a senior points out, "You're sort of on the spot and are forced to think on your feet."

During the senior year, some students, as an elective, serve externships in neighboring hospitals. Treated as interns, and sometimes given full responsibility for a ward, they marvel at this experience. "I had all responsibilities of working up patients, figuring out what was wrong with them, writing orders, keeping up day-by-day, etc.," one enthused. "It was a great experience." The disillusionment is profound, however, upon returning to the teaching hospital to again become "fourth in line."

Amount Learned Per Unit of Time

Because demands made upon students are so great, time is naturally regarded as a precious commodity. Locked into a tight schedule, medical students are herded from one place to another with little opportunity to arrange individual schedules. It is not surprising, then, that they vociferously denounce instructors who waste their time in nonproductive activities.

Basic Sciences

Students are most keenly aware of time pressures when, as freshmen and sophomores, their confidence is shakiest. It is natural, then, for them to praise courses that make productive use of time and condemn the others.

Gross anatomy is singled out as the "best" freshman course, not only because of its obvious clinical relevance, but also because students learn "a tremendous amount" during each session. They like the feeling of accomplishment that the course gives them. "It was so well outlined that we knew what was expected, and we didn't get bogged down in a lot of ambiguous stuff," a freshman explained.

Again, in the sophomore year, pharmacology is regarded as the "best" course because there is little wasted time. "It is concise and jam-packed with pertinent material," a sophomore commented. By contrast, poorly organized courses result in unnecessary repetition and thereby waste valuable time. "When lectures are not well outlined, I spend half my time trying to figure out what I'm supposed to learn," another complained.

By far the biggest waste of time, students agree, is the laboratory work that uses up many afternoons and evenings. Disappointment with this work is almost universal, especially in the freshman year, when students call it "substandard," "pointless," "ridiculous," and "an utter waste of time." "Considering the expenditure of time," one said, "you just don't reap a harvest like you should."

Laboratory time is often spent in routine chores, such as setting up equipment, measuring and pouring substances, washing glassware, and cleaning up. And many of the experiments, students point out, consist of repetitive "cookbook" operations that require little thought. "Once you pipette a couple of times," a freshman complained, "you know how to do it, and I see no purpose in repeating it over and over again." So, students soon come to the conclusion that lab assignments are nothing more than "busywork." "They fill up our schedule to keep us busy," a sophomore charged. "They don't feel comfortable letting us be unscheduled, so they try to make technicians out of us. It's absolutely ridiculous!" Small wonder these students consider independent study the most productive use of time.

Clerkship Experience

Compared with the tightly structured schedule of the basic-science years, training on the hospital floors is, as one upperclassman put it, "a helter-skelter experience." A good deal of time is wasted, students say, by the inefficiency of the hospital routine, lack of familiarity with the hospital system, crowded staff schedules, and periods when the patient load drops off. During these years, nearly half the class complain that too much of their time is spent "sitting around twiddling our thumbs waiting for things to happen."

The most frequently mentioned grievance is waiting for staff members to show up for rounds or other activities. "You're just kind of in limbo," a junior commented. "You can't go off and do something else, so you just stand there." And when the resident does show up, the schedule often resembles a "follow-the-leader" game with students tagging along behind the resident until he or she decides what to do.

Although different services waste students' time in different ways, the effect is the same: frustration. In medicine rotation, for example, a typical student complaint is of "sitting on my ass too long." In contrast, surgery rotation is often described as "standing around a lot":

They don't let you do one thing, except maybe hold retractors for several hours or else elevate the patient's leg until your arms break. Often you don't even get close enough to watch the operation. When it's finished the surgeon says, "Well, that was a good job"—and you haven't seen a thing. You've just spent four or five hours standing there straining muscles and not using your intellectual faculties at all. It's a big waste of time.

Clerkship duty in obstetrics also is described as "a pure unadulterated waste of time." During the duty hours, students sit with women in labor— counting contractions and checking the patient's blood pressure and pulse rate every 15 minutes. "We just sort of hold their hands," a junior remarked. Students feel that the first two or three experiences like this are worth the time, but they do not like repeating these chores over and over again. They feel that they do not learn enough to justify the time required.

Having to do "scut work"—repetitive routine chores that have little instructional value—is a frequent complaint, especially in the third year. Examples are: running errands for the resident (getting X rays, carting "stuff" back from the laboratory, and so on); doing secretarial work that could easily be done by the ward clerk or typist (filling out forms, keeping charts up to date, scheduling X-ray examinations, and the like); starting I.V.s; and doing other "piddly little tasks" that after the first few times have little educational value. At nonteaching hospitals, these menial chores are usually performed by the paramedical or clerical staff.

Fortunately, however, the clinical years have their bright spots, too. Some services are so well organized that they provide a highly productive learning experience with a minimum of time loss. The neurology service is singled out as such an experience:

> They have an excellent schedule planned for us; every day we're really busy, and there is a big variety of patients to work up. I was over there every night pretty late working up patients and doing things. During the day there is something that demands our time almost every hour. The staff members are always teaching us something. They give us the schedule the very first day, and everything is planned to ensure our having worthwhile experiences. I really got something out of it.

Such "cram-packed" learning experiences are highly valued because they give students a feeling of accomplishment, a high yield of learning per unit of time.

SUMMING UP

At the time of this study, the curriculum at the subject institution varied little from the classical curricular design traditionally utilized by medical schools in this country during the previous half century. The teaching techniques at these schools have with few, if any, exceptions consisted of didactic lectures, laboratory work, clinical clerkships and departmental rounds, case conferences, and seminars and grand rounds, as well as assigned reading and individual conferences with mentors. Despite the fact that many schools have recently revised their curricula outlines, these same pedagogical techniques still constitute the primary methods of teaching today's medical students. These are the means by which curricular goals will be realized—namely, transmitting the knowledge, skills, and attitudes basic to the successful practice of medicine.

Being vocationally oriented, medical students naturally value those features of the teaching experience that seem most relevant to their future role, and failure to provide these aspects dominates much of their criticism about the curriculum. It is frustrating to them that much time during the first two years is directed toward pursuits that seem more oriented toward careers in scientific research than to medical practice. Although academic learning may help them achieve high scores on the National Board Examinations, students in loud chorus say that the basic-science emphasis is disillusioning.

Despite recent alterations in curricular offerings aimed to correct this seeming imbalance, it appears unlikely that the educational experiences of future doctors will be significantly different from their predecessors. Some, in fact, view these curricular alterations as only a repackaging and renaming of the same old information, citing the tendency among all human beings, even highly educated ones, to resist change and maintain the status quo. As long as the reward structure of the medical school faculty favors those who excel at research, publishing, and grantsmanship (through promotions and other recognition), the basic scientists will maintain their strong position in the power structure of the institution. After commenting on the federal financing of research and research training, a former dean and president of the Association of American Medical Colleges observed:

> Even forty years ago, the strongest voice in the medical schools was that of the clinician who was in close touch with community practice. Today, the authority in most medical schools resides in the hands of the basic scientists and the full-time, research-oriented clinical investigators. Both of these groups are splendid contributors to the progress of medical science and to the improvement of the scientific foundation of medical education. But neither of these groups is in any sense devoted to presenting to students or house officers the problems of patient care outside the university center and the special kinds of rewards that can be derived from community practice.[12]

So, until the reward structure of the medical center favors good teaching rather than basic research, the formalized curricular structure of the future is, in my judgment, not likely to differ significantly from the past except, perhaps, in peripheral ways.

Regardless of social structure, however, clinicians will continue to be held in high esteem by students and to win their respect through daily application of a thorough and practical knowledge of demonstrable patient care. None can argue the bond of this common ground.

NOTES

1. Concerned about a doctor shortage, the federal government began in the 1960s to subsidize medical education. Since enactment of the Health Professions Education Assistance Program in 1963, more than one million dollars in federal grants have been awarded to medical schools for the purpose of expanding facilities and aiding students. Since then, the number of medical schools has increased markedly. Whereas in 1964 there were 88 medical schools, there are, at the time of this writing, 116 U.S. medical schools with students enrolled ("Datagram," 1977), and there are some that are in the planning stages but have not yet admitted any students. In 1964 there were 7,300 medical graduates. The number rose to 9,600 in 1972, and by 1990 it is estimated that 16,000 students may be graduating. (See Rousselot, 1973.)

2. In the spring of 1971, the Association of American Medical Colleges listed 27 medical schools offering the M.D. degree in less than four years from the date of entry and eight others offering combined premedical and medical education programs leading to the D.S. and M.D. degrees in a minimum of six years. (See Graff and Grossman, 1973.) As of 1975, the minimum number of months required for the undergraduate medical curriculum varied from 28.5 months to 44 months. In 57 schools, the M.D. degree may be earned in less than four years, but only ten require the three-year curriculum. The trend is toward flexibility, with 47 schools allowing options for shortening the curriculum (Crowley, 1975b, p. 1344). A list of schools with three- or four-year options is provided in the *1974–75 AAMC Curriculum Directory* (Association of American Medical Colleges, 1974, p. 281).

3. Evan G. Pattishall, Jr. (1972), has identified the following curricular trends in medical education: (a) the search for relevance; (b) early introduction of clinical medicine and integration of the basic and clinical sciences; (c) an increase in curriculum flexibility with electives, free time, and multiple tracks; (d) the general adoption of the "core" curriculum concept; (e) an increase in enrollment; (f) a decrease in the training time of the traditional four-year curriculum; (g) an increased interest in research on the learning process and the medical student as learner; (h) an increase in self-instruction and independent study; (i) a shift in attitude and preparation of the entering student; (j) an increased interest in the role of human behavior in the training of physicians; and (k) an increased emphasis on family medicine and primary care.

4. While conducting this study, I served for two years on a subcommittee of the curriculum committee specifically assigned to develop relevant ways of

introducing behavioral sciences into the new medical curriculum. This curriculum was later adopted.

5. Performance on the examinations of the National Board of Medical Examiners has been used as an indicator of student achievement as affected by the curricular changes made during the recent decade (Shapiro, et al., 1974).

6. See Goldhaber (1973).

7. According to a study of student attitudes by Rosenberg and Weber (1973), there are three main problems with the old system: (a) tension and anxiety about the educational program, in particular its inflexibility, competition, extreme demands for rote memory performance, and questionable relevance; (b) the shattering of the self-image by a return to academic schedules, heightened feelings of inadequacy, and low status in the medical hierarchy; and (c) reaction to highly charged emotional situations such as death, pain, and euthanasia. These conclusions were drawn from comparing two classes that had participated in the old curriculum with two that had experienced the new.

8. In the year following the initiation of the study, the new curriculum was, with variations, adopted at the school that was the site of my study. This new approach introduced a core curriculum that integrated the basic-science offerings around the organ systems of the body, etc. In other words, my study population was the last to study under the old (traditional) approach.

9. The major drawbacks to this method of conducting rounds are the ease with which abbreviated diagnoses are forgotten or confused, and the rather sketchy training in history taking that is provided prior to internship years. For a critique of this approach and a suggested new format, see Wiener (1974).

10. Content of the "Student Evaluation Form" was originally developed by Donald M. Hayes and Harold Levine.

11. However, federal law now requires that students have, with certain minor exceptions, access to their own performance evaluations (Public Law 93–380 dated August 21, 1974—Title 20 of U.S. Code 1232g).

12. The quotation is taken from John L. Caughey's article, "More Medical Students: The Need and Available Supply" (*Journal of The American Medical Association* 198, December 5, 1966; copyright 1966, American Medical Association).

6. Stressful Experiences: Adaptational Necessities

You continually get your feathers set on fire. But somehow the more you get burned the stronger you become, and the harder it is for them to burn you the next time. (A junior)

THE RIGORS OF MEDICAL TRAINING, especially during the early stages, tend to place a severe strain upon the mental, emotional, and physical well-being of students. A growing body of literature indicates that the number of medical students who experience emotional disturbances is disproportionately large.[1] As mentioned in the Preface, studies conducted at representative schools have shown that 20 to 30 percent of the students come to the attention of faculty psychiatrists at some time during their medical school careers; and it has been suggested that even more students could benefit from psychotherapy.[2]

In my own study, the intense pressures of medical schooling caused 5 percent of the class to withdraw before the completion of the first year; and two out of five students admitted that they had entertained the idea of quitting—some, of course, more seriously than others. The longer students remain in school, however, the less likely they are to consider such action, the primary reason being that they learn adaptive techniques. If students are to survive and otherwise be successful, they must develop the necessary skills and adjustive coping mechanisms.

Professional growth and development can most readily be assessed by first identifying those experiences and situations in the socializing system that challenge—those that are stressful and produce anxiety—and then noting the techniques and processes of personal adaptation. It is my premise that challenge stimulates change. If pressed, a person can withdraw and thereby avoid confrontation, but if that person confronts the situation directly, he or she will develop adaptive skills. Stated in Hegelian terms, new syntheses (in this case, developed skills and adaptive psychosocial mechanisms) arise in response to antitheses (adversity and challenge).

111

Without this stimulation little pressure exists to motivate personal growth. A popular saying expresses this idea well: "If the going's getting easier, you ain't climbing."

Although stress is usually regarded as an evil to be avoided (thereby making us easy prey for drug advertisements that promise to make daily stress more tolerable),[3] stress can be viewed as a necessary, although not a sufficient, cause of personal change. If one is to evolve from childhood into emotional maturity, for example, one must successfully struggle with adversity. Similarly, students cannot be transformed into physicians without encountering problem-solving experiences that, in the initial stages at least, may create considerable anxiety.

In this chapter, anxieties and stressful experiences typically encountered by medical students are explored,* and the subjective processes whereby these adverse experiences become handled routinely are noted. Such observations provide clearer insights into the evolution of laymen into physicians.

REACTING TO CADAVER EXPERIENCE

When a medical student views and handles a cadaver during the first week in school, he or she experiences one of the first lessons in handling stress. How one reacts and adjusts to this experience depends, of course, upon one's emotional makeup. But most students normally feel shock, fear, and revulsion upon seeing a group of dead bodies, lying lifeless and grey on rows of tables. Few, if any, can carry off such a confrontation with complete sang-froid. Rather, the initial reaction is typically marked by

a. nausea triggered by the heavy, pungent smell of formaldehyde;
b. shock, revulsion, and a tendency to recoil upon finding the corpse so unexpectedly cold and rigid to first touch;
c. depression, loss of appetite, and an inability to concentrate for a time after the first encounter.

But no matter how great the initial shock, it apparently wears off rapidly, since most students claim to have adjusted by the second day, with

---

* Information on stress and anxiety endured in medical school was obtained by asking students each year to describe the emotional turbulence they had experienced during the current year. At the same time they were asked to indicate on a seven-point scale the degree to which they had suffered anxiety from specific, typically stressful experiences (as suggested in the literature on medical education). Students were told that 7 on the scale represented a "great deal of anxiety or stress" and that 1 represented "very little or no anxiety and stress." When asked how much anxiety or stress they experienced that year from a specific experience (e.g., the death of a patient), they would indicate a point on the stress scale and then elaborate on their experiences and feelings.

only 5 percent indicating that more than a week was needed.[4] Of the latter, one experienced severe anxiety and others displayed physically related problems. For example, a squeamish student was unable to touch the cadaver without putting on rubber gloves, and a classmate sought medical treatment due to an allergic reaction.

The easy adjustment apparent among the majority suggests a general imperturbability, but a type of "machismo" should not be overlooked. Since the ability to undergo such experiences without betraying disgust or squeamishness is a valued characteristic among clinicians, this may cause students to exaggerate the case with which such discomforting situations are met and, in turn, suppress openness about personal anxieties. In this regard, Lief and Fox (1963) have noted:

> One of the earliest ways in which a first-year student can demonstrate to his classmates that he has the qualities of a good physician is by controlling his feelings in the anatomy laboratory. Apparently, freshman medical students consider it important to prove to each other, as well as to themselves and to the medical faculty, that they are potentially good doctors.[5]

The fact that students who perform their anatomy assignments without too much conscious anxiety sometimes have bad dreams suggests continuing anxiety on a lower level of consciousness.

One's ability to adjust to the cadaver experience apparently relates strongly to the capacity for objectifying or depersonalizing the body so that it is no longer viewed as a human being. Certain laboratory procedures help facilitate this depersonalizing process. For one thing, the cadaver is usually draped so that only the part being dissected is exposed; and the more human dissections such as the face and hands, for example, are reserved until later in the course. Also, instructors can ease the potential anxiety by making the first laboratory experience fairly brief to help students regain composure after the initial shock. If they are not sensitive to the feelings of students, reactions may be more severe and prolonged.

The challenge to the neophyte doctor is, of course, to keep personal sensitivities intact while carving a human body. Humanistically inclined students, those most prone to worrying over the human, moral, and religious justifications of dissecting a cadaver, find relief in the knowledge—a form of rationalization—that patients have willingly donated their own bodies to be used for the express purpose of training medical students.

Relief from inner anxieties is aided by losing oneself in the details of one's work. Pressures to learn myriad body parts in a limited time helps students to lose themselves in the details of the dissection process and in memorizing the scientific names of bones, muscles, nerves, and other body parts. In so doing, they are able to view the body as an object rather than a deceased person, and dissection becomes a mechanistic exercise rather than a humanistic experience.

This absorption in one's work clearly acts as a "psychic counterirritant," to use Lief and Fox's term (1963). Such a coping mechanism is especially important at the institution where the study took place, since the anatomy staff, in deference to those who have contributed their bodies, permits no joking or horseplay, which could, if allowed, provide ready tension relief. So students simply lose themselves in their work as a means of depersonalizing the cadaver experience.

From a socialization perspective it is important to note that, although a vast block of curriculum time is devoted to the anatomy laboratory, not a single hour, as far as I could tell, is set aside to discuss with students the impact of the cadaver experience on their own feelings, or to justify these feelings as a part of healthy career development. This omission, coming early in medical training, no doubt sets the stage for these future doctors to objectify and intellectualize intense experiences while suppressing the emotional aspects of patient care.

WORRYING ABOUT GRADES

In medical schools that use grades as an evaluative tool, students quickly learn that "you have to pass before you can do anything else." Failure to do so may result in being dropped from school, thus shattering dreams and aspirations. So they look upon grades with great apprehension, especially during the freshman and sophomore years when they are most vulnerable.*

Medical school has the reputation of being a very difficult place that attracts only the most able students. Because their classmates are perceived as being brilliant, students have a tendency to become unduly anxious about their own shortcomings. This feeling of inadequacy is exemplified by the freshman who said: "The first realization of my complete inadequacy almost overwhelmed me. I thought, 'What am I going to do? Everyone else is absorbing it and I've hardly gotten anything at all.' "

The first weeks are particularly stressful, since students have no way of measuring their performance. The work load is heavy, and students agonize about the first test. Doubts such as these plague them:

* Bojar (1961) provides a brief description and analysis of the factors in both premedical and medical school training that result in student anxiety over "grade consciousness." My study population indicated on the seven-point stress scale the anxiety and stress that were experienced over grades. Scores of 6 or 7 were rated as high stress; scores of 3, 4, or 5 as moderate stress; and 1 or 2 as being very low stress. Results show that high stress was felt by 25.8 percent of the class during the freshman year, 28.1 percent during the sophomore year, 5.2 percent during the junior year, and 1.8 percent during the final year. Moderate stress was reported by 55.2 percent of the freshmen, 52.6 percent of the sophomores, 46.6 percent of the juniors, and 36.4 percent of the seniors. Low stress was reported by 19.0 percent of the freshmen, 19.3 percent of the sophomores, 48.2 percent of the juniors, and 61.8 percent of the seniors.

Is medical school too big for me to handle? Is there too much to do, too much to learn? Am I smart enough even if I work hard? Can I even pass?

But once the first exam is successfully behind them, pressures usually subside; evidence is furnished that they can make the grade.

Some students are not so fortunate, though. If that all-important first grade is low, they may become almost paralyzed in their learning capabilities.[6] "I just went to pieces and couldn't study," a freshman said. "All I could think about was how far behind I was and how I wouldn't be ready for the next exam; I couldn't pull myself together." This paralysis is sometimes coupled with a state of near hysteria. For example, a freshman who graduated from college *summa cum laude* was distressed to find himself barely passing. "I felt like I was banging my head against the wall, and didn't know which way to turn," he said. "It was quite an emotional experience." Fortunately, he found his way to a psychiatrist's office where he regained his confidence. Talking out his fears helped him realize that he was not unique, that his classmates were having the same troubles. "I thought about that," he said. "Then all of a sudden things started clicking and my grades went up."

Contrary to expectations, advancement to sophomore status does not cause students to be less anxious, for second-year tests, although less frequent in number, are weighted more heavily in grading. "I couldn't eat or sleep for four days before my first exam in pathology," a sophomore admitted. Since each exam is weighted so heavily, students normally concentrate all their energies on the examination that is closest at hand, neglecting other subjects for the time being. The inevitable aftermath is a frantic scramble to recover lost ground in the other courses. When two or more tests occur almost simultaneously, pressure and scrambling become even more frantic. And efforts exerted by those trying to recover from bad grades on the first examination intensify the pressure.

Not only are students worried about the possibility of flunking out or having to repeat a course, they are also concerned with the necessity of maintaining their reputation and self-esteem. After so many years of competing scholastically, achieving good grades becomes an end in itself, an extension of ego. Scholastic achievement has come to be a measure of self-worth. "I hate to make bad grades," one acknowledged. "If you want to know the truth, that is why I study. I don't study for knowledge now."

When grades fall below par, sophomores rarely blame themselves as they did during the first year when preoccupied with their own deficiencies. Instead, they express their dissatisfaction and criticism outwardly—toward the faculty, the curriculum, or their classmates—thereby acquiring the reputation of being a pretty hostile bunch. In reality, they are simply using this coping mechanism to vent pent-up pressures and maintain emotional equilibrium.

Emphasis on grades decreases markedly in the clinical years. Although upperclassmen still view grades as an aid in achieving a good internship or residency assignment, most feel that other things are more important. Showing more confidence, upperclassmen typically feel they are now "over the hump" scholastically and no longer fear failure. "The idea of making that grade, beating your head, just doesn't get you psyched up anymore," a junior explained.

Working on the wards stimulates a desire to learn information for its own sake rather than for acquiring good grades. When one is absorbed in doing a good clinical job, grades are of secondary importance: "If I am able to learn as much about my patients' problems as I can," said one, "then I'm satisfied, no matter what I make on the test."

Moreover, the system used in testing and grading clinical students reinforces the new attitude. Grades are deemphasized and most students see the grading system as "nebulous and subjective." Since test papers often are not returned, students sometimes do not even know what grades they have earned; and this lack of certainty does not worry them unduly.

But for a few upperclassmen it is not easy to overcome the years of concern about grades. "We've been pushed about grades for so long that we're prone to thinking that somebody's always looking over our shoulders," a senior commented. "We shouldn't be worrying about things like this," students remind themselves.

As mentioned in Chapter 5, the functional value of grades is currently a hotly contested issue.[7] Some feel it absurd to grade medical students, thus subjecting these highly achieving individuals to a system that assumes a normal distribution of intellective abilities. By contrast, those who favor grades point to the precipitous drop in board exam scores when traditional grading procedures give way to the pass–fail system. My data indicate that, in order to become adequately motivated, some students require a structured grading system. For most students, however, grades serve no apparent functional value, except perhaps to test stress tolerance and cooperative attitudes (a willingness to "jump through hoops"). From a socialization perspective, then, getting good grades seems more an index of situational adjustment than of long-range career development.[8]

FEARING INABILITY TO ABSORB
AND RETAIN KNOWLEDGE

Medical students are never completely free of worry over their seeming inability to absorb and retain all the information presented to them. Whereas concern over grades declines in the clinical years, worry about assimilation and retention of knowledge remains a persistent source of anxiety throughout all years of medical training.*

Preclinical students complain of having too much to digest in too short a time. "You could study 24 hours a day and not get it done," a freshman complained. "It's just continual study." Seldom can beginning students take time off with a clear conscience, for when away from their books, they agonize about losing ground. "If you slack off even a bit," said one, "you are behind; and while you are still trying to catch up, they are covering new stuff."

These highly idealistic students consider it essential to master all of the assigned materials. Unable to meet these expectations, they naturally feel incompetent and demoralized: "I know I can't absorb it all—no way! It's impossible. I wonder if I should even be here." Slow readers are particularly disadvantaged in trying to keep up with the fast pace. In college, they could get by through putting in longer hours. But in medical school there is no extra time available; everyone is working at maximum.

Anxieties are heightened even more by inabilities to retain the information once it is acquired. The case with which significant facts slip away is disconcerting. "You study this stuff for a few weeks," said one, "and then when you try to recall it, you can't remember it to save your life. It's like you never learned it."

Fortunately, it eventually dawns on most students that their expectations of themselves are unrealistically high and that classmates are experiencing similar difficulties. When upperclassmen acknowledge that they, too, have difficulty retaining information, morale receives a great boost. It is at this time that most students develop adaptive attitudes. This breakthrough results in giving up the impossible task of trying to comprehend everything and, instead, studying selectively. "I don't try to learn everything now as I once did," one said. "Now I try to master the major concepts; some of the other material isn't all that important."

However, some students are uncertain as to the relative importance of the study matter. "Nine-tenths look like minutiae to me," one remarked; "it's hard choosing what is really important." So students listen for cues from the faculty and study with an eye toward what will appear on examinations. Usually this is accomplished by digesting lecture notes. Those faculty members who confuse rather than enlighten or who "fake out" students on "tricky exam questions" are most unpopular.

---

* Students indicated on a seven-point stress scale the anxiety and stress experienced over their seeming inability to absorb and retain knowledge. High stress was noted by 25.9 percent of the freshmen, 40.3 percent of the sophomore class, 27.6 percent of the juniors, and 12.7 percent of the senior class. Moderate stress was felt by 65.5 percent of the freshmen, 50.9 percent of the sophomores, 60.3 percent among juniors, and 61.8 percent of the seniors. Low stress was reported by 8.6 percent of the freshmen class, 8.8 percent among sophomores, 12.1 percent in the junior class, and 25.5 percent of the seniors.

The most idealistic recruits have the greatest difficulty in learning the necessary adaptive techniques. They believe that all materials presented in medical school will play vital roles in their future treatment of and healing of the sick. They think any failure on their part to learn this information might at some future time mean the sacrifice of a patient's life. Small wonder that these students suffer the greatest anxieties. Such apprehensions abound in the second year, as they approach their clinical work. During their first year, some comfort is derived from the knowledge that one more year lies before them as a hedge against the time when they will go on the hospital floors. But when they become sophomores, they see it as their last chance to acquire basic medical facts. The prospect of making a fatal mistake terrifies them. "Heaven help my patients if I've missed anything!" one shuddered.

Once on the wards, however, even these students worry less about their ignorance for they realize that, with the close supervision given them, little chance exists that they will inadvertently harm a patient. They do worry, though, about assimilating pertinent information they will need as interns. Sensing that "the whole thing will be on our shoulders next year," seniors are acutely aware that "time is running out."

However, an increasing number of idealistic students gradually reconcile themselves to the following attitude:

> I can't learn it all anyway, so why get upset about it? I just plug along and remember that I've got an internship and residency ahead. I can't assimilate everything before I get out. In fact, I probably won't learn it all within the first 20 years I'm in practice.

Without lowering self-expectations, such an attitude helps students cope with the gnawing anxiety of not being fully prepared for the clinical road that lies ahead.

ANTICIPATING ERRORS IN DIAGNOSING AND PRESCRIBING

Students reveal considerable anxiety with regard to possible errors in diagnosing and prescribing—an apprehension that continues throughout all four years.* "It scares the daylights out of me!" one confessed. "I think

---

* Again on a seven-point stress scale, students recorded the levels of anxiety and stress they experienced over the possibility of making errors in diagnosing and prescribing. High stress was recorded by 31.0 percent of the freshmen, 26.3 percent of the sophomore class, 13.8 percent of the juniors, and 25.5 percent of the seniors. Moderate stress was indicated by 34.5 percent of the freshmen, 42.1 percent of the sophomores, 51.7 percent of the juniors, and 45.4 percent of the senior class. Low stress was reported by 34.5 percent of the freshman class, 31.6 percent of the sophomores, 34.5 percent of the juniors, and 29.1 percent of the seniors.

about it all of the time; I even go home at night and think about it. Anybody who says it doesn't bother him is a naive fool!"

Preclinical students, most of whom are idealistic and conscientious, cannot condone negligence or stupid errors in treating patients. Such idealism is made clear by the freshman who said, "It seems worse to take a life through stupidity than through premeditated murder." In these inexperienced eyes, "A doctor who is wrong has failed in his job."

As students progress through school and gain experience, it becomes more and more clear to them that a certain amount of human error is unavoidable. Pathology instructors tell them, for example, that "autopsy reports show that about 50 percent of the diagnoses are wrong." Such information helps students become more realistic, but it does little to reduce their anxieties. "Yikes, I could kill somebody if I miss!" one exclaimed.

This anxiety reinforces the tendency to be hypercritical of professors who fail to teach the things students feel are most important. So much instruction, they say, focuses on the obscure and the trivial that when the correct diagnosis should be the common cold, for example, students think instead of "esoteric diseases with weird syndromes." As one student put it, "When we hear hoofbeats, we think of zebras instead of horses."

Every low grade on an exam and each failure on a diagnostic exercise tends to aggravate personal anxieties about clinical incompetence. This aggravation is compounded by students' concern that they will soon be on the hospital floors making critical decisions. "There I am," one imagines, "with 14,000 books in the cabinet and a patient coming in. I look at him and think, 'Good grief! What's he got?' He could be standing there with both arms chopped off and I'd probably have so many things (metabolic disorders, etc.) running through my mind that I wouldn't realize his arms were gone."

Fortunately, such dreaded fantasies are not fulfilled, for, as previously mentioned, rookie clinicians are given little actual responsibility for patient care. "I don't climb a tree if I'm wrong," a junior commented, "because I know somebody is backing me up somewhere." But this doesn't alleviate all stress, especially among those who maintain high idealism. Clinical errors, even though they do not get past the students' notebooks, reinforce anxieties about their lack of preparation and reveal how far distant is the mastery they seek.

Anxiety over the possibility of making errors mounts during the senior year as internship approaches. Students are writing more orders and doing more treating than ever before and several have already narrowly escaped making serious mistakes. For example, one student misplaced a decimal point in prescribing for a patient, causing her to take an overdose of medication. Although the error was not a fatal one, the student was understandably shaken.

Such experiences force students to acknowledge that a certain amount of error is bound to happen. They rationalize, "Doctors are only human like everyone else, you know. They can't be right all the time." Yet many students, even when recognizing their standards are unrealistically high, have difficulty settling for anything less than perfection. Their idealism, though tempered with reality, renders the continuation of stress into their postgraduate years almost inevitable.

FEARING CONTAGION AND LOSS OF PERSONAL HEALTH

Daily activity at the medical center brings students into contact with the ever-present disease organisms that exist there; to some this is a source of apprehension. Nearly half of the freshman class confess at least moderate anxiety about personal contagion or loss of health,* a phenomenon that has been referred to as "medical students' disease" (Woods, Natterson, and Silverman, 1966). These fears result from increased awareness of infectious bacteria, viral agents, and parasites that are studied in the freshman microbiology course. "We've learned that there is more to get sick from," one stated. "Microbiology is showing us all the various organisms, a lot of terrible things that we've never even thought about before."

Anxieties are heightened when course instructors admonish students to use caution when handling slides. "It made me realize that I could easily get those diseases if I swallowed something or if I had an abrasion or cut on my hand," a freshman admitted. Rumors circulating among classmates also add to students' concern. "We've heard stories about medical students who have caught stuff and had to drop out of school," one said. "They might just be stories, but still, it makes me kind of worry about it."

It is natural, then, for beginning students to personalize this new information and to worry, "What if I come down with it?" One student, for example, who had never paid any attention to the lump behind his ear became anxious about the possibility of cancer. Similarly, a classmate who was washing her car barefooted in the backyard became concerned about the possibility of hookworm being in the grass. "It was just a natural reaction," she explained. "I couldn't help it."

Understandably, students having prior histories of poor health or sus-

---

* On the seven-point stress scale, students indicated the levels of anxiety and stress they experienced in regard to their fear of contagious diseases and loss of their personal health. The number of students who reported high stress each year is 6.9 percent in the freshman year, 3.6 percent in the sophomore year, 5.2 percent in the junior year, and 1.8 percent in the senior year. Students reporting moderate stress during each year equal 41.4 percent, 31.5 percent, 39.6 percent, and 23.6 percent, respectively. The number of those with low stress is 51.7 percent, 64.9 percent, 55.2 percent, and 74.6 percent, respectively.

ceptibility to infections are most likely to worry. "My personal health has been erratic," one said. "I've broken bones, had hayfever, and am allergic to poison oak, poison ivy—you name it and I've had it! So, I figure if there is anything contagious around, there is a good chance I'll get it."

Fortunately, anxieties decline somewhat during the second year, despite the fact that course work in pathology keeps awareness of disease organisms current. Only a third of the class report fears about loss of personal health. "We've just got too many other things to worry about now," a sophomore said. Nevertheless, some anxious moments do occur during the second year. One such experience was described as follows: "They brought in a patient for us to see, with some weird kind of contagious skin disease. When the instructor asked us to come down and look at it, I thought, 'Man, I don't want to get close to *that!*'" This student then added, "That's not the way doctors are supposed to think, I guess, but I couldn't help it."

Beginning their clinical clerkships, of course, puts students in direct contact with diseased patients, carriers of such dreaded infectious diseases as tuberculosis, typhoid fever, meningitis, and hepatitis. So, it is not unusual that rookie clinicians should experience apprehension. "I had a lady with a lung problem who was an alcoholic," one said. "After she died, there was some question as to whether she might have had T.B. Believe me, I had some pretty anxious moments during the next few days waiting for the cultures to grow."

After encountering a patient with meningitis, a classmate dashed off to ask the attending physician, "Do you think I need penicillin?" Small wonder that such students are amusingly perceived as hypochondriacs who worry about every little thing and want to run home frequently for showers. At this developmental stage, a third-year student pointed out, there is a tendency to become hypochondriacal: "Because of inexperience, we tend to lose perspective and exaggerate the dangers of potential health hazards."

The majority, however, do not admit to any concern about personal health. One reason is because clinicians fulminate against complainers, hypochondriacs, and "crocks." Thus students, in fear of being so labeled, tend to suppress their anxieties and refrain from talking about their own medical histories. One spoke of apprehension about a growth that possibly could be malignant, but refrained from visiting the student health center to avoid being considered a crock.

Excessive anxiety about personal health is regarded as undesirable at the medical center because it can handicap a doctor in clinical performance. Whatever the risks, a physician cannot be worried all the time; "he or she must go ahead and do the job." In this view, contagion is simply regarded as an occupational hazard, one that clinicians must learn to live with. Having made the decision to pursue a medical career, one must accept the unpleasant consequences of that decision. Among clinicians the feeling is, as Harry Truman expressed it, "If you can't take the heat, stay out of the kitchen."

So students learn to play down the potential personal hazards, displaying instead a nonchalant shoulder-shrugging attitude, as did one who said: "There's no reason to be concerned; if it happens, it happens." Occasionally such a student may go to an extreme in this view, as is exemplified by one who apparently denied his own vulnerability. He maintained optimism by viewing himself as immune, as an exception to the rule. "Most people who find themselves with a tubercular patient run out and get a Vollmer patch test, but I just have a feeling that it couldn't possibly happen to me."

Such an attitude is unusual, however. Instead, most students regard a "reasonable fear" of certain diseases as healthy. There is, they insist, a difference between being brave and foolhardy. "If a person has no respect for the germ theory," one said, "he's going to get in trouble. It's reckless to jump right in without precautions if somebody has a bad disease."

During the senior year, only one out of four students acknowledges even a moderate degree of concern about contagion and personal health. Confidence comes, they say, through having a knowledge of the dangers involved together with an understanding of the necessary precautions to take. If one is alert and proceeds cautiously, they reason, that should ward off troubles. "When patients are in isolation," one said, "we protect ourselves by wearing a mask and gown, and when we have to handle them we put on gloves. So the chance of germs getting in is pretty slim."

It is encouraging, too, when students realize that the odds are in their favor; for relatively few clinicians actually become infected. One said, "It's hard to catch a terminal disease." Still, stressful situations do arise, as a senior witnessed: "I've always been a positive skin reactor, so I have a better chance of picking up T.B. than others. If I take the proper precautions, I'm not afraid of working with these patients; but if I'm in the emergency room and one of them coughs in my face I get pretty upset." As a rule, though, graduating seniors do not expend a lot of energy worrying about diseases; but they have learned to recognize the need for being cautious and alert. In short, they have a healthy respect for disease. After all, they, too, are mortals.

PERFORMING INTIMATE PHYSICAL EXAMINATIONS

Not until the last weeks of the second year are students given the opportunity to conduct physical exams, so it is natural that freshmen and sophomores do not become overly concerned with intimate examinations. Nonetheless, they are aware that before long they will have to perform these examinations regularly. And since it is generally taboo to handle the private parts of others' bodies, they naturally feel some anxiety.*

Nothing in their previous training has prepared students for this experience, so they worry about appearing flustered and clumsy. These fears become realities when they conduct their first physical examinations. "I really didn't know what I was doing," one said, "I didn't know whether what I was feeling was normal or abnormal. I just felt helpless." Such students fear that their clumsiness and lack of confidence will cause patients to be uneasy or embarrassed.

During the first physical exam it took one student three hours, a procedure that later took only 20 minutes. "I wasn't familiar with my tools; I couldn't handle them well; I knew nothing," this student confessed. "I didn't know how to write notes or anything. It was hectic. I kept referring to my little guide to see what to do and if I had missed anything."

Some students write out their questions on cue cards to make sure they do not forget anything, but even this is sometimes embarrassing. Above all, they do not want to appear "green."

One student admitted, "I was so clumsy in handling the stethoscope that I was afraid maybe the patient would get the impression that I didn't know what I was doing or that something was seriously wrong with him if I listened too long. Yet I couldn't hurry, because of the importance of the procedure."

Even after students acquire some experience, intimate physical exams remain a potential source of trouble throughout medical school, especially when the patient is of the opposite sex. There is always the possibility, as some students admit, that when circumstances are right, they can become sexually aroused. Attractive female patients, or those who are deliberately seductive, have the greatest potential of triggering erotic responses in male students. Examining women close to their own age is difficult for them, especially when the patient is also an acquaintance. "When we first went to OB," a senior said, "a couple of girls there had gone to college with us and were friends of my wife; these situations were very awkward."

An unnerving experience with a particularly sexy and seductive patient, reported by a male student, illustrates the problems student-physicians can have:

> She was about 27 and in the clinic because she had just become pregnant. She wasn't married, and she was just as sexy as hell. She was Spanish and had

---

* On a seven-point stress scale, students once more scored the anxiety and stress they felt in regard to performing intimate physical examinations (such as rectal and pelvic examinations). Among freshmen, 6.9 percent reported high stress, while 3.5 percent of the sophomores, 3.4 percent of the junior class, and 1.8 percent of the seniors felt this degree of stress. Moderate stress was indicated by 12.1 percent of the freshmen, 19.3 percent of the sophomores, 32.8 percent of the junior class, and 9.1 percent of the seniors. Low stress was reported by 81.0 percent of the freshman class, 77.2 percent of the sophomores, 63.8 percent of the juniors, and 89.1 percent of the seniors.

an accent and really fiery red hair. She was sitting with the thing draped about her, and the pieces would droop while I was talking to her, and I had to look up and try to keep my mind on what I was supposed to be doing.

What little composure this student had maintained was lost when the patient began flirting with him. "When I asked how old her boyfriend was, she said, 'He's 24.' Then she looked directly at me and said, 'I like them young.'" At this point the rattled student found an excuse to leave the room.

A number of coping techniques are learned by such students in dealing with potentially erotic situations. But when all else fails, students, like the one just mentioned, can extricate themselves from awkward situations by withdrawing. One said, for example, "I try to do the exam as quickly as possible. I don't hang around staring; I just get out of there as soon as I can."

Others, opting for self-control rather than flight, use a variety of means to suppress or block out erotic thoughts. "I just don't let it become erotic," one said. This student then explained that he reminds himself, "This is a patient and not a girl; and I'm here to examine and help the patient." Recalling that doctors are not supposed to be aroused by patients helps the student-physician maintain self-control. Sexual interest in patients is, after all, a violation of professional decorum, and students are anxious to conduct themselves as professionals. Some objectify the patient by separating the person and the body: "I try to consciously make it an organism rather than a person," a male student said. "I try to forget that the breast is attached to a woman."

By concentrating on the details of the examination itself, students keep out erotic ideas. They quickly learn that when they are engrossed in the pathology or details of the examination, erotic impulses do not occur. That is, when trying to conceptualize what is inside the patient, they are able to minimize "outside" distractions. One's fingertips must be fully coordinated with the mind's eye; so it is essential to keep the latter on business rather than on erotic things. This technique is further explained by a senior:

> If you are examining the chest and feeling the breast, you're feeling for nodules, and in your mind you visualize the possibility of a nodule beneath your finger as you palpate. I have found that one of my greatest defenses is that I don't look at the skin. My mind's eye is inside the breast thinking about what I am palpating—a real areolar tissue, ductal tissue, fatty tissue, or what have you. Rather than thinking "Boy, she's really stacked!" I'm saying to myself, "Well, here's such and such a lobe; what would a mass feel like if it were here?" In other words, my mind's eye is inside the patient.

The hospital setting and atmosphere do much to help desexualize the doctor–patient relationship. All the bustling and rushing around act as stabilizers, helping students to keep their thoughts on business. There is usually so much to be accomplished in so little time that one cannot afford to let one's mind wander. Moreover, sterile clothing and antiseptic procedures also minimize sexual stimulation, for they are the very antithesis of erotica. A female patient hardly cuts a provocative figure when draped in sanitary white sheets and propped up on a table in saddle straps. And having a nurse, an impersonal female party, in the room further works against eroticism. All this lends itself to an air of efficiency and authority where dignity and respect are expected by all.

Repeated exposure to patients in such settings tends to desensitize students somewhat to naked bodies. This desensitization begins, according to one student, right from the first day of school. "It's just a gradual thing," she commented. "Previously forbidden words are used as commonly as 'arm,' 'leg,' or any other part of the body; and you see the pictures of private parts put up on a screen in pathology so that they become as routine and commonplace as pictures of the face and back." Regarding this routinization effect, a senior said,

> It's kind of hard to be titillated when you see so many bare bodies. It's possible, and I have been on occasion, but it's kind of like working in a meat market. I hate to say that, but when you see one leg of lamb, it looks a lot like all other legs of lamb.

The surprising success with which students learn to dissociate the erotic from the clinical is illustrated by a male senior who suddenly found himself examining one of the pretty secretaries who worked at the hospital, a young woman he had secretly admired for three years. "When she walks down the halls," he said, "I always look her over from top to bottom. But when she came into the OB suite as a patient, it was entirely different; I wasn't turned on at all." Amazed that such a red-blooded American boy as himself could become so desensitized, he muttered, "It's weird, it really is."

COUNSELING PATIENTS ON SEX AND MARRIAGE

Sex has traditionally been such a taboo topic in our society that talking about it is very difficult for most people, even those who are intelligent and otherwise articulate.[9] Medical students seem to be no less inhibited than others. Yet sexual histories should be taken from patients when physical examinations are conducted. When students first learn of this responsibility they sometimes respond, "Good grief, how can I ask anybody *those* questions?" *

* Students indicated on the seven-point stress scale their anxiety and stress concerning sex and marital counseling. High stress was reported by 5.2 percent of the freshmen, 1.8 percent of the sophomores, 1.7 percent of the junior class, and 5.5 percent of the senior class. Moderate stress was reported by 22.4 percent of the freshman class,

Few, if any, students feel qualified to dispense sex information or counsel, so they worry about giving false advice based on ignorance. What little knowledge they possess comes mostly from books, books that usually emphasize physiological rather than emotional or social aspects. Since most students are unmarried or only recently married, they have only limited practical experience. No wonder they feel so insecure, especially when counseling patients who are older and more experienced than themselves.

Imagine the plight of the rookie clinician suddenly thrust into the role of the sex expert. "It's challenging, to put it mildly," a junior remarked. "It just doesn't come naturally." In such situations, students hope that they will not blush or in other ways reveal how anxious and inexperienced they are. A female student who failed in this regard confessed, "The prostate exam itself wasn't so stressful, but when the patient and I started talking, I was red most of the time; I blush at the drop of a hat, anyway."

It is understandable, then, that students sometimes cope by avoiding the subject. Some simply do not take a sexual history as part of their clinical workup, and they refrain from asking questions that might lead to sexual or marital topics. They justify this stance with the explanation that clinicians have no right to intrude on personal matters. Discussing such topics, they maintain, is an invasion of the patient's privacy. Even those who admit the value of interviewing and counseling patients about sexual topics are often reluctant to initiate sex talk.

Avoidance of sexual talk only adds to the student's anxiety because it adds to the vicious cycle of fears already possessed and gets in the way of gaining needed experience in the art of counseling. Unless one is taken by the hand and pulled through, so to speak, inhibitions will continue to adversely affect relationships with patients. But since many clinical preceptors are as inhibited as their students, a strong probability exists that those inhibitions will be reinforced rather than dispelled.[10]

However, it is difficult for a physician to avoid sex talk in the professional role, for patients often expect help with such problems. And many times there is no one else to whom they can turn for help. Because of their doctor's scientific background and intimate handling of body parts, patients naturally expect physicians to have a knowledgeable, objective, and nonmoralizing approach to sexual problems. When bringing up a sexual or marital problem, patients do not expect the doctor to turn red and change the subject; they anticipate a helpful professional response.

Fortunately, some of the more intrepid students find that talking with patients about their sexual problems is less stressful than they had feared. Some patients, having no one else to confide in and burdened with pressing problems, initiate the conversation or "open up" with very little prompting. One third-year student, for example, who said he "just couldn't

29.8 percent of the sophomores, 44.8 percent of the juniors, and 27.2 percent of the senior class. Low stress was reported by 72.4 percent of the freshmen, 68.4 percent of the sophomores, 53.5 percent of the junior class, and 67.3 percent of the seniors.

do it" at the beginning of the year, changed after seeing how readily patients take advantage of an opportunity to discuss their sex lives:

> When I was on OB, I was amazed that patients would express themselves on the topic and not even be embarrassed, as I was. I started off by saying, "Sex life okay?" as fast as I could, just gunning it by. Before I knew it, the patient was saying, "Well, let me tell you. My husband. . . ." Then I'd sit there for an hour just listening.

Such experiences have a desensitizing effect and help students overcome their reluctance to talk about sex. After awhile, many of them realize that if they are to become effective clinicians they must be able to discuss sexual and marital problems openly and freely. Their ability to do this increases as they gain knowledge and expertise.

HANDLING CHRONIC OR TERMINAL ILLNESS

Although students have only minimal contact with chronically or terminally ill patients in the first two years, many suffer from anxiety concerning the encounters they know are awaiting them.* At this preprofessional stage, personal identification with any doomed patient is strong, especially if the latter is young and/or likeable. Students, when exposed to impending death, often find themselves participating imaginatively in the suffering involved. They have not yet evolved out of the layman's attitude toward illness and pain. In time, they will acquire the detachment and equanimity of the veteran doctor. Even though they realize this, the transition can be quite distressing. Intellectual understanding is one thing, but managing feelings is quite another.[11]

During the first months at medical school, students have such a strong tendency to identify with patients that they find the aloofness and detachment of the case-hardened doctor offensive. For example, one freshman who was given an opportunity to accompany upperclassmen on ward rounds with an attending physician reported being appalled by the "unfeeling way" the physician talked to the group about the terminally ill patient. "I'd sure hate to have the family hear talk like that," the student said. "I suppose the doctor has to be uncompassionate at times, but I wasn't ready for it. It wasn't disrespect; there just wasn't any show of emotion."

The desire to help is so urgent among idealistic students that it is pain-

---

* On the seven-point stress scale, students rated the anxiety and stress that they experienced when dealing with chronic or terminally ill patients. High stress was indicated in this area by 17.2 percent of the freshmen, 8.8 percent of the sophomores, 17.2 percent of the junior class, and 10.9 percent of the seniors. Moderate stress was shown by 34.5 percent of the freshman class, 29.8 percent of the sophomores, 51.7 percent of the juniors, and 45.5 percent of the seniors. Low stress was prevalent in 48.3 percent of the freshmen members, 61.4 percent of the sophomores, 31.1 percent of the juniors, and 43.6 percent of the senior class.

ful to face the knowledge that nothing can be done to cure the terminally ill patient. "It seems as though there ought to be some hope somewhere . . . something," a freshman agonized. "I hate to give up hope; I feel so much emotion, I just choke up!"

Imbued with the concept that the doctor's function is to cure people, entering medical students feel helpless in the face of failure, and this tends to shatter their idealism about the profession. Realizing that there is truly nothing one can do to save a patient is a crushing blow. One acknowledged, "I was really upset and had trouble eating. It was depressing and deflated my ego."

Feelings of personal inadequacy are brought into sharp focus during emotionally charged conversations with patients and their families about incurable illnesses. On such occasions, students typically feel "self-conscious, tongue-tied, and fearful of saying something that will make patients or families feel bad." What can a student-physician say, for example, when a patient or family member pleads, "Isn't there anything you can do?" As they search for appropriate words to use in such situations, students feel acutely inept. Confidence in saying the right thing is minimized by their student status. Not having the authority to act independently and being unaware of how much the attending doctor wants the patient to know makes them feel doubly uneasy. "When I get cornered and they start asking a lot of questions, I don't know what to tell them," a junior admitted. "I'm afraid I'll either hurt them or be way off base."

It is understandable then, that avoidance is often used as a technique for coping with such awkward and stressful situations. For example, when terminally ill patients are presented in clinics, students are hesitant about quizzing them. "We're supposed to ask about the patient's disease," a sophomore said, "but I can't bring myself to ask such questions at a time like that. I wonder, 'What can I say that won't be hurtful?'" To avoid witnessing the suffering of those whose pain they cannot relieve, students sometimes shrink physically or emotionally from contact with such patients. One student became emotionally upset over a little girl who was in constant pain and who feared the white-coated figures whose treatment increased her discomfort. "Finally, I got to where I didn't even want to go in the room to see her," he admitted.

But avoidance is seldom an available or acceptable alternative. More appropriate coping mechanisms must be found. So as a buffer against emotional stress, students gradually develop a philosophical attitude toward incurably ill patients. Some students, of course, take this necessary step sooner than others. Eventually they all learn that frequent exposure to such patients is routine and that, in order to maintain their emotional equilibrium, they must learn to manage their feelings. The emerging attitude is: "You can only do so much for a patient who has a hopeless disease. There's not much you can do about it except offer compassion, so there's no use getting anxious or upset."

But finding a proper balance between detachment and concern is easier said than done. Occasionally, a student is so successful in maintaining detachment from the depressing aspects of a chronically or terminally ill patient that the newly developed attitude itself causes concern. "I've become emotionally isolated this year, which really isn't good," a junior confessed, "and it worries me that I don't feel more than I do." Other classmates have trouble detaching themselves enough. It is easier to control emotions when a patient is comatose or demented; and contact with outpatients or acutely ill patients is usually too brief or irregular to result in much personal attachment. But if the student is on the same service for any length of time, the incurably ill patient can become for him or her a real person, and warm interpersonal feelings make detachment difficult to maintain. Seeing such friends deteriorate before one's eyes and feeling helpless to do anything about it is an emotionally draining experience.

These experiences make abundantly clear the necessity for developing a certain amount of emotional detachment. The following case is illustrative:

> We became great friends because I spent a lot of time with him. I'd give him his medicine and put a little fluid in him every day and he did fine for about a week. Then one day he got real sick and I had to go in and draw blood for a culture and start an I.V. But I couldn't get the I.V. going and I couldn't get any blood from him and he started to cry. The nurse gave me dirty looks, but there wasn't anything I could do. I felt terrible. Then one day when he was sick as a dog in spite of getting all his medicine, he asked me, "Why don't you just shoot me?"

Such experiences naturally have a shattering impact on student idealism. For one thing, it becomes very clear that, as one put it, "the God-complex" is an inappropriate attitude for physicians to have; that is, it is unrealistic to expect to be able to cure everyone. And students also realize that, if they are to become effective clinicians over the long haul, they cannot let themselves suffer personally with each patient. A certain amount of equanimity is necessary and desirable, not only for the clinician but for the patient as well. Yet students are aware that they must still retain the inherent satisfaction that comes from helping people and not become desensitized to the point that they are unable to feel genuine humanistic compassion for patients and their families.

WITNESSING THE DEATH OF A PATIENT

Freshmen and sophomores are only slightly better acquainted with death than the general public, since their contact with it is limited during the first two years. However, they all realize that they must learn to deal with it in all its variations. This often causes an underlying anxiety that stems from the dread of facing close involvement with death throughout their careers.*

Their expectations are often unrealistic. Some regard death as the antithesis of good medical practice. "That's my business," one stated, "to make sure death doesn't occur." And, as previously mentioned, the idea of a patient dying from negligence or lack of knowledge on their part is intolerable. "If I thought a patient's death was caused by my failure," a sophomore emphasized, "I'd feel like I murdered someone."

In performing autopsies in their second-year pathology course, students come closer to experiencing the reality of death. But because these patients are already dead before students see them, such exposure is usually not too traumatic. During the last two years of school, however, most students experience the death of at least one or two patients. The stress of such an event is softened somewhat by the frequent rotation from one service to another. This shuttling back and forth from one hospital setting to another usually does not allow students enough time to form close personal attachments with patients. And there is comfort, too, in the realization that the primary responsibility for patients rests not with themselves, but with attending doctors and house staff. The death of a patient is much less traumatic when one is only an outside observer.

Despite these structured protections, neophyte clinicians experience considerable stress when one of their patients dies. As previously noted, they are initially shocked by the detachment maintained by their mentors and other experienced personnel. In one instance, the first patient of a student died shortly after his initial interview with her. Being unaware of her death, he tried to locate her in her hospital room and was told, matter-of-factly, "She's in the morgue." "That really bothered me," he said. "I went to her autopsy and it made me think pretty deeply for a while."

In another situation, a student was appalled by the detached scientific interest among the staff who attended his first patient, a baby who was unsuccessfully operated on for a congenital cardiac anomaly. "The surgeon was sorry, I guess, but it was kind of a scientific study to him; things like this evidently happen every week or two." Later, during the autopsy, this student was stunned when the pediatric cardiologist was "real excited when the autopsy findings compared well with his own diagnosis."

---

* Students indicated on the seven-point stress scale their anxiety and stress over witnessing the death of a patient. High stress was experienced by 19.0 percent of the freshmen, 7.0 percent of the sophomores, 13.8 percent of the junior class, and 4.5 percent of the seniors. Moderate stress was indicated by 29.3 percent of the freshman class, 29.8 percent of the sophomores, 60.3 percent of the juniors, and 58.2 percent of the seniors. Low stress was recorded by 50.0 percent of the freshmen, 63.2 percent of the sophomores, 25.9 percent of the juniors, and 21.8 percent of the senior class. (Note: Freshmen's and seniors' totals in this instance do not add up to 100 percent. The discrepancy is due to "don't know" responses. This explanation applies to all such tabulations throughout the book.)

Upsetting though these experiences are, students realize, at least on an intellectual level, that the physician's detachment does not necessarily indicate a lack of concern and that, in fact, his or her failure to become emotionally involved may be in the best interest of the patient and the family.

Each experience with death tends to remove students further from their initial idealism and inch them closer to the professional response modeled by their mentors. "It's really hard the first two or three times a patient dies," a senior explained, "so you learn to develop a protective shield to reduce the emotional impact." Consider, for example, the emotional strain that this stressful experience had upon a student who was unprotected by the acquired coping mechanisms of the seasoned professional:

My first patient was a little boy suffering from incurable leukemia. He seemed all right when he left the hospital, but in about two weeks he was brought into the emergency room in shock and died three hours later. I was in the room with him when the attending physician asked, "Who had this patient before?" I told him that I had, so he sent me to look after the mother who was crying in the next room. While the doctor worked on this little five-year-old, I tried to talk to the mother. I really felt terribly inadequate; there wasn't a whole lot I could say to make her feel better. Then we went into the room where they were treating the boy. He was screaming and crying and then he stopped breathing. The mother collapsed and somebody caught her. That experience really got to me!

Such happenings make clear the necessity of developing coping skills that allow medical practitioners to do their work without getting "all wrapped up" in the patients' personal lives.[12] Avoidance is one technique: "I try to keep away from them if I know what's coming so as to reduce the emotional stress." Another coping method is to stop thinking about the patient by busily losing oneself in work. This helps distract or block out stressful thoughts. Depersonalizing patients by thinking of them as "the liver in Room 214" also serves as a protective shield. "If one doesn't get personally involved with the patient," a senior points out, "death can then be almost as neutral as reading the obituary section of a newspaper."

Although humor or lightheartedness in the midst of such painful human drama seems inappropriate, it is also used at times by seasoned clinicians to reduce the emotional tension and strain created by such stressful circumstances, thereby allowing them to perform their responsibilities more effectively. Rationalization, such as thinking the patient is better off dead than alive, also helps to soften the death experience. For instance, when the patient is old or has been sick for a long time with no hope of improvement, it is even easy to wish the release of death for him.

Although students usually achieve some success in managing their feelings when a patient dies, dealing with the family is always difficult. Knowing what to say and how to act with relatives is a constant worry. "It's an overwhelming experience," a senior points out. "You go through it a hundred times and never get used to it. You're expected to be a pillar of strength for them to lean on and turn to for advice, so it can be very uncomfortable."

To help themselves through such awkward encounters, students develop communication skills that serve as a coping mechanism. One is the frequent use of technical language in referring to death. These terms tend to insulate and isolate death by classifying it as a medical event—an event occurring in professional life rather than personal life—and thereby permitting easier and freer discussion. Indirect reference is also utilized to soften discussion of stressful events. "The situation" or "the incident" is often used to refer to death. Because such speech is vague, oblique, and elusive, it reduces the anxiety by an overly bald or too frequent reference to death. Euphemisms, used in the same way, also conceal the stressful event. Clinicians speak of patients who are "not going to make it" and who are "on a hopeless decline." "Critically ill," while not a euphemism, functions as one when it is used in referring to a patient who is dying.

Latin derivative terms also appear to reduce stress and to make discussion of difficult subjects easier. "To pass on" or "to expire" are identical in meaning with "to die," but neither has the immediacy or the emotional force of the Anglo-Saxon term. So, although Latinate terms function differently from euphemisms, the effect created is the same—a softening or concealing of fact. As George Orwell (1954, p. 173) stated, "Inflated style is itself a kind of euphemism. A mass of Latin words fall upon the facts like soft snow, blurring the outlines and covering up all of the details."

Such techniques, acquired through experience and role modeling, help clinicians maintain a professional demeanor and retain emotional composure while rendering compassionate medical care. This balanced attitude has been labeled "detached concern" (Lief and Fox, 1963).

SUMMING UP

Examination of student adaptation to stressful training experiences most clearly demonstrates the process of professional career development. When confronted with such personally challenging circumstances, students cannot remain unchanged. They must either go forward and confront these events squarely or they must retreat. In either case, they will never be the same again, because their choices will influence decisions throughout the remainder of their careers. When challenges are successfully met, adaptive skills emerge to minimize the emotional shock and discomforts of such experiences. Repeated incidents shape responses so that the old is left behind (the layman's viewpoint and response) and the new is begun (the professional's attitude and behavior). Viewed in this way, medical school is not only a teaching institution where knowledge and professional doctrines are disseminated, but it is also an obstacle course where stressful situations frequently require recruits to prove their adaptive ability.

From a socialization perspective, the hurdles and emotional obstacles that lie along the career path serve as rites-of-passage for participants to prove their ability, their dedication, and their emotional vigor. Although stressful to endure, these hurdles, when successfully overcome, enhance a sturdy product. By comparison, medical school is not dissimilar from military boot camp where, it is claimed, boys are changed into men. These experiences also approximate the rigorous initiation rites of preliterate tribes, such as bringing back a bear claw in order to establish one's readiness for the adult role. In a similar way, medical recruits, in order to prove their mettle, must successfully confront stressful obstacles.

The functional usefulness of challenge and stress, when observed in this manner, may be appreciated; but the price in failure and psychic distress must also be assessed. If the traveler of this career path arrives victoriously at the destination in full possession of physical, emotional, and marital health, all well and good. But it is bitter irony when a student loses out on the very goals being sought for others.

Many medical recruits who withdraw from medical school do so not because they are academically incompetent but because they succumb to adversity and emotional strain. And those who remain sometimes do so only with the aid of psychiatric help. In this regard, it is important to realize that in addition to these stressful professional experiences, medical students also face formidable problems of a personal nature. Female students, especially, face major adjustments when bucking the tide of tradition concerning female roles. Not only must they find a personally acceptable balance between traditional and contemporary attitudes about womanhood, but also they must work within a profession that has for generations been male dominated.

Similarly the traditional norm for American adult males is to settle down by marrying, obtaining a good job, and then acquiring a family, home, and material goods. The typical male student, however, remains in a relatively dependent, adolescent-like situation until he approaches the age of 30.[13] Because the medical curriculum is so demanding and leaves so little time for earning money, dating, or engaging in other social and recreational activities, many students feel isolated, lonely, and frustrated.

When students marry, their domestic relationships are usually not ideal. Traditionally, a husband is defined as breadwinner, and male medical students, being fiercely independent, covet this role. Their financial dependence upon others is understandably galling to them. Moreover, at an age when the sex drive is strongest, even married students complain about deferred sexuality.

Medical school is no less stressful for married women. Not every husband may be willing to assume household tasks that have been customarily defined as the province of the female while his student wife studies, or to shoulder the extraordinary financial burden that is entailed. And, how many male egos can deal with the probability of eventually having lower occupational status than their wives?

Clearly, the path toward physicianhood is a steep, uphill route marked by obstacles that must be hurdled if one is to continue onward. Those who achieve the goal must possess personal dedication, a willingness to sacrifice, and physical, mental, and emotional stamina.

In balance, then, what seems to be needed is not fewer challenges and obstacles, for these can serve a positive function, but more awareness and sensitivity among socializing agents (the administration and faculty) to the plight of the struggling student. To a newcomer, one of the most striking features about medical education is the scant attention given to the basic psychosocial aspects of the socialization process, specifically the urgent anxieties that confront medical students. Scientific detachment and objective rationality reign supreme at the medical center, so that, for the most part, recruits are left pretty much on their own to deal with their own fears and inner conflicts.

Although many beginning students are anxious and profoundly disillusioned, rarely can they talk openly about their feelings without risking the appearance of being weak or unsuccessful. "You figure," one said, "if I tell this person my troubles he might say, 'What's wrong with *you?*' " So, unless students find their way to a staff psychiatrist, each one must, for the most part, resolve his or her own anxieties and doubts. And, in so doing, the fledgling physician is quite apt to wonder, "Gee, what *is* wrong with me?"

Even when students successfully work out their situational adjustments and make it to graduation, the long-range results are not always healthy. When utilizing avoidance or suppression as dominant coping techniques, for example, the budding physician may cover up or deny vitally important subjective feelings. From a socialization perspective, this may yield dysfunctional results that will hinder rather than benefit the doctor in performing the clinical role.

Although the medical school product may be technically competent and represent the school well by scoring high on board exams, he or she may be inadequate to deal freely and openly with the subjective features of medical care. How is a practitioner to deal successfully with emotions and feelings of patients and their families when personal doubts and inner feelings have not been successfully dealt with? It is this dimension of the doctor's performance that is most often overlooked, allowing unfinished professionals to step into the world of patient care where the fully rounded physician is so sorely needed.

NOTES

1. See Strecker, Appel, and Braceland (1936); Levitt (1966); Hunter, Prince, and Schwartzman (1961); Pitts, Winokur, and Stewart (1961); Blaine and McArthur (1961); McGuire (1966); Adsett (1968); Woods, Natterson, and Silverman (1966); Funkenstein (1961); Saslow (1956); and Bojar (1961). For additional information on stress in medical education, refer to Lief (1971), Chapter 2; and Coombs and Boyle (1971b). Also see Coombs and Boyle (1971a), and Boyle and Coombs (1971).

2. See Levitt and Rubenstein (1967), and Lief, Lancaster, and Spruiell (1963).

3. For a discussion on media enticement, refer to Chapter 1, "Mass Inducements" in Coombs, Fry, and Lewis (1976).

4. Similar findings have been reported by Lief and Fox (1963). See also Becker, et al. (1961, pp. 103–106), and Fox (1959, p. 110).

5. The inclination to deny unusual sensitivities in anatomy laboratory is also noted by Rosenberg (1971).

6. For a discussion of anxiety related to classroom examinations, see Nichols and Spielberger (1967).

7. For the student view on the value of grades, see Martire (1969).

8. Regarding the relationship between grades and future clinical performance, see Wingard and Williamson (1973).

9. For a discussion of sex as a forbidden topic, refer to Coombs (1971a).

10. Stimulated by the prodding of psychiatrist Harold I. Lief and some of his colleagues, medical educators have recently come to acknowledge a deficit in the training of medical students in the area of human sexuality. For discussions of this topic, see Coombs (1968a) and Pauly and Goldstein (1970).

11. Medical schools currently offer little formal instruction on the issues that face the doctor and the dying patient. For further discussion of this critical omission, see Barton (1972) and Olin (1972).

12. For a review of literature pertaining to the various coping mechanisms used by hospital staff, see Coombs and Goldman (1973).

13. Medical training, requiring so many years, may prolong adolescence longer than any other career. Eriksen (1959) has said ". . . college education is probably the greatest organized postponement of adulthood, emotionally speaking, that could be imagined." See also Bojar (1961) for a discussion of various problems in the medical student's personal life within the overall context of a prolonged period of dependency during training.

PART IV
EMERGING OUTCOME

7. Patients

Patients can sense when a doctor is nervous and scared. From the second I walk into a patient's room, he is sizing me up and assessing how well I am handling myself. So I tell myself over and over again, "I'm not scared; I know what I'm doing." (A junior)

SINCE PATIENT MANAGEMENT is the essence of medical practice, the future physician must learn the proper attitudes and techniques for handling this career aspect with professionalism and diplomacy. The science of medicine is learned primarily from lectures, books, and laboratory work; but the art of relating to patients is acquired chiefly through imitative role modeling, intuition, and trial and error.[1] Views about patients and ways in which these attitudes change as students gain clinical experience are explored in this chapter.

GAINING CONFIDENCE OF PATIENTS

As the quotation above suggests, playing the doctor's role when one is not yet an M.D. can, at times, be an uncomfortable experience. Patients are interested in being cured, not in having novices study them; and they may have misgivings about receiving physical examinations from young and obviously inexperienced clinicians.[2] Even though students generally are attired in white coats, carry black bags, and conspicuously display a stethoscope and other medical paraphernalia, patients sometimes learn that they are not fully qualified doctors. For example, when one unsure student was drawing blood from a patient for the first time, he asked, "Are you all right?" Recognizing the student's inexperience and insecurity, the patient replied, "Yes, I am, but how about you?"

Even when professional techniques are faultless, patients who are aware of the hospital hierarchy seem to be able to spot students. Some of the more arrogant and assuming patients—usually V.I.P. types who demand

139

treatment only by private physicians—ask "now-what-are-you?" type questions, apparently expecting students to trot out their credentials.

Naturally, students try to prevent such experiences whenever possible. To learn how they do this, I inquired about their techniques for winning the confidence of patients. At first students try to maintain a confident facade, as one said, ". . . by keeping my mouth shut and just standing there and watching."* The time soon comes, however, when silence will not suffice, when the patient must be interviewed as part of the clinical work-up. Then students must make an effort to gain the patient's trust and confidence through varying approaches.

Acting Confidently

Many students believe that one way to secure a patient's confidence is to give the impression of self-assurance and competence.† Even though quaking in one's boots, a student must project the image of the calm and confident physician from the moment of entrance into a patient's room. "That initial impression is really important," a senior said. "You can't look shaky and jittery." Specific techniques used to create an aura of self-confidence are summarized as follows:

a. Look the patient squarely in the eye and keep him busy answering questions.
b. Never hesitate; always be doing something; just move ahead, a step at a time.
c. Assume an air of authority; never seem timid or allow yourself to show that you feel inferior; act like you've done it all a thousand times before; remember that you're in the driver's seat and, most important, the patient *wants* to believe in you.
d. Refrain from talking too much.
e. When stuck, don't panic; leave the room after giving a plausible reason, reorganize, then come back with your plan clearly in mind.

Rather than letting the patient know they are novices, some students would rather act like they know what they are doing even if they do not. They feel there is no harm in doing this, provided it poses no danger to the patient. So many students eagerly seize the opportunity to listen to a heart murmur even though they may have little idea of what they are

---

* Freshmen do not usually know how to gain the confidence of patients; 33.9 percent of the freshmen admitted this when asked "How do you go about winning the confidence of patients?" But the proportion who replied "I don't know" dropped to 15.8 percent in the sophomore year and to 3.4 percent in the junior year. The percentage jumped back to 7.3 percent in the senior year.

† This response is given by 35.6 percent of class during the freshman year, 50.9 percent during the sophomore year, 53.4 percent in the junior year, and 40.0 percent in the final year.

hearing or to examine a patient's eyes through the ophthalmoscope without really knowing what they are looking for.

An example of the bluffing and role-playing that go on is provided by a sophomore who was learning to do a venipuncture. His patient showed him her arms, which were black and blue as the result of one of his classmate's unsuccessful attempts to find a suitable vein the day before, and then stated emphatically that she did not want any more of that. To this the student replied, "We try to keep the beginners out of here." "I couldn't tell her I was a beginner, too," he rationalized; "she would have died on the spot!" Fortunately this story had a happy ending; the vein was contacted on the first attempt, and the technician who was standing by was not needed.

Students take comfort in the fact that most patients do not differentiate between medical students and doctors; and few students feel the need to clarify the difference. In fact, some even introduce themselves as "Dr. _____," reasoning that, after all, hospital staff call them by this title. They know that in a teaching hospital the title "Doctor" is more of a functional label than an indication of formal credentials. Thus, these students suffer few pangs of conscience. If patients regard them as doctors, why shake their confidence by telling them otherwise?

Demonstrating Competence

Better than simply acting and appearing competent, of course, is being competent. "There is nothing like a job well done," a senior commented, "to inspire confidence on the part of the patient, not to mention the boost it gives your own self-esteem." A confident appearance is of little use unless it is backed up by competent performance. Results speak for themselves.*

Students realize the impossibility of being proficient in the entire spectrum of clinical tasks. They know all too well the boundaries of their own knowledge. Although these parameters are constantly enlarging, a wise student is satisfied to proceed within his or her particular limits and discuss with each patient only subjects in which a solid foundation of personal knowledge is established. When ventures into uncertain areas are made in order to impress a patient, the rookie clinician is treading on dangerous ground and may end up with the patient's faith badly shaken, not to mention potential cracks in a fragile professional self-image.

At times the distinction between showing off and demonstrating real competence becomes a bit blurred. Some students give tacit approval to the practice of asking patients leading questions in order to steer them into

---

* The percentage each year who try to gain the confidence of patients by displaying professional competence is as follows: 10.2 percent, freshmen; 14.0 percent, sophomores; 29.3 percent, juniors; and 27.3 percent, seniors.

familiar areas where the students can exhibit their knowledge. This enables them to speak with authority rather than hesitating or giving vague answers. In all fairness, this is not an out-and-out exhibitionist technique; rather, it can serve as a confidence-building mechanism. A third-year student provides an example of how this practice can have a dual beneficial effect, that of strengthening the patient's faith in the student and helping the latter feel more self-assured. Having read a patient's history and being familiar with his symptoms, he said, "You're having some nausea and vomiting, aren't you?" The patient was immediately impressed with his perspicacity and said, "Yes, that's right, I am." Similarly, a classmate became a hero to an OB patient who, because of an injection of novocaine into her spinal column, had lost all feeling in her legs and feet. He predicted that she would regain the lost feeling in her extremities by the next morning. Sure enough, the student's prophecy came to pass and his reputation in that patient's ward was assured. He explained, "You can tell patients what to expect when you are darned sure what the outcome is going to be; then they get the idea that you really know what you're doing."

Being Honest

There is a definite line between the above confidence-building tactics and delibrate misrepresentation of oneself as a physician with greater competence than one really has; and stepping over that line seems blatantly deceptive to some students. To them, casually using the title "Doctor" in a teaching hospital is a far cry from deliberately fooling patients by assuming the air of authority expected of a seasoned veteran. One student described the latter behavior as "snowing patients by pulling the wool over their eyes." Such actions are decried as adversely affecting a clinician's credibility.*

The approach recommended by such students is "to act normal and not hide behind a facade." When patients ask them questions they cannot answer, they simply say, "I don't know, but I'll see if I can find out for you." These students, usually upperclassmen, tell a patient the truth by explaining, "I am a student physician and in the learning process." This approach, they say, usually meets with acceptance and understanding. Rather than losing confidence, patients seem to respect them even more. Some patients, in fact, seem flattered by the opportunity to participate in the educational process and go out of their way to help students who are unequivocally honest. "Most people can sense a false front," a sophomore commented. "They can usually tell when you're trying to be something you're not, and they respect you more for being honest."

---

* The proportion of the class who try to obtain the confidence of patients by being strictly honest with them is: 0.0 percent, freshmen; 1.8 percent, sophomores; 17.2 percent, juniors; and 20.0 percent, seniors.

This latter approach becomes more popular as students near graduation, but even then it remains a minority viewpoint. During the first two years, only one student mentioned honesty as a technique. The most prevailing approach is to simply play the doctor's role as competently as possible and let the patients' assumptions suffice.

Showing Concern

Demonstrating or pretending technical competence are not the only ways of securing the patients' confidence. Taking an interest in them and showing true concern is another technique.* Advocates of this approach warn that pretense is dangerous, for its path is fraught with potential pitfalls. Problems are frequently encountered that can get one in over one's head. Moreover, trying to impress patients with technical competence may backfire if in so doing an image of cold professionalism is projected. An upperclassman said, "A patient feels safer with a student who has a good bedside manner than with one who comes in and tries to play God, rattling off fancy terms and showing off his knowledge for the patient's benefit." Genuine expressions of concern help a patient bear uncomfortable treatments, but to maintain trust and goodwill these students agree that such solicitude should not be used to deliberately divert attention from unpleasant but necessary procedures.

The elements of a "good bedside manner," as students call it, come intuitively and informally by osmosis rather than by formal indoctrination. "It's something you kind of feel your way into," a sophomore explained. Taking time with patients, showing friendliness and personal interest, being sensitive to their concerns and viewpoints, and using reassurance and gentleness all enter into the ideal bedside manner. Most patients assume that their clinicians are competent, but they yearn for one who is concerned.

DEFINING IDEAL PATIENT BEHAVIOR

Because medical recruits, like most young adults in the middle and upper consumer brackets, have at one time or another been patients themselves, they have internalized fairly standardized ideas of how patients are expected to act. These acquired concepts are brought to medical school and apparently little is done there to alter them. Few students show any appreciable change from year to year in the ways they define "good" patients and "bad" ones.[3] Overwhelmingly, students at all stages say that

---

* The proportion of students who gain the confidence of patients by showing concern for them is: 5.1 percent, freshmen; 19.3 percent, sophomores; 24.1 percent, juniors; and 23.6 percent, seniors.

the chief virtue of good patients is a cooperative attitude. As the following discussion indicates, however, there are variations in the ways patients demonstrate cooperativeness.*

Being Motivated and Concerned About Own Health

One characteristic of cooperative patients is taking an active interest in their own health and willingly participating in the healing process. A good patient seeks the physician's aid because of a genuine desire for help, not because a nagging spouse or somebody else makes the appointment. When a patient blusters that there is nothing wrong and that the whole idea of seeing a doctor is sheer nonsense, the physician is placed in the uncomfortable position of having to promote both self and services much as a salesman does. It is much more comfortable for a clinician when a person is already motivated to make use of the services provided.

Displaying Pleasant Disposition

Students naturally prefer to deal with patients who have pleasant personalities. As in any social situation, those who are good-natured, cheerful, optimistic, and uncomplaining are enjoyable to work with, especially if they have a sense of humor. "Grumbling old biddies," who constantly make a big production when some procedure causes minor pain or discomfort, make clinical work an ordeal. "It is just impossible to please some people," a junior observed. "For them nothing is ever right; nothing satisfies them."

Good patients realize that they are not the only ones needing the physician's attention. Bad ones feel that they are entitled to special consideration and frequently make inconvenient, unreasonable, or impossible demands. "They try to monopolize all of your time," one senior said. "They want to be treated like they're on a pedestal." These patients expect the doctor to be at their beck and call and to respond to their every demand.

Good patients are also appreciative and never fail to say, "Thank you, doctor." By contrast, bad patients are not only unappreciative, but also may actually feel they are doing the doctor a favor through their patronage.

Trusting the Doctor and Following Directions

Another characteristic of good patients is trusting and having confidence in the healing powers of the clinician. They do not doubt motives or

* When asked "What are the characteristics of a good patient?" eight out of ten students during each year replied, "He is cooperative." Similarly, when asked about the characteristics of bad patients, three-fourths replied, "He is uncooperative."

challenge clinical judgments. Such patients may ask questions about directions or procedures, but these questions are motivated by a legitimate curiosity or interest rather than by mistrust. Skeptical patients who adopt a doubting attitude challenge the already shaky authority of student-physicians and thereby undermine self-confidence. "When they question your ability and don't respect your opinion," a sophomore testified, "it doesn't do too much for your ego."

Good patients cooperate by answering the doctor's questions readily and honestly, neither concealing information nor distorting facts. Furthermore, they follow instructions faithfully, taking medication as directed and returning for checkups on schedule. If advised to stop smoking or to follow a certain diet, they comply. In short, they realize that the doctor can help them only if they follow the advice given.

By contrast, bad patients adopt the attitude: "Here I am; fix me up." Or else, feeling that they know more than the doctor, they diagnose their own disease and dictate the treatments; for example, "This is what's wrong with me; give me this pill; I prefer that drugstore." Other patients may be noncompliant because of religious beliefs ("It's more important to submit to God's will than to obey the doctor") or because, as students express it, "They're not intelligent enough to understand the doctor's instructions."

Worst of all is the hostile patient who dislikes doctors and hates to submit to their authority. One such patient, when interviewed by a student about his malady, sneeringly replied, "You're the expert; you tell *me*." A patient like this, who has a chip on his shoulder, creates a difficult interpersonal situation.

Since student views concerning proper patient behavior remain stable during medical school training, it seems clear that the societal role definition corresponds with that of medical educators. At all stages of training, patients are expected to cooperate with the doctor. This is demonstrated by recognizing and accepting authority, trusting clinical judgment, and then cheerfully and gratefully following directions.[4]

HANDLING UNCOOPERATIVE PATIENTS

Although medical school does little to change preexisting concepts of proper patient behavior, the same cannot be said about student approaches to managing difficult patients. Although two out of five freshmen have no idea at all about how to deal with difficult patients, this number declines with each year in medical school. Increasingly, patience and persuasion constitute the most popular approach; the proportion of the class who advocate this technique increases from 37 percent in the freshman year to

65 percent in the senior year. Although considerably less popular, avoidance as a way of dealing with troublesome patients increases in favor during the first three years, and then drops in the last year. Firmness as a technique is less enthusiastically advocated during the clinical years than in the first two years.

Students receive little, if any, formal instruction on the techniques of handling noncompliant patients.[5] This skill seems to be acquired by observing role models at work or by personal trial and error. When probed about the techniques for managing these difficult patients, this sophomore's reply was typical: "I don't know. They've never told us and I haven't yet had enough experience to develop any techniques of my own." That 16 percent of the seniors still cannot pinpoint any recommended techniques for dealing with such patients reinforces the idea that such learning is subtle and informal.*

Patience and Persuasion

Fortunately for patients, a favored approach—especially in the senior year—is one of acceptance, patience, and kind persuasion. Each year an increasing number of students adopt the view that "tender loving care" works best with troublesome patients as well as good ones.† Most students come to feel that harshness, although it may squelch an annoying patient, is likely to alienate him and cause him to reject the treatment he really needs. Therefore, most students conclude that, as a general rule, it is better to "keep your cool, be as courteous as possible, and don't let them bug you." So, when exasperated by a troublesome patient, they try to suppress their irritation and cultivate an attitude of patience.

A good clinician tries to gain the trust and confidence of the uncooperative patient by providing reassurance and emotional support. One approach, for example, is to say, "You seem to be a little bit anxious," or "You look like you have the blues today." A student who had utilized this approach remarked, "I've been surprised how often patients will open up and dump out a lot of problems. Once they've done this, they're more cooperative, and, in many cases, their organic symptoms decrease in number and severity."

Another approach is to sit down and talk with patients about fishing or gardening or whatever they enjoy. "It opens them up so that when you

---

* When asked about the techniques of handling difficult patients, 37.3 percent of the freshman class could think of none. This percentage declined to 22.8 percent in the sophomore year, 22.8 percent in the junior year, and 16.4 percent in the senior year.

† The percentages of those who advocate patience and persuasion in handling uncooperative patients are as follows: 37.3 percent, freshmen; 43.9 percent, sophomores; 45.6 percent, juniors; and 65.4 percent, seniors.

try to get a medical history, they are helpful," one said. "You've got to show patience and win their trust before you can assert yourself with them."

Taking time to explain in simple language a necessary procedure or treatment goes a long way toward motivating patients, as does the practice of answering questions. To convince a doubting patient that he really was sick and needed to comply with medical instructions, one student lent her stethoscope to the patient so that he could hear for himself that one lung was not working. When this approach failed to convince the patient, the student showed him the X rays and results of the laboratory tests. In this way, the patient began to accept the seriousness of his condition and agreed to return for checkups. Taking time to "coax patients along" generally produces the desired results. "With patience," one said, "they usually come around."

Avoidance

It is probable that most students, like most doctors, consciously or subconsciously avoid troublesome patients whenever possible (Coombs and Goldman, 1973). However, relatively few admit to deliberately employing avoidance as a technique.* But the number who do so increases significantly during the third year when students are trying out their clinical wings. When patients are disagreeable—"nasty, smart-alecky, or disrespectful"—students try to stay out of their way. Consequently, such patients may receive only minimal personal attention. "You do what is necessary, but in as little time as possible," a junior remarked. "They usually aren't asked to return for a checkup, either."

Indirect methods, such as utilizing family members as go-betweens, are among other avoidance techniques used, especially with ornery children or old people. Such techniques, learned through trial and error, sometimes help clinicians cope with troublesome patients.

Firmness

A firm approach is sometimes necessary, some claim, for dealing with the troublesome patient.† This approach is defined in several different ways, but most students use stern, authoritarian methods of handling pa-

---

* Only 8.5 percent of the freshmen, 12.3 percent of the sophomores, 26.3 percent of the juniors, and 16.4 percent of the seniors mention avoidance as a technique in dealing with difficult patients.

† Firmness as a technique for dealing with difficult patients is mentioned by 28.8 percent of the freshmen, 28.1 percent of the sophomores, 21.1 percent of the juniors, and 21.8 percent of the seniors.

tients as a last resort, only after patients become intolerable and other approaches have failed.

The firm approach lets the patient know that the doctor is in charge and that cooperation is required. "There isn't any sense in fooling around with belligerent patients," a sophomore explained. "You just have to lay it on the line with them. When they start talking back and acting nasty, you need to cut them down. If you let them get away with it, they are not going to respect you."

The analogy of a parent–child relationship is used by advocates of this approach. "Patients require a strong personality in the doctor," a fourth-year student points out. "Just as children must be disciplined or spanked at one time or another, patients sometimes need a back-of-the-hand or hairbrush type of handling." "Casper Milquetoast" doctors, these students say, are ineffective. "It pays to tell patients where they stand and even blow your top occasionally," one said. "When they give me a lot of trouble, I just let them know that if they don't cooperate I won't play ball." On one occasion, such an approach got quick results from a belligerent patient in the emergency room. After putting up with his behavior for some time, the student finally said, "If you want me to help you, you are going to have to shut up and cooperate!" The patient did.

DEALING WITH "CROCKS"

The term "crock" is common parlance among physicians when talking about certain patients. But a large majority of freshmen are unfamiliar with the term. Only 17 percent of the first-year class correctly define the word as pertaining to patients whose physical complaints have no discernible organic basis. But it does not take long for them to catch on. By the second year, only 15 percent of the class were unsure of the connotation of the term, and a year later the number dropped to 2 percent.

Attitudes about crocks are acquired through informal interaction with more advanced clinicians.[6] The only formal course work dealing with this topic, even peripherally, is in psychiatry lectures on psychosomatic illness. Most psychiatry professors deny the crock concept and deplore the tendency to label and stereotype patients in this way. Thus, students are subjected to two opposing influences: the "hard-core M.D.," who resents these patients because they waste precious time by pretending to be sick when, in fact, they are not; and psychiatrically inclined physicians who decry the use of this label, yet have a lot of "fancy names" for people like them. The resulting confusion is shown by this student's comment: "I don't know what to believe. One group of faculty members tells you that half the patients you will see are crocks, and the other group says there is no such thing."

It is not surprising, then, that attitudes about crocks vary markedly from student to student. Like their mentors, some come to reject these patients outright as malingerers and fakers; others tolerate them; and still others express interest in them and enjoy the challenge of helping them. Most students, however, try to be tolerant; but with increasing clinical experience, more and more admit their frustration in dealing with such patients.

Tolerant Attitudes

Most upperclassmen, nearly two-thirds of the class, try to maintain an understanding and compassionate view of psychosomatic illness, realizing that "you can't just write these patients off." There is danger, they say, in labeling any patient as a "crock." As a junior pointed out, "A lot of people tagged as 'crocks' actually have something wrong with them. You've got to be absolutely sure and adopt the attitude that everyone is sick until proven otherwise."

These students maintain that pain or discomfort, whether actual or imagined, is real in its consequences and therefore must be adequately dealt with. They view pain as an emotion, not strictly a physiological event, and feel that the physician who practices good medicine must try to help all patients, regardless of what their laboratory tests show. "Illness is illness either way," a senior pointed out. "If people have problems, they need to be treated regardless of whether the cause is organic or functional." "The word 'crock' is a bad term," a classmate added, "something invented by the doctor to explain away a patient who is not understood and difficult to deal with. We put the designation of 'crock' on patients because of our own inadequacies." Such students, instead of running the patient off, take a little more time, listen attentively, provide emotional support, and perhaps suggest referral to a physician who is better qualified to deal with the emotional component of the problem.

When time is precious, however, it is not easy to maintain idealism and patience toward such patients. Students, like physicians, are on the horns of a dilemma in trying to maintain a balance as competing demands are thrust upon them.[7] They must take time to listen and maintain a caring attitude, yet still keep up with all that needs to be done.

So, idealistic students sometimes feel guilty on becoming frustrated and annoyed with patients who, in more relaxed settings, would win their sympathies. "I really hate to admit it," one confessed, "but I've gotten more impatient this year. When I have a patient who ties up all my time when I need to be seeing others, I get irritated and a little bit hostile. I know I shouldn't feel this way, but when it takes all morning to run laboratory tests on a patient with vague complaints without finding anything, I feel affronted because my time has been wasted." Then, with a sigh, she reminded herself, "Yet every crock will be sick enough to die sometime, so I've just got to make sure this isn't the time."

Rejecting Attitudes

By the senior year more than a third of the class give up all pretense of being tolerant with crocks and admit that these patients give them "a pain in the neck." Adopting the attitudes of their "hard-core M.D." mentors, these students regard crocks as "spooks," hypochondriacs, and fakers —people who complain of excessive pain or disability when medical procedures indicate nothing physically wrong. "Every minor ailment is completely magnified out of proportion," a junior stated. "They're really not sick at all."

Two types of crocks are defined by students, although the line between them is not always clear. First are the neurotics who, because they believe they are sick, actually develop symptoms or pain. Second are those who more or less consciously feign sickness because they seek some secondary gain, such as escape from work, unemployment compensation, insurance benefits, personal reassurance, or sympathy and attention:

> For a lot of them, coming to the clinic is a big social event. It's like going to church. They enjoy themselves by talking with others about their aches and pains. They talk about how many doctors they've seen, what they think of each one, what is done for them, and so on. When they see the doctor, they go through the same thing and enjoy all the attention. Every little thing the doctor says or does gives them something to go on. They have more fun than if they were at a movie.

Crocks are also annoying because of the diagnostic problems they present. Ego rewards come from accurately diagnosing and effectively treating the patient. Because crocks have a lot of odd symptoms and usually cling to them in spite of all therapeutic measures, they are frustrating patients to deal with.

Clinical pride is hurt when patients fool the doctor. After a student had spent a great deal of time with one patient, a resident laughingly said, "This one is a crock." "It's no fun being made to look like a fool," the student remarked. So, to avoid such embarrassment, clinicians learn a sign language to alert each other to patients suspected of being crocks. For example, one may say to another, "Maybe we ought to do a porcelain [as related to crockery] test."

A variety of tricks are also learned to outmaneuver crocks or discourage them from wasting the doctor's time. One is to trick them with placebos as "cures." Another is to deny them the sympathy and attention they seek by keeping them waiting for long periods in an isolated room. Some even suggest use of dull needles when giving shots in order to make the experience as unpleasant as possible. The hope is that the patient will eventually come to the conclusion: "Good grief! It's terrible to be a patient; I'd rather be home."

PREFERRING VARIOUS TYPES OF PATIENTS

No two patients, of course, are entirely alike, and students are exposed to all types during their medical training. Children and adults, for example, can present striking contrasts, as do men and women and patients from different socioeconomic backgrounds. Similarly, the organically ill and the emotionally ailing differ, just as do the acutely ill and the chronically or terminally ill. And among all these patient types, some talk a lot and ask many questions while others are quiet and accepting. The question to be addressed here is how student preferences for these different patient types are influenced by medical school experiences.

Adults Versus Children

Most medical students would rather work with adults than with children. This preference—pronounced at the beginning of medical school— becomes even stronger during each succeeding year. The proportion who initially prefer children and of those who hope to work with both age groups shows a corresponding decline. As they neared graduation, only 7 percent of the class still preferred children and 9 percent had no preference, wishing to work with both types.*

Preferring Adult Patients

A few freshmen frankly admit that they just do not like children. Most students, however, generally prefer adults for other reasons. For one thing,

---

* When asked "Which would you prefer as a patient, a child or an adult?" 49.2 percent of the freshmen, 54.4 percent of the sophomores, 72.5 percent of the juniors, and 83.6 percent of the seniors said they would prefer adults. The percentages preferring children were 22.0 percent of the freshmen, 14.0 percent of the sophomores, 10.3 percent of the juniors, and 7.3 percent of the seniors. Those who indicated no preference for either group were 20.3 percent of the freshmen, 24.6 percent of the sophomores, 10.3 percent of the juniors, and 9.1 percent of the seniors. The remainder gave a "don't know" response, preventing the other percentages from totaling 100 percent.

medical school experiences seem to promote greater confidence in dealing with adults. "Almost everything we've learned so far has been related to adults rather than children," a senior remarked; "I've learned a lot more about adult medicine than I have about pediatrics or adolescence."

Exposure to pediatric clinics simply tends to convince students that young patients present more difficult problems. For one thing, the child's small size complicates matters. "It's a lot harder to hear and interpret the beat of a child's heart," a junior commented. Children are also more vulnerable to infection, and their response to drugs and other treatment is more unpredictable. "Their problems are so much more acute than adults," a senior notes, "that if you don't act fast you may run into real problems. They can go silent on you and die so quickly it's frightening."

The more tenderhearted students hope to avoid children because the sight of a suffering child unnerves them. "I can't stand to see kids sick," a senior commented. "Just going on the pediatric wards bothers me. There are all these screaming kids who are sick or maimed. I try to stay away from it."

Others prefer to avoid pediatric patients because they find them un-cooperative or otherwise difficult to work with. In the first place, children are often afraid of doctors. "Kids just go bananas when they see people in white," a senior commented. "They're afraid you're going to stick a needle in them if you get half a chance." The resulting screams and tears are nerve-racking. Remaining calm in the presence of a howling child is no small challenge. It is exasperating to wrestle with a child in order to complete a physical examination; and the situation is made all the worse when anxious parents stand over them and further upset the child. This senior's experience is illustrative:

> I was trying to get the confidence of a child when the mother spoke up and said, "Johnny, if you're not good, the doctor's going to give you a shot." And I said to myself, "Oh hell, lady! How am I going to deal with this kid when you're telling him things like that?"

Obtaining an adequate medical history is also more difficult with children. A child's memory is often sketchy or undependable, and his vocabulary and comprehension are limited. So the doctor must couch questions in simple language and coax the answers out of a small patient. Recognizing that he had neither the talent nor the patience to do this, a male student said, "I'm not the 'coochy-coochy-coo' type; I just don't have the technique."

Even when the doctor succeeds in getting some sort of response from a young patient, the results are not always satisfying. Catching on to what a two-year-old means requires a special skill. For, as one student notes, "If you ask a child, 'Does your tummy hurt?' the child will mutter, 'Hurt.' If you say, 'Does it hurt all the time?' all the kid says is, 'It hurts.' " Consequently, clinical students must rely heavily on their own intuition and hunches. "You poke here and you poke there, almost working by the seat of your pants," a senior said. "You just have to be blessed with a special gift to sense where the problem is."

Depending on parents to provide information—a necessity when working with small children—is less than ideal, since the history is secondhand. Unfortunately, no observer, even one as intimate as a parent, can adequately describe how another person feels. And the problem is further complicated when parents give conflicting interpretations.

Aside from the fact that adults are easier to examine and give a more satisfactory history, work with adult patients is, for most students, more rewarding in other ways. "Adults are smarter," a junior observed; "they know more, they've been around, and you can talk to them. They're more stimulating and entertaining." Consequently, most students feel more comfortable with adults and fail to acquire the art of dealing with children.

Preferring Children as Patients

Despite the inherent problems, a few students still prefer to work with children. "I really like kids," one said. "I just enjoy being around them." These students enjoy the innocence of children and their lack of contamination by the "corrupting influences of adult society." Unlike guileful and practiced adults, children are seen as open, honest, trustworthy, and forthright. "They are just delightful creatures," a sophomore commented; "I like the child's mind—the curiosity, the inquisitiveness, the implicit faith they will have in you if you are careful with them. I find them refreshing."

One advantage such students see in working with pediatric patients is that their illnesses are seldom complicated by an overlay of emotional problems. It is easy to get to the root of the problem, because children, being straightforward and "transparent," rarely fool the doctor. "It's easy to tell when they're putting you on," a junior observed. Another advantage is that children consistently accept the doctor's authority. "They don't give you all the back talk that adults do," a senior said. "When they leave the office, they are less likely to say, 'I don't think the doctor is right. I'm going to do what I want to anyway.' "

Nurturing instincts are also aroused by the vulnerability and helplessness of children. Helping a child in need can bring a warm glow of personal satisfaction, as this sophomore witnessed: "It is a million times more rewarding to see a child smile or stop crying than to have an adult patient say, 'Thank you.' " And saving a child's life may add 60 years or more to a life span, whereas saving an adult may mean the gain of only a few years. But, although one in five freshmen shares this view, their idealism about children wanes progressively as they advance through school. In the end, only a handful retain a preference for children.

Men Versus Women

A large majority of students—about two-thirds of the class—hoping to have a medical practice composed of both sexes, have no preference for either male or female patients. This point of view is dominant among entering freshmen and becomes even more pronounced during subsequent years. For nearly eight out of ten graduating seniors, it is an irrelevant question.*

Preferring Male Patients

Among the minority who express a preference for one sex or the other, male bias exists that persists throughout the four years of training. A male junior's comment is typical of this group: "It's a lot easier to deal with a guy," he said, "because I have more in common with him and can talk on his level. With a girl, it's harder to strike up a conversation." Such male students feel that men are more direct and to the point than women; they simply say what is needed without a lot of extraneous talk. One advantage of this directness and economy of speech is that it shortens the time required for taking a medical history. "It's a pain in the neck," a junior commented, "when patients talk on and on about irrelevant things and you have to keep cutting them off."

Men patients are also perceived by this male segment of the student body as being more logical and rational and less emotional than women, although it must be mentioned that this perception may be a result of life-long conditioning. In the same vein of reasoning, men are believed to have an admirable tendency to "keep a stiff upper lip" and to be more stoical, whereas women are perceived as being more "whiny, complaining, hypochondrial, and 'crocky.' "

Aside from personality stereotyping, the physical examination presents more problems for male students when the patient is a female.[8] Although anxieties decline with added experience, male clinicians do not stop worrying about the female patients being nervous, uncomfortable, or irritated

---

* Students were asked: "Would you prefer dealing with men or women as patients?" The overwhelming majority of this predominantly male cohort had no preference: 64.4 percent of the freshmen, 59.6 percent of the sophomores, 69.0 percent of the juniors, and 78.2 percent of the seniors. Of the remainder, 27.1 percent of the freshmen, 33.3 percent of the sophomores, 27.6 percent of the juniors, and 18.2 percent of the seniors preferred men rather than women patients; only 8.5 percent of the freshmen, 3.5 percent of the sophomores, 1.7 percent of the juniors, and 3.6 percent of the seniors preferred women as patients.

about being examined by a series of men. "When I'm the third or fourth guy to do a pelvic exam," a junior said, "I'm afraid the patient will feel she's being molested or something."

Also, the elaborate precautions that must be observed when examining female patients are troublesome. It takes time to hunt up a chaperon and many nurses resent the intrusion on their time. "The chaperon often has an attitude of 'You're wasting my time, buddy.' " But to examine a patient of the opposite sex without a chaperon involves an element of risk, perhaps "getting dragged into court for something." None of this fuss and worry is necessary when dealing with men, so these male students prefer to avoid female patients.

Preferring Female Patients

Only a handful of entering students in this male-dominated class prefer female patients, and this number decreases during medical training. Those who maintain a preference for women view them as being less demanding and more docile and cooperative than men. Because many men associate illness with unmanly weakness, they seem more resistant to the doctor's efforts. "Men don't like to see doctors, and they want to leave as soon as they can and get back to work," a junior complained. "They are more restless and assertive." By contrast, women are seen as more amenable to seeking and accepting a doctor's counsel.

Middle-Class Versus Lower-Class Patients

A wide range of socioeconomic classes is represented among the patient population at this teaching hospital—the very rich, the very poor, and those in between. Large numbers of poverty-level patients, both blacks and whites, are designated as "service patients" and receive free physician care. As a rule, these patients are not as popular with students as middle-class patients. Only 10 to 15 percent throughout the four years of medical school prefer dealing with the poor, whereas nearly half favor middle-class patients. But it is interesting to note that more than 30 percent of the class enjoy working with patients from both income brackets and dismiss class differences as irrelevant. Student attitudes regarding class differences show little change during four years of training.*

* The question asked was "Which would you prefer to deal with, middle-class or lower-class patients?" In making this comparison, students generally preferred middle-class patients (49.2 percent, freshmen; 40.4 percent, sophomores; 48.3 percent, juniors; and 49.1 percent, seniors). Fewer students preferred lower-class patients (15.2 percent, freshmen; 10.5 percent, sophomores; 17.2 percent, juniors; and 9.1 percent, seniors). However, a sizable percentage had no preference at all (35.6 percent of the freshmen, 47.4 percent of the sophomores, 31.1 percent of the juniors, and 40.0 percent of the seniors).

Preferring Middle-Class Patients

Because the large majority of students are from middle-class homes, most find it easier to relate to middle-class patients. Rapport develops most easily in familiar territory with those having a common bond of similar values and interests. "You can do much better with people your own speed," a junior remarked. "You can joke or kid with them and they understand what you're talking about; they catch the subtleties."

As this student indicates, easy communication is an important factor in developing good relationships with patients. Because low-income people have had strikingly different experiences and educational backgrounds, it is sometimes difficult for students to catch the meaning of their expressions or even to understand their vocabulary or dialect. "We don't even use the same language," a freshman commented. "There is a real communication barrier." The patient, of course, has equal difficulty in understanding the clinician, and this causes frustration. "You ask a question, and they don't even know what you're talking about," a junior complained. Frequently the clinician must rephrase his question several times before the patient can grasp the terminology.

A few students interpreted these communication problems as indicating inferior intelligence. ("They're not very bright and can't talk sensibly; some of them can't even write their own names.") Most students, however, recognized these problems as resulting not from lack of intelligence but from differential experiences and limited educational opportunities.

Managing men from the lower classes can be challenging to middle-class clinicians. While lower-income women are considered generally docile and easy to handle, student doctors note that men of this background often resist treatment because they feel it is unnecessary or demeaning, that the sick role is incompatible with their sense of masculinity.

Preferring Lower-Class Patients

The few students whose family backgrounds are more lower class than middle class naturally identify with low-income patients and feel they are "good, good people right to the core." "Unlike so many middle-class people," one said, "there is nothing false or pretentious about them."

But among middle-class students, humanitarian motivation is the principal reason for finding enjoyment in working with lower-class patients. "They're the ones who need the most care," one said. Such students feel compelled to do their bit to correct social inequities. And because these patients have so little to begin with, they are often more appreciative of the little things the doctor does for them.

But less noble motives can also influence student preferences. For example, the neophyte physician who is insecure in the clinical role may feel more comfortable and confident with lower-class patients, since the latter tend to be more accepting and powerless. Unlike middle-class patients, their expectations are not high, so they are less critical, demanding, and questioning. They seem to have more faith in the doctor and, in addition, often mistake students for bona fide doctors. So lower-class patients are preferred, not for their intrinsic qualities, but because they boost the student ego. This point is made clear by a senior who frankly acknowledged, "While I'm at the learning stage I prefer lower-class patients because I'm insecure in my role, and with a lower-class patient I'm not as nervous when I make a mistake starting an I.V. or something."

Informed middle-class patients are more critical of possible errors in technique and are apt to recognize that the clinician is a student, not a doctor. They resent being used as experimental guinea pigs when they are paying for the services of a private physician. So insecure students may view such patients as being arrogant, critical, and demanding.

Organically Ill Versus Emotionally Ill Patients

Overwhelmingly, students prefer to deal with organically ill patients rather than those with emotional disorders. Eight out of ten freshmen express this preference, and the feeling becomes even more pronounced as graduation approaches. By the senior year only 2 percent of the class expressed a preference for emotionally ill patients; and 6 percent maintained an attitude of "no preference." All the rest hoped to avoid such patients.*

Preferring Organically Ill Patients

Lacking confidence in their ability to treat emotional illnesses, most students feel ill at ease with these patients. Lack of knowledge and expertise accounts for much of their discomfort. "We've been taught just enough to know that, unless you really know the ropes, it's dangerous to deal with this type of patient," a sophomore stated. "It's easy to blunder and harm the patient." More extensive psychiatric training is needed, students feel, before this kind of problem can be tackled confidently.

Because emotional disorders are more abstract and nebulous than physical ones, clinical students complain of "never being able to grab onto anything concrete." There are "no handholds," a senior observed,

---

* When students were asked, "Would you rather deal with an organically ill or an emotionally ill patient?" the majority emphatically chose the organically ill patient (79.7 percent of the freshmen, 71.9 percent of the sophomores, 82.4 percent of the juniors, and 92.7 percent of the seniors). Those who had no preference at all (13.5 percent, freshman; 17.5 percent, sophomores; 7.0 percent, juniors; and 5.5 percent, seniors) exceeded the number who actually preferred emotionally ill patients (5.1 percent, freshmen; 8.8 percent, sophomores; 7.0 percent, juniors; and only 1.8 percent, seniors).

"no readily detectable set of symptoms all laid out." Organic problems, by comparison, are generally more clear-cut and concrete; diagnosis is much easier, since measurable test results can be obtained; and, in most cases, treatment brings quick results. When students are struggling for self-assurance in the clincial role, quick results are understandably preferred.

Emotionally ill patients rarely respond rapidly. Their treatment is often a long drawn-out process, and discernible improvement is slow. For neophyte students, this is demoralizing. Emotional disorders seem pretty hopeless. "There's very little you can do to treat them," one commented.

But avoiding patients with emotional problems is not always possible since many illnesses have an emotional overlay. So, as one senior observed, "It's like getting two for the price of one." When organic problems have an emotional component, diagnosis can be much trickier. It is difficult and time-consuming to obtain a reliable medical history when such patients "keep getting off the subject, rambling, or going back to their childhood days."

Such experiences reinforce the preference for "scientific medicine" rather than psychiatry. Although conceding that psychiatry is an interesting study, few students have a desire to explore it; and some admit a strong bias against psychiatry, which, at its present stage, they believe to be "comparable to alchemy," and against psychiatric patients, whom they term "weaker people for the most part." They find these patients depressing and nerve-racking.

Preferring Patients with Emotional Disorders

The few students who enjoy working with the emotionally disturbed find them to be a fascinating challenge. Not repelled by the complexities and practical difficulties of emotional problems, these students instead find stimulation and enjoyment. "Anyone can work with an organically sick person," a sophomore observed, "but it's more challenging with the emotionally ill. There's more personal interplay, and you have to do a lot of off-the-cuff reasoning."

So, for them, dealing with physical maladies is far less interesting and rewarding than complex emotional problems. The psychosocial aspects of illness hold a special intrigue for such psychiatrically inclined students. And, as a freshman points out, "There's just no limit to what can be done to help these people."

Acutely Ill Versus Chronically Ill Patients

Preferences for dealing with the acutely ill or chronically ill change very little during medical school. A substantial majority of incoming students (more than three-fourths of the class) prefer the acutely ill, and this preference remains constant during subsequent years of medical school. A very few students prefer chronically ill patients, and about one out of six indicates no preference for one type or the other, feeling that each type of illness presents special challenges.*

Preferring Acutely Ill Patients

In medical school it is "drilled into our heads," as one student put it, that the doctor's job is to restore the patient to health again. But with chronically ill patients, relatively little can be done toward accomplishing this goal.

Being young and action-oriented, as well as ambitious to succeed as doctors, most students naturally prefer working with patients who respond rapidly to treatment. Visible positive results provide immediate gratification for the fledgling doctor and help build self-confidence. "It does great things for my ego to see the patient change because of me," a senior acknowledged. But chronically ill patients require a long demanding period of maintenance and support. Such patients just keep coming back and back again. Those with acute illnesses, on the other hand, usually get well quickly and go home. Seeing patients improve rapidly fulfills the young clinician's need to do something for the patient.

A greater variety of problems and procedures are usually involved in dealing with acute illnesses, so they provide students with superior learning opportunities. "It's something new and different all the time," a senior said. "But with chronically ill patients, it gets boring because you're not learning anything from them."

The drama associated with acute illness also provides excitement and challenge. "It's more fun being where the action is," a junior points out. "The whole atmosphere is different." In acute cases, students sometimes get the chance to make the original diagnosis, for there are no old charts to read and no set regimen already worked out. Because the problem must be diagnosed from scratch, students can test their acquired knowledge. So, as one said, with such patients "You either flunk or pass; the patient either dies or gets better."

Because acutely ill patients expect to improve and usually do, they are typically more optimistic and grateful than the chronically ill. In the

* In response to the question, "Would you rather deal with an acutely ill patient or one who is chronically or terminally ill?" the majority of students unhesitatingly chose the acutely ill patient (76.3 percent during the freshman year, 72.0 percent during the sophomore year, 75.0 percent during the junior year, and 81.8 percent during the final year). A small percentage had no preference (18.6 percent, freshmen; 19.3 percent, sophomores; 17.9 percent, juniors, and 16.4 percent, seniors), while only a limited few actually preferred the chronically or terminally ill (1.7 percent of the freshmen, 5.3 percent of the sophomores and juniors, and 1.8 percent of the seniors).

student view, the latter sometimes become "soured—the whole world seems to be coming down on them." And, because they are also more dependent, they may require an exceptional amount of the clinician's time. They return again and again, so the doctor's patience sometimes wears thin.

All this adds up to the fact that most students find it depressing to deal with chronically ill patients. The desired feelings of elation and fulfillment that come from seeing patients progress and recover are seldom experienced with these patients. Instead there is a discouragement and futility, especially when the illness is terminal. "You try and try, but they just keep dropping off," a senior lamented. "It's like butting your head up against a wall." Even the satisfaction of prolonging life is blunted when the patient has suffered much and wishes to die. In these situations the clinician may agonize over the advisability of fighting on. As one expressed it, "It's just a crummy feeling."

Preferring Chronically or Terminally Ill Patients

The few students who prefer chronically ill patients seem to lack confidence in their ability to deal with acute situations where life hangs in the balance. For them, emergency situations like the following produce too much anxiety: "Somebody comes running in and is losing blood. You hesitate and wonder, 'Wow! What shall I do for him? He's dying!' " In such situations, of course, diagnosis and treatment cannot wait until the clinician reads up on the case. So, because they are not yet good at thinking on their feet, these students prefer chronically ill patients who do not require snap judgments that may affect their lives.

With the chronically ill, "everything is usually pretty standard," yet satisfaction can sometimes be found in prolonging the lives of these patients or in helping them feel better as they are "going out."

Talkative and Questioning Versus Quiet and Accepting Patients

Student attitudes reveal a preference for the talkative and questioning patient during the first, second, and fourth years. Indeed, only one in six students prefers the quiet and accepting patient. A temporary reversal of attitude sets in during the third year.* The relative popularity of quiet

---

* "Would you rather deal with a talkative and questioning patient or one who is quiet and accepting?" When students were asked this question each year, approximately half of them, over time, said they would prefer talkative and questioning patients (55.9 percent of the freshmen, 50.9 percent of the sophomores, 40.4 percent of the juniors, and 49.1 percent of the seniors). Those with no preference numbered 27.1 percent, freshmen; 28.0 percent, sophomores and juniors; and 32.7 percent, seniors. Those preferring the quiet and accepting numbered 13.6 percent, freshmen; 15.8 percent, sophomores; 29.8 percent, juniors; and 18.2 percent, seniors.

patients at this time is probably due to the fact that students begin full-time work on the hospital floors and, being clinically inexperienced, feel less threatened by quiet patients who are not likely to question them and force them to reveal any areas of ignorance.

Preferring Talkative and Questioning Patients

Most students agree that talkative patients are easier to diagnose than docile ones. The garrulous patient is preferred to one who just sits there saying "yes" or "no" and making the doctor drag information out of him. A patient's comments and questions may provide valuable clues as to the nature of his problem and anxieties; and this information can ultimately be of more value than a routine medical history.

Other personal benefits accrue to the student-clinician when dealing with talkative and questioning patients. For one thing, the burden of asking all the right questions is lifted when patients spontaneously volunteer information. And challenging questions also enable students to see areas where their own knowledge is deficient, so that they can take steps to fill in the gaps.

In dealing with quiet patients, however, the clinician is never quite sure how much is being understood. Good two-way communication helps the clinician determine how well instructions are grasped. When "yes" or "no" is the only comment offered, the clinician may wonder how much he or she is getting across. "After all, you can't be a mind reader," a sophomore points out.

Clinicians are sometimes uncomfortable about patients who have little to say. A senior said, "I worry about what the quiet patient is thinking. Is he quiet because he's resentful or because he's afraid? Is he a stoic who's hurting like hell but doesn't want to complain? Or is it that he just doesn't care? When he is talking and asking questions, at least you know what's going on in his mind."

One of the more taciturn students suggested that two introverts make for bad company. "I'm basically a listener rather than a talker," he said. And students at the other end of the spectrum, who love to talk, find talkative patients much more interesting and easy to "connect with."

Preferring Quiet and Accepting Patients

For those who disagree with the majority viewpoint, talkative and questioning patients seem to pose a threat, making students feel anxious and uncomfortable. Recognizing their lack of authority, these students feel uneasy in pronouncing medical opinions when queried by patients. "It really puts me in a bind when they ask a lot of questions," a junior commented; "I wouldn't mind it if I were the intern in charge of the patient, but for a med student it's different." When unable to answer a patient's questions, a student's already shaky confidence may be undermined. "When I don't know the answers, I feel inept and uncomfortable," a junior remarked, pointing up the prevalent third-year feeling. "It's just impossible to have all the facts at your fingertips."

Sometimes insecure students perceive questions as motivated by a desire to assess the clinician's competence. For instance, a third-year student said, "When they ask a lot of questions, I sense that they don't really have any trust in me as a doctor." So for these students, a docile patient who simply does what is requested without comment is much less threatening. The ideal patient, according to such a student, "listens to what you tell him to do, does it, and then says, 'thank you.' "

Patients who refrain from "flapping off at the mouth," some say, are usually more direct and to the point. They tell the doctor what is necessary, without burdening him or her with a lot of "superfluous junk." A senior commented:

I like a patient who will give you a simple "yes" or "no" answer when you ask if blood has been coughed up. Some patients have to go into a long story about what the circumstances were that day, whose birthday it was— just a whole lot of totally unrelated information.

The talkative patient forces the clinician to sort out the needed facts, making it hard to get at the root of the problem. Beginning clinicians sometimes become confused when too many facts are presented, for it is not easy to keep one's train of thought amidst constant chatter.

Because they want to be polite and pleasant, students are usually reluctant to interrupt loquacious patients. Consequently, they can lose control of the interview. One junior, for example, found herself looking at pictures of a patient's children. "Pretty soon she was running the interview," she said.

Limited time is another factor. When clinicians are hurried, as they generally are, talkative patients can be a nuisance. Gracefully extricating oneself from a patient who asks a lot of questions is an art that comes from experience.

SUMMING UP

The primary function of medical training, is, of course, to equip future health practitioners with the pertinent knowledge and technical skills necessary to help patients with their health-related problems. In medical school, potential doctors are heavily indoctrinated with the scientific principles that underlie health and illness. But when abruptly confronted with living patients, each of whom has individual problems, students learn that human maladies are not neatly classified as they are in the textbooks. The lawfulness of patterns and the uniformity of symptoms presented in classroom and laboratory settings seldom manifest this simple orderliness among live patients. Coming face-to-face with those seeking medical help, students confront many untried, untested, and unknown areas that they must deal with primarily by intuition. No matter how scientific and objective they have become about patient ills, students soon find there is no escape from the subjective aspects of patient care.

To enhance the probability of clinical success, student-physicians usually prefer certain types of patients—those who are most easily dealt with from both a medical and an interpersonal standpoint. Although variations are influenced by student background and personality, most rookie clinicians are more comfortable when dealing with adults rather than children, patients from middle-class rather than the lower-class backgrounds, the organically ill rather than the emotionally ill, and the acutely ill rather than the chronically or terminally ill. During the course of medical training, few lasting changes occur in these preferences except that, in some cases, they become even stronger.

Regardless of patient type, the greatest challenge for beginning clinicians is obtaining the patient's full trust and cooperation. But since medical students are not yet real doctors, they naturally fear that patients will not accept them or behave as desired. It is not surprising, then, that students often bluff their way through initial patient encounters by creating an impression that they already have the M.D. degree. But as they move closer to graduation and obtain greater confidence, there is less role playing and students feel freer to reveal their true status. As their experience expands, they come to expect, as do their mentors, that patient cooperation is their due. After all, the M.D. degree is nearly a reality.

Not all patients, though, conform completely to the ideal expectations, and neophyte clinicians must develop ways of dealing successsfully with this nonconforming group. Unfortunately, little formal training is offered in medical school for developing the interpersonal skills of patient management. Instead students are left pretty much on their own to work out these techniques, to discover by trial and error what works best for them. Of course, learning can and does occur through imitation and role modeling. Rarely, however, do mentors openly discuss with students their own feelings of frustration, anger, etc., which commonly occur when encountering difficult patients and stressful circumstances. It becomes amply clear to students that if they are to become like their mentors, they must be stoical about revealing personal feelings. The status structure of the academic medical center expects emotional control and rewards scientific and technical excellence.

Nonetheless, a range of attitudes does exist among faculty and house staff about problem patients, and this influences students who would emulate them. Some faculty members obviously have great breadth of interpersonal understanding and possess an impressive ability to establish rapport; others are emotionally aloof and even fail to recognize the legitimacy of psychosomatic components in illness. Fortunately, most students retain much of their initial idealism about patients, holding to the view that, no matter how irritating or troublesome, all patients should be treated with patience and kindness. However, continuous exposure to annoying individuals can easily wear thin their idealism.[9]

Clearly medical students are better trained in the science of medicine than in the art of patient care. Although much time is spent on the rote mastery of inanimate sciences, a relatively small amount of formal instruction is devoted to the interpersonal aspects of patient welfare.[10] Accordingly, professional socialization regarding patient care does little to alter common-sense assumptions about patients. The learning process primarily involves intuition, imitation, and trial and error. In other words, students must resort to feeling their way as they press forward along the clinical road to physicianhood.[11]

Such a path may incorporate, probably more often than not, a subconscious carryover from earlier, growing-up years, for medical school does not by any means mark the beginning of the socialization process of the doctor–patient relationship. Probably as far back as he or she can remember, the medical student has, from time to time, played the role of the patient and has, presumably, learned how the latter is expected to act. Thus, students come to medical school with these preconceived ideas and very likely may continue to function on the basis of premises that have come to be known as natural until they are able to adjust their responses in the light of a more mature understanding of the related process.

NOTES

1. A study of Schumacher (1968) of the opportunity for student–patient confrontation during clerkship (the presumed goal) indicated a comparatively small investment of student time in patient contact (13 percent) and a rather large investment in laboratory activities (35 percent).

2. For an analysis of how patients and hospital functionaries interpret the facts of social life in the hospital, see Coser (1962).

3. Geertsma and Stoller (1966) have also reported that impressions of ideal patient behavior are not greatly influenced by medical school training, indicating that since students have been patients themselves, they bring acquired concepts to medical school.

4. Davis (1971) has demonstrated a relationship between the quality of professional interaction between doctor and patient and the willingness

of the patient to follow the doctor's advice after leaving the consultation room.

5. For a discussion of patient noncompliance and the need for greater recognition of this important feature of medical practice, see Senior and Smith (1973).

6. For an interesting discussion of medical school conditions that promote negative attitudes among students toward "crocks" and emotionally disturbed patients, see Stoller and Geertsma (1958).

7. For an excellent discussion of the tightrope-like situation that clinicians must face in physician–patient relationships, see Merton, Reader, and Kendall (1957, pp. 74–75), where competing "pulls" are listed, such as the necessity for remaining emotionally detached while at the same time having a compassionate concern for the patient.

8. Refer to Chapter 6 for a discussion regarding the embarrassment experienced by male students when dealing with taboo areas of the female body during physical exams.

9. See Lewis and Resnik (1966) for an interesting study comparing medical and nursing students' attitudes toward patients as measured by descriptive adjectives. Medical students were found to be more negative and were primarily disease-centered and biologically oriented, whereas student nurses showed positive attitudes, were patient-oriented, and were more concerned with social factors.

10. Recently many medical schools have initiated courses on patient interviewing or have allowed underclassmen to follow at least one patient longitudinally. Such a course, "Introduction to Patient Interviewing," was initiated at the study institution the year after my study was begun. Recently a similar course has been incorporated into the curriculum of the Chicago Medical School, where students interview patients in hospitals six weeks after they enter as freshmen (*Los Angeles Times*, 1975). Judging from the *1974–75 AAMC Curriculum Directory* (1974), these courses are still a rarity, however. For a sample description of such courses, see Pollack and Manning (1967).

11. For a critical discussion of deficiencies in medical education and proposed solutions, see Engel (1971).

8. Doctors

I used to think that doctors are all Albert Schweitzer types going about helping the world. But now I realize their image is slipping: The doctor is falling off his pedestal. (A sophomore)

PHYSICIANS have a highly visible occupation. They are presented to children in primary school as community heroes. This idealized image is subsequently reinforced by romantic television dramas about doctors and news coverage of medical breakthroughs destined to improve the lot of mankind. Beyond this public view, however, exists a private domain, the realities of which may differ markedly from the stereotyped view. How are medical recruits affected when they see the inner workings of this world and become apprentice doctors? Does constant exposure behind the scenes change student views about the doctor's status and role? Such questions are addressed in this chapter.

PUBLIC IMAGE

Most freshmen, nearly 60 percent of the class, imagine the public view of the doctor to be one of general respect and admiration.* "They occupy the highest status possible," one said, citing a survey that ranks physicians "just below Supreme Court judges." When patients place their physical well-being in their doctor's hands, it is natural to want to be trusting and to hope for more than human qualities. For this reason, the public tends to regard the doctor as a "superhuman person." Or so it seems to idealistic freshmen.

By the second year, however, students' views change dramatically. Instead of perceiving the masses as generally respectful of doctors, they

---

* In the freshman year, 40.7 percent say that, generally speaking, doctors are viewed with respect; and an additional 16.9 percent, the most idealistic students, think that physicians have unqualified public admiration.

begin to see the public as critical, suspicious, and resentful. That is, they become aware of public ambivalence toward the doctor.[1] When first realizing that laymen do not always have positive feelings toward the medical profession, students are quite surprised. Illustrative of this attitude is an experience recounted by a freshman who, when working at a summer job during his premedical years, was queried by his fellow workers about his long-range career plans: "When I told them I was studying to be a doctor, I immediately began hearing about everybody's bad encounters with doctors. I didn't realize people felt that way."

During the sophomore year four times as many students as in the previous year viewed the doctor's status as declining.* "Other professions are moving up," one said, "but the medical profession is moving down; the doctor is looked upon now as just another professional, not anything special."

Reasons for the doctor's declining status are, students say, as follows:
a. High Cost of Medical Care—The most frequently cited cause of popularity decline is the allegation that doctors are increasingly charging outrageous fees, thereby earning excessive amounts and getting more than their share of the wealth.
b. Impersonal Relations with Patients—Doctors who do not make an effort to learn the names of patients, remember their faces, or interact warmly with them contribute to public alienation. Their lack of effort destroys the feelings of intimacy and trust that once characterized the doctor–patient relationship.
c. Dissatisfaction with Medical Care—Failure of the medical profession to deliver adequate health care to the entire citizenry has caused public disenchantment with the doctor. The profession has been hurt by the American Medical Association's resistance to the idea that health is a basic right of all mankind, not just a privilege for those who can afford it.
d. Malpractice Suits—Public awareness of professional incompetence has come to light with the publicity surrounding malpractice suits. Such information exposes the fallibility of the doctor.
e. Increased Layman's Knowledge—Because today's patients are more sophisticated and better informed about medical matters, the mystery surrounding medicine has diminished and the awe and veneration once enjoyed by practitioners has inevitably declined. No longer can doctors count on ignorance to safeguard them against criticism.[2]

---

* Of the sophomores, 57.9 percent indicate that the doctor is admired less than formerly; an additional 22.8 percent perceive a public attitude of suspicion and resentment. During this year only 14.0 percent think doctors are generally respected; an additional 10.5 percent still regard the public as having unqualified admiration for physicians.

Students have different reactions to such censure. Some sympathize with the public view, feeling that criticism will have a beneficial effect by "keeping the doctors on their toes." Others, however, see physicians as being overworked, imposed upon, and unfairly judged. "They expect too much from doctors," a sophomore said. "They lose sight of the fact that doctors are human, too, and need some consideration."

Following the sophomore year, there is a slight increase in optimism about the public view. One out of three now perceive public respect for the doctor. Nonetheless, most upperclassmen are generally pessimistic.* Some of the latter realize, though, that although the public may typically react negatively to the medical profession, as individuals they still look up to their own doctors, especially during times of illness. "Everybody I know gripes about money-hungry doctors," a senior commented, "but by and large people are still thankful that they have a physician they can turn to." Then he added, "When they're sick, there is nobody greater. But when they're well, look out!"

CAREER MOTIVES

The traditional stereotype of physicians as being motivated by benevolent humanitarianism has often been portrayed in the popular media. Yet, contrary to expectations, fewer freshmen attribute humanistic motives to the doctor than at any time thereafter.† Also surprising is the fact that the largest number of comments about the doctor's humanism come in the sophomore year when students become most keenly aware of negative public sentiment.

A potential explanation for these unlikely findings is that beginning students, still fresh from the screening processes of admission committees, have wearied of inquiries about benevolent motives. Even after gaining admission to medical school there is no letup from people who ask, "Why do you want to be a doctor?" "It's embarrassing," a freshman said, "to be asked to reveal your deepest thoughts and motives to just anybody." So, to cope with such motive-meddling, students often develop a standard response, giving, as they put it, a "bunch of hogwash about wanting to save the world."

---

* In the senior year, for example, 29.1 percent say the doctor is viewed with general respect and an additional 5.5 percent think this respect is actually uncritical admiration. However, 32.7 percent say the doctor is regarded with less respect than formerly and an equal number (32.7 percent) think doctors are regarded with suspicion and resentment.

† When asked, "What motives attract people to careers in medicine?" only 28.1 percent of the freshmen mentioned humanitarian motives. This compares to 59.6 percent during the sophomore year. The junior and senior year percentages are 42.1 and 43.6, respectively.

That more humanitarianism exists among doctors than meets the eye is made clear from the comments of a female student about her male colleagues. "A lot of people," she said, "especially men, have tender feelings of benevolence, but they don't want you to know it; they think it's just not masculine." Since "the humanistic business" is embarrassing and has been so thoroughly overworked, many freshmen cannot bring themselves to describe doctors in this way.

By the time they become sophomores, however, students' idealism surfaces—undoubtedly in defense of the clinician who seems under critical attack, not only from the public but also from basic-science professors. Whereas only 28 percent of the freshman class describe doctors as being primarily motivated by humanistic concerns, 60 percent of the sophomores do so. After two years of being saturated with basic-science classwork, students yearn to get into clinical medicine. This no doubt contributes to an idealizing of the physician's role. In subsequent years, however, as students gain daily contact with clinicians, their descriptions of doctors are somewhat less generous, and comments about benevolent motives drop from the sophomore peak.

While benevolence probably plays an important role among most doctors, the actual motives for being in the medical profession are elusive. It is not easy for students to fully identify their own motives, much less recognize and understand those of others. Most students agree, though, that rarely does a single motive dominate. For most doctors it consists, students say, of "a whole collection of things."* Doctors are attracted to the field, as are careerists in any line of work, by assessing the basic rewards and liabilities of such a career.

REWARDS AND LIABILITIES

Understandably, the rewarding aspects of medical practice are much more apparent to medical recruits than are the negative features. Most students talk at length about the attractive features of the profession but have little to say about the undesirable ones. In fact, one out of six freshmen failed to perceive even one negative aspect.

* Other motives mentioned in response to my question regarding doctors' careers are: (a) satisfying work (38.6 percent of freshmen, 50.9 percent of sophomores, 43.9 percent of juniors, and 54.5 percent of seniors); (b) financial rewards (40.4 percent of freshmen, 49.1 percent of sophomores, 47.4 percent of juniors, and 47.3 percent of seniors); (c) status and prestige (29.8 percent of freshmen, 33.3 percent during both sophomore and junior years, and 34.5 percent of seniors); (d) interpersonal rewards (17.5 percent of freshmen, 8.8 percent of sophomores, 14.0 percent of juniors, and 14.5 percent of seniors); and (e) gratified emotional needs (7.0 percent of freshmen, 1.8 percent of sophomores, 12.3 percent of juniors, and 12.7 percent of seniors). (See also Table 11–1 concerning career motives.)

Rewards

At all stages of training, medical practice is seen as an interesting and challenging career that offers ample ego rewards and an opportunity to work with people in a most important way.

Interacting with People

Person-to-person contact in one's own work is regarded by students at all stages of training as the most desirable benefit of a medical career. During the freshman, sophomore, and junior years, two-thirds of the class mention the desirable aspect of working closely with people; but the percentage drops to 40 percent in the final year.*

Initially, student altruism evolves around "serving mankind," although, as mentioned, students are often reluctant to discuss their humanistic feelings. "The last thing I tell people is that I want to help people," a freshman admitted. "That sounds too melodramatic. But that is what I want to do; that *is* my reward."

But as students advance through school they learn that patients, too, have something to give. So during the clinical years some students acknowledge that in meeting the needs of others they are also satisfying their own needs. In other words, as they become conscious of the importance of personal gratification, their earlier idealistic altruism shows signs of being tempered with self-interest. "When I first came to medical school," one junior commented, "I used to think it would be great to help people, but now I'm not so sure—I'm leaning more toward my own interests." Nonetheless, even for fourth-year students, the opportunity to work closely with people remains a major factor.

Feelings of Accomplishment

Although recognizing that other occupations may offer prestige and related rewards, students bask in the knowledge that doctors are engaged in worthwhile activities that no other profession can perform. This perception contributes to a feeling that physicians are indispensable. The keen sense of worthwhile accomplishment inherent in the medical profession, of being engaged in "providing services that can't be bought on the market anyplace else," comes to a peak during the third year when students have left the classroom for their clinical clerkships. At this time one-half of the class express pride in the profession's involvement in

---

* When asked, "What are the most rewarding aspects of a medical career?" 62.7 percent of freshmen, 70.2 percent of sophomores, 64.9 percent of juniors, and 40.0 percent of seniors mentioned the opportunity to interact with people.

something of unmistakable value:* "It's exhilarating to play a major role in doing something that's important for mankind. Giving a person health and life is just about the greatest thing you can do."

Interesting, Challenging Work

Because medical practice is stimulating, exciting, and challenging, there is little possibility of boredom or loss of interest. Doctors see a variety of people with a wide range of problems. "Every patient is a separate case," a junior points out. "Even if the person in the next bed has the same disease it has different implications for each patient."

Moreover, the intellectual demands of medicine require constant learning and testing of one's mettle. "It isn't like some careers where you learn it all and then sit back and take it easy," one said. There is little possibility of stagnation when one is constantly confronted with problem-solving situations involving the complexities of the human body. A continual intellectual challenge and a need to apply one's knowledge in an artistic fashion keep the practitioner constantly alert." †

Independence and Responsibility

Medical trainees enjoy the thought of being self-employed and determining the conditions of their own work. After being under the thumb of supervisors so long, student doctors, especially seniors, look upon freedom from restraint as a significant benefit offered by a medical career.‡ There is no time card to punch and no boss to direct the work in private practice. One can be his or her own boss.

Parenthetically, it should be noted that when entering freshmen are asked to rank a list of seven possible motives for selecting medicine as a career, independence is ranked fifth in importance. But as students progress through school, the value of independence increases in importance until at the end of the senior year it becomes first priority. (Refer to Table 11–1.)

Having had little opportunity in school or part-time jobs to exercise control without someone standing over them and telling them what to do, medical students relish the future opportunity to become independent and

---

* A feeling of worthwhile accomplishment is considered rewarding by 22.0 percent of the freshmen, 19.3 percent of the sophomores, 50.9 percent of the juniors, and 27.3 percent of the seniors.

† Work that is interesting and challenging is seen as a reward by 23.7 percent of the freshmen, 24.6 percent of the sophomores, 31.6 percent of the juniors, and 18.2 percent of the seniors.

‡ Having the independence and responsibility of being one's own boss is not as important during the first three years (freshmen, 13.6 percent; sophomores, 17.5 percent; and juniors, 12.3 percent), but increases in value during the last year (seniors, 34.5 percent).

assume full clinical responsibility. "Right now it's a little scary," one admitted, "but if handled well, responsibility can be the greatest thing in the world."

Income, Status, and Prestige

Mention of income and financial security as career advantages remains low throughout medical school, varying between 8 and 14 percent.* Bald references to the size of the doctor's income seem to cause embarrassment when one's own motives are discussed. The same is also true when discussing status and prestige. Rarely are they mentioned separately or emphasized; instead these rewards are referred to in a passing way without elaboration.†

But when describing doctors' motives in general, rather than their own, students are much more willing to mention status and pecuniary considerations.‡ During each year of school nearly half the class mention financial inducements as motives for going into medicine. A medical career offers a good living and the possibility of enjoying a comfortable life. As one freshman wryly observed, "I've never seen a doctor starve to death."

Liabilities

The sparsity and brevity of student comments about the disadvantages of medical practice indicate that relatively little thought is given to this subject. At least, students do not express much concern about the negative aspects of the profession.

Demanding Nature of Work

Most frequently mentioned as a liability are the long hours of a doctor's work. This drawback is noted by more than half of the freshmen, increasing to three-fourths of the class by the senior year.§ The demands on a doctor's time "can eat up your entire life," one said. Since people do not always get sick at convenient times, doctors are on "command performance" 24 hours a day, and students do not relish this prospect. Fourth-

---

* Few students mention the physician's substantial income as a major personal reward: freshmen, 8.5 percent; sophomores, 10.5 percent; juniors, 8.8 percent; and seniors, 14.5 percent.

† Status and prestige rank about the same as income as a personal incentive: freshmen, 8.5 percent; sophomores, 8.8 percent; juniors, 15.8 percent; and seniors, 7.3 percent.

‡ See note on page 169 for statistics regarding perceived financial and status motives among doctors in general.

§ The demanding nature of the work and the long hours of the physician are named as by far the greatest liabilities by 54.2 percent of the freshmen, 68.4 percent of the sophomores, 64.9 percent of the juniors, and 74.5 percent of the seniors.

year students are particularly vocal in expressing annoyance over calls that occur in the middle of the night, especially when they are for trivial matters. As one said, "This will require some getting used to." [3]

Some concern is also expressed about the hectic pace and the constant pressure resulting from emergency situations. The possibility of failing the patient, making a fatal mistake, is a terrible prospect that places strain and fatigue on the doctor. "We've been told that we will kill somebody before we get through," one shuddered.

The endless detail involved in running the business end of medical practice is another area presenting constant demands on the physician's time. Although clinical students are given only a small taste of paperwork, they learn early that the multiplicity of insurance claims, legal documents, medical forms, and birth and death certificates required by governmental agencies and insurance companies, aside from being a nuisance, takes them away from more urgent matters; and they object to being "bogged down" in this way. They also consider the more routine aspects of clinical work, such as lab work, cleaning up, starting intravenous infusions, and other jobs that can be done efficiently by technicians to be "scut work" or "dirty work."

Intrusions on Personal Life

A disagreeable feature of practicing medicine is the intrusion of work on personal life. Freshmen are most sensitive to this area, since they are stunned by the demands that heavy workloads make on their time. Nearly a third of them complain about the inroads that a medical career makes on the doctor's private life.* "If you give 100 percent to medicine," one said, "you can't give much more to anything else."

The irregularity and unpredictability of doctors' long hours minimize opportunities for leisure. A junior stated, "Opportunities can come when you have a day off and can get out of town, but you'll never know about it very far in advance." Something like an influenza epidemic can always interfere with a vacation. As important as medical practice is, students also recognize the need for some free time for themselves and their families.

Problem Patients

Working with certain types of patients is sometimes seen as an unpleasant aspect of medical practice.† Some students, for example, hope to

---

* Those considering intrusion in one's personal life as a major liability of being a physician include: freshmen, 30.5 percent; sophomores, 14.0 percent; juniors, 19.3 percent; and seniors, 16.4 percent.

† Only a few students believe that problem patients are a drawback in medical practice: freshmen, 6.8 percent; sophomores and juniors, both 14.0 percent; and seniors, 5.5 percent.

avoid terminally ill patients so they can be spared watching these helpless people suffer. Others worry about having to deal with the families of such patients: "I'm sure I will never get used to telling the families that a case is terminal," one said.

Certain behaviors and attitudes of patients also irk students. Most annoying are uncooperative patients who will not follow the prescribed regimen, unappreciative or ungrateful patients, and inconsiderate ones who make unnecessary demands at inconvenient times. Nonetheless, students take such patients in stride and do not fret over these negative concerns, for they are greatly outweighed by the benefits offered by a medical career.

"GOOD" AND "BAD" DOCTORS

Even before entering medical school, students have had considerable exposure to physicians, in real life as patients and over the air waves and in print as recipients of the mass media. Almost without exception, students and their families as well have preconceived ideas as to the characteristics of a successful physician. So freshmen have little difficulty describing the qualities of both good and bad doctors; and their views change very little while progressing through school. Naturally, they all hope to become good doctors, and it is with this ideal in mind that they express views about the various qualities that distinguish good and bad physicians.[4]

Technical Competence

Most freshmen regard competence as an essential trait of a good doctor, and in later years an even larger number hold this view.* Rarely, however, is competence mentioned as the only quality of a good physician; for although an unquestioned prerequisite for success, it must be accompanied by other qualities if a doctor is to be effective. Nonetheless, without basic technical competence, all other qualities are like the "frosting without the cake."

Each year more than one-third of the class define a bad doctor as one who is technically incompetent, one who is incapable of administering good medical care. No matter how compassionate or how noble motives

---

* A good doctor is described as technically competent by 54.2 percent of the freshmen, 59.6 percent of the sophomores, 70.7 percent of the juniors, and 61.8 percent of the seniors. Technical incompetence is seen as characteristic of bad doctors by 50.0 percent of the freshmen, 36.8 percent of the sophomores, 46.6 percent of the juniors, and 52.7 percent of the seniors.

may be, the doctor is not a good one unless symptoms can be skillfully recognized and correctly diagnosed.

In addition to diagnostic ability, a good doctor must also have the necessary skills to perform competently. A surgeon, for example, must be skillful as well as knowledgeable about surgical procedures or the patient is in trouble. A doctor must continually refine his or her knowledge and skills by keeping abreast of new developments. Those who are rigidly set in their ways, who have a set routine or approach to handle every person who comes in, are viewed as lazy and lacking in dedication.

Being careful and meticulous are also characteristic of the good doctor. One who measures up in these respects gives attention to every detail, asks significant questions, and performs complete examinations. The "sloppy doctor," on the other hand, is considered negligent or careless in work performance. Haphazard in approach, this doctor says, "It looks like a case of such and such and proceeds on that assumption, promptly ruling out other possible diseases."

Technically competent doctors realize and acknowledge their own limitations of knowledge or skill. This observation, foreign to freshmen, is increasingly brought out as students progress through school. As an upperclassman remarked, "The bad doctor may not have tumbled to the fact that the approach is wrong." But blindness is more often due to complacency and intellectual conceit than to dull-wittedness. "The bad doctor," a junior remarked, "is just cocksure, knows all the answers, won't listen to anyone else, and is unwilling to admit the possibility of being wrong or making mistakes."

At just what point do such doctors enter the never-never land of "quackdom," where professional status and respect are denied and where the healing arts, effective or not, must be practiced on the outer fringes of respectability? During each year, more than a third of the class define a quack as "an incompetent," a person "who is dealing with problems without knowing how to handle them" or one "who doesn't know what to do." * Although students may single out non-M.D.s as quacks, a licensed physician can also be a quack if poor techniques are practiced, for such lack of technical know-how leads to wrong diagnoses and ineffective treatment. Quacks, whether licensed in a pseudo-medical service or not, are seen as being more interested in relieving patients of their money than their ailments. "They are out for a fast buck," said one student.

* By far the most prevalent description of a "quack" is incompetency, according to 48.3 percent of the freshmen, 43.9 percent of the sophomores, 41.4 percent of the juniors, and 36.4 percent of the seniors. Quacks are also viewed as unauthorized practitioners (freshmen, 36.2 percent; sophomores, 22.8 percent; juniors, 27.6 percent; and seniors, 40.0 percent), and as unprincipled practitioners (freshmen, 19.0 percent; sophomores, 24.6 percent; juniors, 27.6 percent; and seniors, 16.4 percent). Only a small number of students define "quacks" as "chiropractors and other non-M.D.s": freshmen, 10.3 percent; sophomores, 15.8 percent; juniors, 12.1 percent; and seniors, 12.7 percent.

Relationships with Patients

Although a doctor must obviously be competent to practice medicine successfully, this is of little value unless patients are dealt with effectively. What good is an abundance of technical ability if the patient's cooperation is not elicited? Each year more than 60 percent of the class say that interpersonal skills are essential to being a successful doctor;* in fact, these qualities are mentioned more often than technical competence. More than any other skill, students say, the ability to handle patients stratifies doctors in terms of clinical effectiveness.

Varying opinions exist as to what constitutes a good patient relationship and what qualities are needed to achieve it. Some picture a benign figure who is kind, sympathetic, courteous, patient, and tolerant, one who relates to patients simply as one person to another and never lords it over them. A contrasting view is the aloof doctor who relates to patients in a gentle but firm and forceful manner so that respect is not lost by becoming too friendly with them.

More consensus exists, however, about other interpersonal traits, such as taking a personal interest in patients and showing concern for their problems. A successful doctor sees the person, not just the patient, and is sensitive not only to the patient's complaints but to his total needs: "Rather than treating a liver," one said, "the doctor treats a person with liver disease." Thus, the overall picture is considered—the patient's total lifestyle and the particulars of his economic, family, and social situations.

To be a truly great doctor requires a concern for the patient's needs and an empathy for personal feelings and anxieties. "While the patient is with you," a senior remarked, "you must show that you care and that he or she is a very important person to you." Anyone lacking this fundamental quality cannot be considered a good doctor, for knowledge and technical competence are no substitute for concern. To put it succinctly, proficiency in one's craft is not sufficient; there must also be concern for patients.†

A successful doctor is also ethical and honorable, offering thorough and conscientious care to all patients regardless of their station in life. This kind of physician never takes advantage of another simply because of that person's dependence. And good doctors retain humility and a sense of hu-

---

* Maintaining good relationships with patients is seen as the most important characteristic of a good doctor by 61.0 percent of the freshmen, 68.4 percent of the sophomores, 72.4 percent of the juniors, and 61.8 percent of the seniors. Conversely, poor relationships with patients contribute to bad doctoring according to 20.7 percent of the freshmen, 12.3 percent of the sophomores, 31.0 percent of the juniors, and 23.6 percent of the seniors.

† Lack of concern for patients is singled out as typical of the bad doctor by 56.9 percent of the freshmen, 70.2 percent of the sophomores, 53.4 percent of the juniors, and 61.8 percent of the seniors.

manity, always remembering that they are not almighty beings, nor are they supposed to be. Instead of acting like "the big muckamuck," a good doctor communicates with patients in such a way that they do not feel they are being talked down to. Such a physician is friendly and pleasant with all types and can "talk with a garbage man as easily as with another professional."

Inability to communicate effectively with patients labels doctors as inept. For example, an inarticulate doctor may be disquieting to a patient; if he or she is silent all the time, the patient may have lots of questions unanswered and may leave the doctor's office with them still unanswered. In reverse, a doctor can talk too much. A junior reported that, while on ward rounds, an attending physician discussed a patient's condition as though the patient were not present:

> This doctor walked right up to the patient and asked another doctor, "Are you sure this is a stroke? Have you ruled out a brain tumor? Do you think it will recur again more severely?" No respect at all was shown for the patient's feelings.

Such doctors, being insensitive, increase patient fears. To allay patients' anxieties, a good doctor must tune in to their feelings and reactions, but also must let them know what is being done and why.

So, throughout all four years, there is a tendency to define a good doctor as "just being a good person," that is, one who has "qualities of the heart"—not an egotistical-type person who is cold and unfriendly. The good doctor has warmth and humility. Having a social conscience, such physicians are concerned about humanity in general.

Management of Time and Money

Good doctors are also distinguished by their attitudes and values relating to those precious commodities: time and money. One characteristic of the good doctor is a willingness to spend adequate time with each patient. "The overly busy doctor can't be a good doctor," one student said, "because patients' emotional needs can't possibly be met when a doctor is hurried." Developing rapport and gaining an understanding of their problems require adequate time. So, as another expressed it, "physicians who find ways of spending a little more time with patients are the ones who become really successful."

Students condemn the doctor who seems more interested in the number of patients who can be seen rather than those who can be helped, who runs an office like a factory—the larger the output, the larger the financial return. Such doctors will not give more than the allotted time to any patient because the cash register will not ring as often. "Patients are just run through and separated from their money," one student stated, "with no worry wasted on them."

Of course there are also potentially good doctors who, due to patient demand, become overextended.

> I know a doctor who is really a decent guy, but he has brought such a heavy case load on himself that he hardly sees patients except when they're on the operating table. I think he's a good technical man, but not a very good physician.

Doctors who do a "nine-to-five job" are also considered bad doctors. "They can hardly wait to get out of the office and go home," one said. The involvement of this kind of doctor consists of worrying whether the patient's chronic appendicitis will recur at about the fifteenth hole." Even if there is a real emergency, there is an unwillingness to make house calls and the response to late phone calls is, at best, grudging. For such a physician, medical practice is just a job, not a calling. "Patients are just walking illnesses that can be given a few pills and charged a fee."

The good doctor takes time and effort to explain what is being done and why. "After all," a senior stated, "it is the patient's body. Information should be given freely on anything affecting it." Even when a diagnosis is unclear, students say, it is better for the doctor to be truthful about the patient's condition.

In short, the good doctor does not evade answering the patient's questions; it is better to say, "We don't know yet." This opinion is formed through observing situations like this:

> We have a patient right now who's been in the hospital for several weeks or longer and no one knows what's wrong with him. He keeps asking, "What have you found? What do you know?" but the doctors just avoid answering him. He's getting so depressed that they're thinking of giving him some mood-elevating drugs to pep him up. I feel they ought to tell him the truth—"We're still running tests to find out." A doctor is human and shouldn't pretend to know everything. It takes real courage to admit that one is stumped.

The good doctor is also sensitive to patients' financial capabilities and does not initiate tests and procedures without making sure patients understand what is happening and can afford them. Such a doctor avoids running up excessively high bills for the patient.

Unprincipled practitioners are also viewed as deliberately preying on the citizens of the community, especially those who are ignorant or desperately ill. "It is a big psychological racket," a student observed. "They play on people's emotions and promise cures when little can be done in a medical way. They knowingly take advantage of the 'susceptible ones' and deliberately hoodwink the public."

Unlike the quack, good doctors refer patients with problems beyond their competence to other physicians. The unethical practitioner will not refer a case because of fear of losing it and the monetary gain as well. Or such a doctor can hold patients back so that colleagues will not recognize his or her inability to handle certain cases.

Admittedly, some doctors are preoccupied with money and prestige, and this type of doctor is denounced by some students. They see this approach to medicine purely as a business proposition to make money: "They're in it for what they can get out of it and don't really give a damn about what happens to the patients."

It is interesting to note, however, that in the senior year not a single student censured the money-grabbing and prestige-seeking doctor, whereas up to one-fourth of the class had done so earlier.* This change may indicate that clinical students have become more personally concerned about money, hence show reluctance to criticize doctors who evidence interest in the financial aspects of medicine. It would be a mistake, however, to interpret this as meaning that students are greedy. When considering the number of years spent in school at tremendous cost, it is not surprising they are concerned with financial matters. Clearly, their idealism regarding the patient's welfare is not lost. By contrast, entering freshmen seem naive about money, and only as they approach graduation do they assume a more realistic view toward monetary affairs. This shift may account for their reluctance to label as "bad doctors" those practitioners who are noticeably concerned about money.

Nonetheless, a large number of students still perceive the good doctor to be dedicated in sacrificing time and money and personal conveniences in order to resolve patients' problems. From two-fifths to one-half of the class describe such doctors as service-oriented, "putting their patients first." And this altruistic outlook remains high—held by half the class—even in the senior year.†

SUMMING UP

There is little uncertainty in the minds of entering medical students about the doctor's status and role. Since infancy they have been regularly exposed to doctors, and these personal experiences, spanning the entire length of their lives, have promoted clear ideas about the profession, concepts that are widely diffused throughout American society.

---

* A bad doctor is seen as overly concerned with money and prestige by a few students during the first three years (freshmen, 12.1 percent; sophomores, 24.6 percent; and juniors, 8.6 percent), but not by any during the final year of medical school.

† A good doctor is viewed as service-oriented and dedicated to patients' welfare by 39.0 percent of the freshmen, 49.1 percent of the sophomores, 41.4 percent of the juniors, and 49.1 percent of the seniors.

With these concepts so well imbued before training is launched, it is not surprising that student views about doctors change so little during the sojourn in medical school. Seniors define the characteristics of good and bad doctors essentially the same as they do as freshmen. At all stages of training, good doctors are described as being technically competent, dedicated to their patients' welfare, and maintaining good relationships with them. By contrast, bad ones are viewed as lacking technical competence, having little concern for patients, maintaining poor relationships with them, and being overly concerned with money and prestige.

The only qualification to this no-change generalization is that seniors are less likely to define bad doctors as being unduly interested in money and prestige. This, no doubt, reflects a growing awareness of their own financial needs. After all, they have struggled long and hard to reach graduation, and the prospect of finally earning a little money and achieving some recognition is a happy thought indeed.

Similarly, few changes occur in the way students perceive the rewards and liabilities offered by a medical career. And, through all four years of medical training, they see the rewards as clearly outnumbering the liabilities. The former include: (a) a chance to interact with people, (b) feelings of personal accomplishment, (c) interesting and challenging work, (d) opportunities for independence and responsibility, (e) sizable financial income, and (f) considerable status and prestige. The only perceived liabilities are: (a) demanding work, (b) potential intrusion of work into personal life, and (c) problem patients.

Nor do students' views change regarding the motives that attract individuals to medical careers. Seniors, in about the same proportion as freshmen, describe these motives as satisfying work, generous income, status and prestige, interpersonal rewards, and gratified emotional needs.

Humanitarianism, another motive, is minimized by freshmen, whereas a year later it is emphasized. This change is probably due to the fatigue that incoming students experience after being queried so frequently about their own humanism. Following application interviews, such commentary sounds trite and corny. But idealism surfaces again in the second year when students are most aware of criticism about the medical profession. Other than these limited shifting views, however, it is striking how few attitudes change throughout medical training regarding the doctor's status and role.

NOTES

1. In their essay entitled "Sociological Ambivalence," Merton and Barber (1976) provide a theoretical framework for understanding how the medical profession, like other professions, can be an object of ambivalence (i.e., of

praise and all manner of positive feelings and yet also of censure and all manner of negative responses).

2. See Wax (1962) for an interesting interpretation concerning the disenchantment that the public has with the medical profession.

3. Of course, night calls for trivial matters are pretty much screened out these days by telephone answering services. Also, doctors in individual practice usually band together, having one of them "on call" during night hours and holidays, thus banishing the 24-hour duty of old times. In addition, few doctors allow their home telephones to be listed.

4. For a discussion on success in medical practice and a review of research on this topic, see the article by Carl M. Cochrane (1971).

9. Medical Specialties

When I came to med school I had a pretty clear idea about which specialty I would choose. But as I've rotated through the different services, I've changed my mind about ten times. For one thing, all the specialists try to court you into their own line of work. What makes a specialty look good or bad is the people in it; their personalities really sway you. (A senior)

THE SELECTION OF A MEDICAL SPECIALTY is, of course, a momentous decision, for it sets the future course of one's career. No decision since the original plan to study medicine has such potential for influencing the doctor's future. In its personal impact, this choice is akin to selecting a marital companion; both can profoundly affect the course of one's life.

How do medical students, all of whom share similar courses and educational experiences, come to decide on divergent specialties? What factors influence that final choice? This chapter addresses these questions and provides, as well, a developmental perspective of students' views of various specialists.[1]

HOW A MEDICAL SPECIALTY IS SELECTED

For nearly a third of the class, the preference for a specific branch of medicine had been crystal clear from the outset; each of these individuals is now practicing in an area of medicine initially preferred upon entering medical school. One said, "I wanted to be a psychiatrist before I wanted to be a doctor. Medical school was only the means to an end."

For many students, however, the choice of a specialty is a more gradual process that is not resolved until the final year of medical school (21 percent of the class) or until their internship (23 percent).* Although orig-

---

* To obtain information on specialty choices, I asked the following question each year: "If you were to select a branch of medicine now, which would it be?" If a student's

inally having definite ideas about a preferred specialty, they frequently change their minds as they progress through school.[2]

Eventually, 28 percent of the class became surgeons (19 percent general surgeons, 5 percent ophthalmologists, and 4 percent otolaryngologists), and 22 percent specialized in internal medicine. The next most popular fields were pediatrics and family practice, each selected by 7 percent of the students. Obstetrics/gynecology, psychiatry, radiology, and general practice each became the choice of 5 percent of the class. Three percent chose anesthesiology; in addition, pathology, neurology, and dermatology were each selected by 2 percent of the class.*

The decision process varied somewhat among students. For some, like one senior, it consisted primarily in "taking a good look at myself, analyzing my talents and skills, and then funneling these into the most appropriate field." Others, however, placed less emphasis on rational decision-making, believing simply that "you'll know it when you get to the thing you are really good at and like." Among such students, it is a gradual settling in: "You just play it by ear until you stumble into an area you enjoy. You kind of feel your way until something clicks; you find yourself more comfortable, enjoying the work and the people—and off you go."

The choice of a specialty is usually a complex process. Students seeking the one that will best fit them for the rest of their lives must weigh some hard practicalities and balance them against the intangible qualities they also want from the world. They are likely to settle on one, only to change their minds perhaps several times as they go through the various clerkships. The decision will be influenced by countless factors and, although impressive numbers of students make their selection each year, the pathway to that choice is indeed unique for each individual. Some of the many forks in the road are now examined.

Process of Elimination

Career decisions can be influenced by repelling forces as well as attracting ones.[3] "Certain specialties just sort of turn you off," a senior remarked, "so you narrow down the range of possibilities by eliminating these fields. They're so dry they turn you off immediately and you can't remember any of that stuff."

response remains the same in subsequent years and matches his or her final choice, the decision is considered as having been made at the time the response was first given. Results indicate that decisions were made by 31.0 percent of the freshmen, 8.6 percent of the sophomores, 10.3 percent of the juniors, 20.7 percent of the seniors, and 22.5 percent of the interns.

* The information regarding eventual specialty choices was obtained by writing the subjects after they left medical school and were about to begin their residency training. At that time, 1.7 percent were still undecided, and the clinical practices chosen by 5.2 percent of the class who did not respond are not known.

The prerequisites for entering a particular specialty may be repugnant. For example, one aesthetically inclined student who had considered a career in plastic surgery where he could utilize his artistic talents had to change his mind when he realized that he could not stand four years of the prerequisite residency in surgery. He finally ended up in psychiatry, a seemingly unrelated field.

Areas of medicine in which students feel incompetent or uncomfortable are, of course, sooner or later dropped from consideration. For instance, neurosurgery was eliminated by one student who realized: "I just don't have the hands for it; surgery is not the specialty for a person who requires three hands to tie a knot."

Forces That Attract

Specialties having most appeal are those that provide intrinsic satisfactions and utilize personal abilities. Those that meet the first criterion, as one said, "just automatically interest you and lead you to think, 'This is for me!'" There is a natural tendency to gravitate to fields that hold the most interest, to "the one that you go back to when you are off duty." Those who enjoy children, for example, automatically lean toward pediatrics.

Personal aptitude and ability, the second criterion, are also prevailing factors. After being weighed down by the overwhelming amount of information to be learned, it is satisfying to find a specialty area that is compatible with personal aptitude and skills. For example, one said, "Right now I'm attracted to urology because I understand the anatomy of that area best. I also like general surgery because the area is large enough for me to feel confident; it's not like surgery of the eye."

Types of Patients and Interpersonal Relationships

Students having a strong preference for certain types of patients (as discussed in Chapter 7) are naturally attracted to certain specialties. Psychiatry, for example, has little appeal for those who dislike "crocks," just as obstetrics and gynecology offer no attraction for male students who feel uncomfortable with women.

The length of time required to deal with patients is another factor—whether the relationship is long-term and psychologically intimate or brief and impersonal. "You have to choose something that fits you best," one said. "If you like to get in quickly, get instant results, and then have the patient go home, then surgery is your bag. But if you like to listen to people rehearse their problems for hours on end, then psychiatry is your thing. Everybody has a personality for a certain area."

Those who feel uncomfortable with patients of any kind can settle into research or laboratory-oriented specialties. By contrast, those who enjoy a variety of patients can choose a field such as family practice. "That's why I want to go into ENT," one said. "It offers a broad spectrum of patients—all types."

Influential People and Experiences

Rotation through the various clinical services of the hospital provides an opportunity to size up each area. "You see firsthand the good and bad points of each," one said. "It really opens up a lot of doors and helps you find out what you like best." And, as pointed out at the beginning of this chapter, the attending and resident staff of a particular service significantly influence student opinions.[4] "The personality of a good resident or staff person can really influence you," one said. "That alone can make the specialty look good." So, the most appealing clinical services are those where the house staff takes a special interest in students, explains a lot, gives clinical responsibilities, and treats them well. "When staff members go out of their way to make you feel part of the team, you naturally like that area," a student remarked.

The overall status of the clinical department is also influential.[5] Certain specialties have a reputation because the faculty is outstanding; so there is a general tendency to be inclined toward these fields.

Externships in other clinical settings or the summer jobs at the hospital also influence choice of specialty. "I've been surprised how many people who had summer jobs in hematology, radiology, or the like, now want to go into these areas," a junior commented. "It's the first thing they've been exposed to, and they want to stay in it." Such opportunities offer in-depth exposure to a particular branch of medicine and make students feel part of the clinical team. The personalized association with these specialists also fosters loyalties and enhances identification.

Practical Considerations

Increasing awareness of the practical advantages offered by specific specialties also influences choice. Questions such as the following are considered:

How much money and prestige are there in this specialty?
How hard must I work for how many hours per day?

What type of work schedule is involved?
Are there night calls?
Is there time for family and personal life?
How long is the residency training?

Such considerations are evaluated in terms of personal needs and preferences. For some, fatigue is a factor; for others, pride. "By the time you
have finished ten years of training," one said, "you're fed up with being
everybody else's lackey." Disruption of family life can also be a consideration. "Night calls never bothered me before," a recently married student
pointed out, "but they do now that I'm going to have a family."

In summary, then, a variety of factors interact to shape specialty preferences. As students progress through their training, they eliminate some
specialties while considering others as distinct possibilities. Eventually each
clinician reaches a decision that constitutes a commitment to a particular
type of medical practice.

PERSONALITIES AND SPECIALTIES

Laymen usually view doctors as being essentially alike, regardless of the
specialty, and often attribute to them noble qualities of personality and
motivation. Medical practitioners, however, rarely if ever possess these romantic opinions and, in fact, are often sharply critical of one another.
Within the medical profession, unseen by the outsider, a differentiated and
fiercely competitive world exists.

When asked to describe the types attracted to different specialties,
freshmen usually reply as laymen do, expressing idealistic appraisals or uncertainty. Upon gaining greater exposure to the inner world of medicine,
however, student judgments, like those of their mentors, become more
critically delineated.

Views of the various personality types drawn into the different branches
of medicine increasingly reveal definitive appraisals.[6] My procedure was to
ask each year, "What type of person is attracted to general practice?" and
then to repeat this question for each of the following specialties: internal
medicine, surgery, obstetrics/gynecology, pediatrics, psychiatry, pathology,
radiology, neurology, dermatology, and anesthesiology.

General Practitioner

The lack of hesitancy with which freshmen describe the general practitioner (G.P.) suggests previous contact with this type of physician. Only

8 percent of the freshmen said, "I don't know," when asked to describe the G.P., fewer than any other specialty.*

Initially, the general practitioner is seen as a "small-town doctor, somewhat backward and slow moving, the antithesis of the big-city specialist—not at all flashy." In the freshman view, the G.P. is a remnant of the old-time country doctor who "runs around in a buggy during freezing weather helping people." As such, he or she is also seen as compassionate, altruistic, and dedicated, a "basically humanitarian person who is one hundred percent devoted to helping people." Having a missionary-type personality, such doctors are "willing to sacrifice for the patients' benefit." †

Adjectives used by freshmen to describe the G.P. include: friendly, congenial, outgoing, warmhearted, genuine, companionable, generous, good-natured, and happy. In short, this doctor is viewed as being a pleasant person, one who gets along well with others.‡

Nonetheless, at the time of my study, there was an initial tendency to view such physicians as being less bright or not as ambitious as other doctors. This opinion was, no doubt, due to the fact that G.P.s did not complete the three-to-five-year residency training required for becoming a board-certified specialist. However, there is no longer a factual basis for that opinion, as there are now an American Board of Family Medicine and a three-year residency program in some 250 places around the country. But even at the time of my research, such early deprecating views were often replaced with awe when students, struggling to master the basic-science materials, realized the wide variety of clinical problems with which the general practitioner must deal. Despite this impressive clinical mastery, though, some still retained their initial view of the G.P. as an "academically unexceptional person." Among such students, the G.P. was thought to have "a lot of guts to step out into scary situations with such limited training." §

* "Don't know" responses are given by 8.5 percent of the freshmen, 3.5 percent of the sophomores, 3.4 percent of the juniors, and 7.3 percent of the seniors.

† More freshmen (23.7 percent) perceive the G.P. as being service-oriented than possessing any other single characteristic; this trend continues, almost but not quite exclusively, for the remaining three years (sophomores, 26.3 percent; juniors, 25.9 percent; and seniors, 29.1 percent). Many students, however, emphasize the personal benefits of general practice: freshmen, 20.3 percent; sophomores, 17.5 percent; juniors, 22.4 percent; and seniors, 16.4 percent.

‡ The general practitioner is described as pleasant and sociable by 18.6 percent of the freshmen, 24.6 percent of the sophomores, 13.8 percent of the juniors, and 18.2 percent of the seniors.

§ In the first two years, an identical number of students (freshmen, 11.9 percent; sophomores, 19.3 percent) view the general practitioner as having unexceptional academic ability as do those who see the G.P. as being knowledgeable and capable. Opinions change markedly in the last two years, though; 15.5 percent of the juniors and 23.6 percent of the seniors see the general practitioner as having unexceptional academic ability, while only 10.3 percent of the juniors and 9.1 percent of the seniors see the G.P. as being knowledgeable and capable.

The freshman's view of the G.P. as a vestige of the old-time country doctor evolves, in the senior year, to a more updated awareness of family practice, a specialty that combines the old with the new.* In contrast to the "vertical" training in one particular area, as required in other specialties, family practice offers "horizontal" training in the usual medical, surgical, sociological, and psychological ills of families, and "vertical" training in the usual and commonplace illnesses that plague the greatest number of people.

By the senior year the most typical impression is that G.P.s simply prefer primary patient care; that is, they like having the total care of patients and their families over a long period of time, working with them on a more intimate basis.† Such a relationship confers a certain amount of status, especially for those who value this type of practice. For them, medical specialties hold little appeal when involving narrowly defined areas of treatment, short-term care, and depersonalized patient contact. The treatment of nothing but ear, nose, and throat ailments, for example, without involvement in the patient's overall situation, is too much a segmentalized, assembly-line operation for such individuals.

The general practitioner is seen by seniors as being on "the first line of defense against disease." As such, he is a "medical traffic director," who screens a large variety of people and refers them to the appropriate specialist when something serious arises. "G.P.s are the initial protectors of the people's health," one said. "They can take care of 80 percent of those who come to them and make early diagnoses of the other 20 percent and refer them to specialists."

So, although those who aspire to general practice are not thought by my cohort to be the flashiest classmates in academic display, they are generally regarded as being solid, down-to-earth, very stable persons who perform an important role. Nonetheless, those aspiring to prestigious medical specialties cannot resist looking down their noses at them just a little.

Internist

The internist, unlike the general practitioner, fails to project a well-defined image. The label "internal medicine" does not convey a distinct impression. The word "internist" is easily confused with "intern," and

---

* The four-year period is marked by a definite decline in those who describe G.P.s as rural and conventional: freshmen, 22.0 percent; sophomores, 15.8 percent; juniors, 13.8 percent; and seniors, 9.1 percent.

† The number of those saying that a general practitioner is the type of person who enjoys primary care increases steadily during the four years in medical school include: freshmen, 18.6 percent; sophomores, 24.6 percent; juniors, 27.6 percent; and seniors, 36.4 percent.

"medicine" is associated with all doctors. So, many entering students have little idea about the kind of person who becomes an internist. One-third of the freshmen have no insight at all about characteristics of such specialists; instead, they typically describe the internist's role. But by the second year, relatively few are unable to describe their personality traits.*

The image ultimately taking shape is pieced together from comparisons with general practitioners, who are seen as similar,† and surgeons, who are viewed as dissimilar.‡ A substantial number of freshmen, one-third of the class, view the internist as performing "a glorified brand of general practice." One said, "He probably would have become a general practitioner, but didn't feel competent enough, so he took a couple more years to get his confidence." In the senior year, this same view is expressed by nearly half of the class. "There's not all that much difference between the two groups," one said. "They both have the same sort of problems, the same face-to-face contact with the patient; and they both get to know the patient in his entirety and become involved in total patient care."

Just as internists are seen as playing a role similar to the general practitioner, they are also viewed as pleasant, service-oriented people who achieve emotional enjoyment from their personal contact with others. The adjectives used to describe the internist—nice, easygoing, understanding, gentle, popular, dedicated, interested, helpful, and devoted—are similar to those of the G.P.

But as students progress through school, a growing number note differences between general practitioners and internists.§ For one thing, the internist has better job advantages—more prestige, better pay, fewer hours, and greater security.‖ But the main distinction, discerning students point out, is that internists have more training, and therefore their knowledge of disease processes is more extensive. For this reason, they say, the in-

---

* Students who have no opinion of the type of person who becomes interested in internal medicine include 35.6 percent in the freshman year; the figure then drops down to 7.0 percent in the sophomore year, 10.3 percent in the junior year, and 9.1 percent in the senior year.

† Internists are described as being similar to general practitioners by 33.9 percent of the freshmen, 47.4 percent of the sophomores, 39.7 percent of the juniors, and 43.6 percent of the seniors.

‡ Internists are perceived as being dissimilar to surgeons by 3.4 percent of the freshmen, 8.8 percent of the sophomores, 15.5 percent of the juniors, and 12.7 percent of the seniors. (Even though relatively few reported this perception during the interviews, it was very clear in my informal conversations with students that they were aware of this dichotomy. This comparison is frequently mentioned by practitioners at the medical center.)

§ Those students who describe internists as dissimilar to general practitioners number 11.9 percent in the freshman year, 24.6 percent in the sophomore year, 24.1 percent in the junior year, and 32.7 percent in the senior year.

‖ Specialty-related factors, such as those mentioned in the text, are given by 8.5 percent of the freshmen, 22.8 percent of the sophomores, 25.9 percent of the juniors, and 23.6 percent of the seniors.

ternist is a much more astute and academically inclined diagnostician than his G.P. colleagues.

Generally speaking, internists are seen as being intelligent and analytical.* "I've heard that the internists are drawn from the top quarter of the class," a freshman remarked. "You know they are a lot more intelligent than the others." One out of four freshmen makes such comments, and by the senior year 40 percent of the class similarly describe internists as "intellectuals who have broad interests, enjoy variety, and relish the challenge of puzzling out tough diagnostic problems." A senior observed, "They find satisfaction in making astute observations about minor clinical phenomena and then putting the whole thing together in one diagnosis; the more complicated the puzzle, the happier the internist." In fact, some seniors view internal medicine as the most intellectually challenging of all specialties. "The internist has to know just about everything," one volunteered.

As earlier noted, the contrast between internists and surgeons is apparent, for the latter are viewed as being less reserved and reflective, not the type who like to read or meditate. In this regard a senior said, "Internists sit around and theorize but surgeons like to hurry and get at it." The competitive feeling that often exists between surgeons and internists is captured by a surgical mentor who told one student, "Internists are the type who like to sit around and mentally masturbate."

Surgeon

An aura of magic and power surrounds the surgeon perhaps more than any other specialist. On television and elsewhere, surgeons stand at the top of the medical status hierarchy and their authority is generally unquestioned. Still, one-fifth of the entering class had no idea about the type person attracted to this specialty; but by the second year only 5 percent remained uncertain.† The emerging picture is a colorful one and becomes sharper each year as students gain closer personal contact with surgeons.

Because surgery obviously involves manual dexterity, the first impression of these practitioners centers on their technical and manual inclination; and this remains a prominent view throughout all four years of medical training.‡ Seen as individuals who enjoy working with their hands,

---

* Internists are described as being intelligent and analytical by: freshmen, 27.1 percent; sophomores, 33.3 percent; juniors, 36.2 percent; and seniors, 40.0 percent.

† Of the freshmen, 20.3 percent give "don't know" answers when asked about the type of individual who becomes a surgeon; in the sophomore year, only 5.3 percent give this reply, and in the junior and senior years, 3.4 and 3.6 percent, respectively.

‡ Surgeons are viewed as being technically oriented and manually inclined by 27.1 percent in the freshman year; 26.3 percent, sophomores; 32.8 percent, juniors; and 23.6 percent, seniors.

surgeons are called the plumbers, the carpenters, or the mechanics of the medical profession. They are, a senior remarked, "demolition experts who like to change the structure of things; they actually rebuild the body, taking things out and putting them back in." Because surgeons "prefer concrete problems that have no mystery," they are sometimes seen as antitheoretical, or even antiintellectual. "They get so wrapped up in surgery," a senior said, "that they forget there are things that can be done short of wielding the scalpel."

Increasingly, surgeons are viewed as people who like quick action and immediate results, the type who prefer to cure patients by "getting in and taking it out in a hurry." Only 8 percent of the freshmen describe surgeons as activated in this way, but the number increases steadily; by the senior year more than half the class hold this view.* It becomes increasingly clear to these students that delayed gratification is not compatible with the surgeon's personality. As fast-moving people of action, they are impulsive individuals who like absolute diagnoses and immediate return, where the problem can be solved by surgery in one morning or afternoon. "Why mess with a pill," one said, "when you can whop it out and have it fixed?"

Since it is commonly known that surgeons must continually confront acute life-and-death situations, beginning students naturally see them as "more confident persons than most doctors." But as students evaluate surgeons firsthand, their perceptions shift and they begin to see them as being domineering, aggressive, and egotistical rather than simply self-confident.† Increasingly they are described as "cocky and arrogant—a self-centered bunch that likes to dominate the scene; domineering people who have a very high opinion of themselves and believe they are always right." It is claimed that surgery attracts egotistical and domineering personalities — "blowhards who need to be in command of the situations as 'king of the castle' " — and, in fact, that the specialty reinforces these qualities:

> The training program itself causes surgeons to become arrogant and cocky. It's not a congenial atmosphere like that of medicine. Most surgeons are hard; they work long hours and they'll jump all over you and chew you out. In such an environment you develop that compulsive, rat-race, competitive, aggressive personality.

Even a first experience in the surgeon's role makes clear how one can feel powerful and superior, thereby getting drunk on one's own juices.

---

* The number of those who describe the surgeon as being action- and result-oriented increases dramatically after the first two years: freshmen, 8.5 percent; sophomores, 14.0 percent; juniors, 34.5 percent; and seniors, 56.4 percent.

† Student perceptions of the surgeon as being domineering and egotistical take a sharp upturn after the freshman year (11.9 percent); 29.8 percent of the sophomores, 31.0 percent of the juniors, and 40.0 percent of the seniors hold this view.

For example, a senior recalled how his ego was inflated upon successfully removing the top of a cat's head:

> It was a perfect operation, the way I removed the cranium with minimal bleeding. I felt like stepping back and saying, "The rest of you peons now do what you want." It really gave me a tremendous feeling of power.

This sense of power is also enhanced by the way the internist hands his patient to the surgeon for an operation and then asks, "What was wrong with him?" Such a relationship reinforces the surgeon's feeling of authority in medical matters.

Another interesting change in student views may be noted. Freshmen tend to picture surgeons as "thorough and meticulous." By the fourth year, however, they no longer describe surgeons this way. Instead, some see them as having an excessive orderliness and a driving perfectionism and hang on them the psychiatric label "obsessive–compulsive."* However, realizing that many, if not most, doctors have such traits, students label the surgeon as "super-obsessive–compulsive." They have to be to drive themselves the way they do," a senior explained.

As energetic and dynamic personalities,† surgeons seem "the most hardworking, physically speaking, of the medical profession, intensely 'gung-ho,' manifesting a kind of perpetual motion with an inability to relax. They seem to be more aggressive and unable to sit back and enjoy life." Some students attribute these traits to the life-and-death tensions encountered in the operating room. Others, however, see the surgeon's obsessive work habits as resulting from a strong ego that requires high status, a driving urge to get to the top. For this reason, some speculate that underneath the surgeon's brash confidence lies an insecure ego which prompts the choice of this ego-inflating specialty.

But, whatever the motives, most students agree that surgery is a more athletic type of medicine, one that attracts highly egotistical and dynamic individuals—those who are aggressive, have good manual dexterity, an abundance of energy and physical endurance, and are more interested in action and results than in interpersonal relationships.‡

---

* With increased exposure to surgeons and to psychiatric labeling, students change markedly in their views of surgeons as obsessive–compulsive personalities: freshmen, none; sophomores, 7.0 percent; juniors, 15.5 percent; and seniors, 21.8 percent.

† Surgeons are described as energetic and dynamic by 5.1 percent of the freshmen, 21.1 percent of the sophomores, 20.7 percent of the juniors, and 12.7 percent of the seniors.

‡ Each year a small number of students portray the surgeon as one who is cold and aloof (an "iceman"), is hard to communicate with, and has a disengaged attitude toward patients. (The surgeon is viewed as preferring limited emotional involvement by 8.5 percent of the freshmen, 7.0 percent of the sophomores, 6.9 percent of the juniors, and 12.7 percent of the seniors.) According to one student, "The surgeon is apt to stride into the patient's room and announce, 'I'm going to take out your appendix—you're scheduled for tomorrow,' with little consideration for the patient's feelings."

Obstetrician/Gynecologist

The failure of the obstetrician/gynecologist (OB/GYN) to have a well-defined image reflects the students' lack of personal exposure to this specialty. This is understandable since most of my study population are young men and, therefore, have not patronized these physicians as patients. Initially, nearly 40 percent of the class have an ill-defined image of the OB/GYN, and this persists throughout all four years of school.*

Among freshmen venturing an opinion, the most typical view of these doctors is that they are pleasant people. Obstetricians, they say, are "warm, outgoing personalities who are concerned, sympathetic, and easygoing, sort of happy-go-lucky types who like to joke around a lot." But this viewpoint becomes less and less popular in ensuing years. By the senior year, the initial view of the obstetrician as "a fat, jolly person, a Santa Claus in white—just a good guy or gal with no bad qualities" is all but extinguished.†

Since OB/GYN practice deals with women, it is logical to conclude that these specialists enjoy contact with them.‡ Female students may be stimulated by a common bond of understanding and sympathy. However, the motivations of male students may be more complex. Some, like the following, see this in a positive light:

> Obstetricians understand the female psychology. They are patient and have the ability to inspire confidence. They can put apprehensive and embarrassed women at ease. These doctors can also deal with sexually charged topics without increasing female anxieties or appearing lecherous.

But the male obstetrician's interest in women causes other students to imagine that attraction to this field is due to psychosexual problems.§ Underclassmen, using hearsay evidence, suggest that the male obstetrician's interest in females is due to a sublimated voyeurism. "They are the kind of guys who like to peep through keyholes or bathroom windows," one said. "They get delight in seeing the private anatomy of others; when examining a female body, they think 'Whoopee! Look what I'm looking at!' "

In the clinical years, remarks about voyeurism are replaced with com-

---

* Thirty-nine percent of the freshmen, 36.8 percent of the sophomores, 36.2 percent of the juniors, and 29.1 percent of the seniors have no opinion about OB/GYN.

† Pleasant personalities are seen as characteristic of those who enter the OB/GYN specialty by 18.6 percent of the freshmen, 14.0 percent of the sophomores, 3.4 percent of the juniors, and only 1.8 percent of the seniors.

‡ The number who describe the obstetrician/gynecologist as being interested in women are: freshmen, 5.1 percent; sophomores, 19.3 percent; juniors, 8.6 percent; and seniors, 5.5 percent.

§ Personality quirks in the male obstetrician/gynecologist associated mostly with psychosexual disorders are perceived by 13.6 percent of the freshmen, 22.8 percent of the sophomores, 13.8 percent of the juniors, and 20 percent of the seniors.

ments about "sexual athletics." Male obstetricians, they say, tend to be "playboy types" who go "ape over sex." A senior commented, "They're the ones in the class who are always preoccupied with their dating plans for the weekend. They're really nuts on sex." In contrast to this Don Juan image, however, other students see obstetricians as inhibited, sexually frustrated individuals who get their kicks vicariously. "They are the ones who have problems getting dates or have hangups in their social lives," another observed:

> They are little guys, psychologically speaking, who like women to look up to them and be dependent upon them. Look at the power this guy has! He sees 12 to 20 women a day and gets a great feeling of power by doing pelvics and telling women what's wrong with them—I mean, baby, there's something wrong with *him!* You get the impression that he is trying to prove his masculinity.

Aside from sexual pathology, a happier theme running through all four years is the idea that obstetricians are simply people who prefer the sunny side of medicine.* Rather than dealing with the sick and diseased, these doctors prefer well patients. "Their patients tend to be a happier crew," a senior remarked. "Most are nice, healthy women, many in the prime of life."

In obstetrical practice, sad moments are relatively scarce. Instead of dealing with death and its attendant problems, obstetricians typically participate in life-creating processes. Expectant mothers may experience some pain during birth, but generally there is joy and happiness all around. "Birth gives most people a thrill," one said, "including the doctor, who is a key participant. It's all smiles then; everything is well and good." And to make things even better, patients usually go home thinking of their doctor as "the greatest person in the world." In some cases they even name their children after their obstetrician. "Brother," exclaimed one student, "that's rewarding!"

The fact that obstetrics is a narrowly limited field and therefore comparatively simple to master appeals to some candidates; but it repulses others. "There aren't that many unusual things to see or that much to learn," a senior pointed out. "In fact, you become kind of a tradesman in delivering babies—and hysterectomies aren't that difficult to do." So, students say, this field appeals to those who enjoy being free from the challenge of having to make a lot of critical decisions. Yet, from the perspective of those impressed with this field, obstetrics offers the best of all worlds—a chance to do a little surgery, to practice a little pediatrics, and,

---

* Those who describe the obstetrician/gynecologist as one who prefers a happy work atmosphere in medical practice number 16.9 percent in the freshman year, 12.3 percent in the sophomore year, 19.0 percent in the junior year, and 14.5 percent in the senior year.

while doing so, to enjoy rewarding associations with grateful patients over an extended period.*

Pediatrician

Since almost everyone has at one time or another been to see a pediatrician, this practitioner's image is very clear. Only 12 percent of the freshmen had difficulty describing the pediatrican, making this specialist a close second to the G.P. in clarity of impressions.† And student descriptions change very little during subsequent years.

Nearly two-thirds of the freshmen describe the pediatrician as one who simply likes kids, and this image is retained by more than half of the class throughout the ensuing years of medical school.‡ "Kids really turn them on," students observe.

As "fatherly or motherly types," these specialists are the kind who like working in children's summer camps or promoting peewee baseball teams. "They are the nurturing type who have kind of a sixth sense," one student remarked; "it's an inner feeling for children that enables them to understand and communicate with little kids who usually make more noise than sense to others."

During all years of medical school, students view the pediatrician as having a pleasant personality—outgoing, warm, and friendly. More than any other specialist, he or she is described as a "nice person." "Pediatricians seem to be easygoing people who are very responsible and easy to get along with," one said. "They are a little more relaxed, freer, and happier than others."

Especially prevalent among students is an admiration for the pediatrician's patience, tolerance, and imperturbability.§ "They have nerves of steel," a senior exclaimed. "A tornado couldn't rattle them. You could shoot off a cannon right next to them and they'd just let it go by without batting an eye." They must be this way, students say, if they are to survive the tumult in pediatric clinics:

---

* The number of students who describe the obstetrician/gynecologist as being attracted by practical advantages of the job (namely, a delineated field that is easy to master) increases dramatically from 3.4 percent in the freshman year to 19.3 percent in the sophomore year, 20. 7 percent in the junior year, and 23.6 percent in the senior year.

† Those who have no opinion about the type of student who goes into pediatrics number 11.9 percent, freshmen; 10.5 percent, sophomores; 22.4 percent, juniors; and 16.4 percent, seniors.

‡ Those who say that pediatricians enjoy children and select this specialty for that reason include: freshmen, 62.7 percent; sophomores, 56.1 percent; juniors, 50.0 percent; and seniors, 52.7 percent.

§ Personalities that are pleasant and imperturbable are seen as characteristic of pediatricians by 25.4 percent of the freshmen, 36.8 percent of the sophomores, 17.2 percent of the juniors, and 23.6 percent of the seniors.

Kids are always crying. They rant and rave and kick and bite and carry on so you can't make a decent diagnosis. While they yell and scream and otherwise are uncooperative, the parents are on you. And the little monsters are always getting sick at night—it's a hard, trying life. You've got to be tolerant. Boy! You've really got to be tolerant!

Needless to say, the pediatrician's quiet, unruffled approach is greatly admired, as is the ability to interpret information from young patients, many of whom cannot talk. In this regard, pediatricians are described as "the veterinarians of the medical profession."

To voluntarily submit to such difficulties, some students reason, pediatricians must surely be a "dedicated and compassionate bunch."* "They're probably the most humanistic of all groups," a senior commented. "They're the kind who would stop and help anybody in trouble. This field is definitely not the one for you if you want an eight-hour day and lots of money. So you really have to have a strong interest in people."

But pediatrics also has its rewards.† For one thing, it offers an opportunity to deal with the "whole person" and his total family milieu. In this regard, these clinicians are described as "the general practitioners for children." Yet, like internists, they encounter great challenge in difficult diagnoses. So the specialty is sometimes called "a subfield of internal medicine applied to children." And, like OB/GYN practice, pediatrics offers opportunities to practice preventive medicine with basically well people, for there are relatively few hopelessly ill and dying patients.

The main attraction, though, is clearly the satisfaction that comes from the direct honesty of children and their delightful ways and the gratification of watching them grow up to become healthy, normal people. For those students so inclined, the greatest thing in the world is helping a little child grow up.

Psychiatrist

Although more students have a clearer idea of the psychiatrist's role than that of some other specialists,‡ they rarely display much empathy toward these practitioners, and these initial sentiments are not altered by medical training. Only a few students in my cohort gave serious thought to psychiatry as a career. Clinically oriented and fatigued from the hard

---

* Pediatricians are viewed as service-oriented by 10.2 percent of the freshmen, 15.8 percent of the sophomores, 15.5 percent of the juniors, and 3.6 percent of the seniors.

† Practical rewards that attract individuals to the field of pediatrics are mentioned as motivating factors by 8.5 percent of the freshmen, 22.8 percent of the sophomores, 20.7 percent of the juniors, and 18.2 percent of the seniors.

‡ Those who had no opinion of the kind of person who becomes a psychiatrist number 20.3 percent in the freshman year, 8.8 percent in the sophomore year, 20.7 percent in the junior year, and 16.4 percent in the senior year.

work of medical school, they could not fathom why anyone would elect to end up in a field seemingly set apart from actual medical practice, unless, they speculate, it is because there are so few emergencies, late hours, or dirty work. "Let's face it," one said, "it's a pretty soft life." *

Generally speaking, psychiatrists are seen as "a breed unto themselves." For one thing, they seem repelled by organic disease and the physiological aspects of medicine—"guts, needle-jabbing, blood samples, urine tests, etc." † "They're the ones who are turned off by all of the bioscience stuff in med school," a sophomore explained.

More than any other specialty, psychiatry is singled out as attracting "weird people"; and the number who maintain this opinion does not dwindle significantly.‡ According to this view, those with psychological problems—the insecure, uncertain, disturbed, and troubled—gravitate into psychiatry in order to understand their own problems. "Psychiatrists need a psychiatrist," one student said. "They are a little bit screwy and as zoned out as the people they are treating. Psychiatry is a 'do-it-yourself specialty' for those needing psychological help."

A corollary view is that although such persons may be psychologically healthy before beginning psychiatric training, they tend to become strange after practicing in this field. That is, they get all mixed up in other people's problems and thereby become mixed up themselves. One student, reflecting the opinions of some classmates, described the end result as:

> . . . an extremely nervous person, but when with a patient this M.D. suddenly becomes a psychiatrist (super-cool so that the patient will think he or she is all right). But at 10 minutes to the hour when the patient has left, the doctor becomes a shriveled little person sitting in the fetal position waiting for the next patient. (Here the student demonstrated by putting his thumb in his mouth and assuming the fetal position.)

This particular description was presumably offered with tongue-in-cheek, since the one who gave it eventually became a psychiatrist. But at least one classmate withdrew as a psychiatry candidate, fearing he might become psychologically unbalanced.

There is an underlying tendency among students to feel uncomfortable around psychiatrists and to distrust their methods of introspective probing —and this uneasiness may contribute to the view of the practitioners as being psychologically odd. Students often have the nervous feeling, as one

---

* The practical benefits of psychiatric practice are mentioned as reasons for choice by 1.7 percent of the freshmen, 5.3 percent of the sophomores, 5.2 percent of the juniors, and 12.7 percent of the seniors.

† Those who see psychiatrists as being repelled by organic procedures are: freshmen, 13.6 percent; sophomores, 7.0 percent; juniors, 17.2 percent; and seniors, 18.2 percent.

‡ Psychiatrists are mentioned has having personality quirks by 13.6 percent of the freshmen, 19.3 percent of the sophomores, 22.4 percent of the juniors, and 18.2 percent of the seniors.

said, that the psychiatrist is "psyching me out, prying into my inner thoughts as if I were his patient. I feel like the mouse the cat is toying with."

Psychiatrists are frequently described as "people-watchers"—"psychology or sociology majors tripped off to medical school"—the kinds of persons who have a question for everything that comes up.* Rather than dealing with just the organic components of health and illness, these practitioners like to "dig deeper" to understand the inner person, to figure out what makes the patient tick. Instead of patching up the patient's body like a car when it breaks down, the psychiatrist likes to "get inside" and study the underlying personality and total life situation.

Because psychiatric practice deals with complicated emotional problems not easily or quickly resolved, the psychiatrist must be well endowed with patience, tolerance, empathy, and a deep sensitivity for others. Unlike the surgeon who notes a quick improvement after removing an appendix, the psychiatrist rarely experiences dramatic cures. Interaction with psychiatric patients often extends over considerable time.†

And because emotional illnesses, unlike most organic disorders, are not concrete or easily definable, the psychiatrist must have a capacity for ambiguity and theoretical thinking. In this regard, one-fourth of the senior class describe psychiatrists as "thinkers—philosophically oriented people who seek explanations and enjoy dealing with abstraction." ‡ They are seen as analytical persons who think on a more conceptual plane than other doctors:

> Psychiatrists are people who are interested in lots of theory and unresolved speculative issues; they can mold their own thinking into the profession. In other words, they can take a particular type of patient and project themselves into the therapy and work up a patient through philosophical rather than technical means. This is an art.

But this proclivity for abstract thinking is not admired by all students. Some, in fact, distrust psychiatrists as "free thinkers" or "hippie doctors," people who have "weird ideas" and "strange thought processes." They are, as one put it, "a little off in the woods."

But despite the fact that many students have trouble relating to psychiatry, they acknowledge the need for someone to look after the emotionally

---

* Interest in human behavior is mentioned as being characteristic of psychiatrists by 20.3 percent of the freshmen, 33.3 percent of the sophomores, 29.3 percent of the juniors, and 18.2 percent of the seniors.

† Psychiatrists are seen as enjoying in-depth patient contact by 20.3 percent of the freshmen, 26.3 percent of the sophomores, 15.5 percent of the juniors, and 27.3 percent of the seniors.

‡ In the freshman year, 15.3 percent describe psychiatrists as being theoretically and philosophically inclined. This number increases to 24.6 percent in the sophomore year, drops to 13.8 percent in the junior year, and once more increases to 27.3 percent in the senior year.

ill and are glad that a few of their classmates are so inclined. They see psychiatrists as the ones willing to help patients whose lives are so "messed up" that they have no one else to turn to.

Pathologist

Freshmen have little familiarity with the pathologist; more than a fourth of them look upon this practitioner with uncertainty. However, following the pathology course, their "don't know" responses decrease and many descriptive comments emerge.*

As with some other specialists, students sometimes attribute characteristics symbolic of their patients to the practitioners themselves. Knowing that pathologists perform autopsies, a few students each year visualize them as "morbid characters" who work in "ghoulish atmospheres" and enjoy "closing out the books on people." "They must have some kind of hangup to enjoy constant contact with the dead," a sophomore said. "They must get some kind of morbid pleasure from conducting autopsies and working with the deceased."

Encounters with pathologists reinforce earlier images of preferences for limited interpersonal involvement. Slightly over 27 percent of the freshmen characterize pathologists this way, and, by the senior year, the number increases to nearly 60 percent.† This is because, some students say, the pathologist is a recluse—insecure, uncomfortable, ill at ease with others, and inept in interpersonal communication. They see this specialist as shy, introverted, aloof, and cold—a "loner who sits back in a corner alone." A senior put it this way: "If you can't deal with people or don't want to, then pathology is the thing for you."

Other students, however, view pathologists as normal people who are simply trying to beat the "hassles" of everyday medical practice.‡ This specialty is not only economically rewarding; but also it permits a regular schedule minus emergencies and a heavy workload. Cited as evidence of these advantages are several pathology residents who were previously in general practice. "They simply got tired of dealing with patients and having total responsibility for them," a senior explained. "They were worked to death, and it was just too much for them." For such doctors, pathology offers a haven from the "rat race."

* The number who express no opinion about the pathologist are: freshmen, 27.1 percent; sophomores, 8.8 percent; juniors, 10.3 percent; and seniors, 18.2 percent.
† Pathologists are described as disliking interpersonal involvement by 27.1 percent of the freshmen, 36.8 percent of the sophomores, 53.4 percent of the juniors, and 58.2 percent of the seniors.
‡ Practical benefits of pathology as a motive for entering this field are not mentioned by freshmen; but 19.3 percent of the sophomores, 13.8 percent of the juniors, and 29.1 percent of the seniors recognize specialty-related motivations.

But the most prevalent explanation of the pathologist's antisocial tendencies is preoccupation with scientific matters.* "It's not that they don't like people," a student explained. "They'd much rather be involved in scientific activities." The science of medicine is much more enjoyable to these specialists than the art of medicine. Analyzing diseased tissue in a quiet laboratory holds more intrigue than chatting with patients about their maladies. Thus, pathology offers the ultimate opportunity—to be a physician and a scientist at the same time.

Pathologists–scientists are seen as being very literate, "bookish" persons with large vocabularies. Although the dictionary hardly makes exciting reading, it is, students say, a favorite among pathologists. And when it comes to analyzing a problem, these practitioners are "very exact, real bugs on specifics." As textbook-oriented perfectionists, they like to "pinpoint things down to the finest detail, cataloging every minute thing with great precision."

In this regard, pathologists seem to be at the opposite end of the spectrum from psychiatrists. Rather than dealing with the subjective, the abstract, or the ambiguous, pathologists like precise and concrete factual evidence.† "They love absolutes," a senior explained. "They like to get their hands on the facts and to know exactly what is going on. Everything must be down pat, laid out before them in a clean-cut manner, cut and dried, exact! They demand straight 'yes' or 'no' answers with nothing in between—real 'all-or-nothing' types."

Having the concrete facts thus assembled, the pathologist then becomes the final authority, the absolute diagnostician. A senior explained, "While patients wait on the operating table, specimens are sent to the pathologist to see if the tissue is diseased or not. That decision will determine what the patient will receive and whether an organ will be removed, etc. What the pathologist says is rarely challenged." Having such diagnostic power is, of course, very ego rewarding, an aspect that does not escape the attention of students. One said, "Pathologists like to give the conclusive verdict, the ultimate word. They regard themselves as the 'father of medicine' type who has the final answer on everything. It is very satisfying to say, 'This is it!' and have that be the last word." Being in such a strategic position, the pathologist can, if so inclined, take great relish in ridiculing another physician who has erred in a diagnosis, for this establishes him or her as the authority among authorities.‡

---

* Pathologists are described as being scientific and research-oriented by 44.1 percent of the freshmen, 61.4 percent of the sophomores, 53.4 percent of the juniors, and 47.3 percent of the seniors.

† Those who perceive pathologists as having a dislike for ambiguity are: freshmen, 13.6 percent; sophomores, 24.6 percent; juniors, 5.2 percent; and seniors, 1.8 percent.

‡ Although no freshmen mention the pathologist's preference for final diagnostic authority, a few members of the class do later: sophomores, 10.5 percent; juniors, 8.6 percent; and seniors, 5.5 percent.

Radiologist

The radiologist seems to be a mystery to 39 percent of the entering freshmen. They profess to have no opinion about the type of person who wants to become a radiologist.* But to almost 29 percent of the same beginning class, he or she is a true scientist and diagnostician. The remainder see this doctor as possessing a melange of desirable and objectionable traits. However, those who share the "scientist" image tend to be awed by the radiologist's ability to practice nuclear medicine and apply space-age knowledge to patients. "By picking up clues from X-ray pictures, it is possible to diagnose a person's trouble without even laying a hand on him," one first-year admirer marveled. This specialist is seen as "the Buck Rogers of the medical profession, a wizard who sees things through instrumentation that no one else can see." †

However, as the training years progress, these students find much of their high regard for scientific activities in medical school all but extinguished. Aversive experiences in the basic-science course work contribute to their devaluation of research-oriented activities and the formation of a new description of radiologists as "medical cop-outs." This loss of esteem was verbalized when a third-year student said, "All radiologists do is snap their pictures and then look at the dopey things to see if they can find some darn thing that nobody else can see." Their fall from grace is assisted by a perceived departure from the medical ideal of being clinically oriented and personally dedicated.‡ Because they shoulder so little primary care for patients and have short, convenient working hours, radiologists are increasingly seen as the antithesis of the student ideal. "They don't give of themselves the way others do," a senior explained, "and knowing how to interpret pictures doesn't qualify them as doctors by my definition of medicine."

Each year an increasing number point to money, good hours, and an easy life to explain why some select this specialty. "That's where all the money is," a senior remarked. "Radiologists are money-grubbers — persons interested in making a pile." Although such comments are made by only 7 percent of the freshmen, by the senior year 6 out of 10 students express this view.§ Radiologists, they say, are people who look for the

---

* In the freshmen year, 39.0 percent have no opinion about the type of person who becomes a radiologist. But this number decreases to 24.6 percent in the second year, to 10.3 percent in the junior year, and to 9.1 percent in the final year.

† Although 28.8 percent of the freshmen describe radiologists as being scientifically and diagnostically inclined, this figure drops to 22.8 percent in the sophomore year, and then to 15.5 percent and 12.7 percent, respectively, in the final two years.

‡ Radiologists are described as socially and clinically detached by only 13.6 percent of the freshmen, but this number increases to 31.6 percent in the sophomore year and 53.4 percent in the junior year, and drops slightly to 45.5 percent in the senior year.

§ Practical advantages as motivation for becoming a radiologist are seen as significant by only 6.8 percent of the freshmen, but this factor steadily increases over the remaining three years: sophomores, 33.3 percent; juniors, 36.2 percent; and seniors, 60.0 percent.

most lucrative branch of medicine, one that does not have much responsibility or take much time:

> They stroll in about 9:00 and leave the office by 4:30 or 5:00 o'clock, and they don't like to be bothered until the next morning, either. They're like business executives who sit at their desks and wait for work to come in. Their attitude is, "If you have a problem bring it to me—but not after 5:00 p.m."

As evidence of this view, a senior points out, "Whenever I ask one how the interest in radiology came about, the answer is usually, 'The hours are good.' It always comes out, one way or the other."

Radiology is increasingly seen as presenting few emergencies or stressful circumstances. "Radiologists are people who don't want to make a lot of decisions," a student commented, "especially the split-second kind that will determine whether somebody will die or not. They just like to look at X rays and not have to worry about things."

Because there are so few night calls, these practitioners also have ample time for personal pleasures. "Humanitarian dedication is definitely not a requirement," an upperclassman said. During all four years only one student suggested that radiologists have any interest in helping people. Incidentally, this student aspired to a career in radiology.

Because of their clinical detachment and preference for the scientific, technical,* or academic aspects over direct patient care, radiologists are sometimes compared to pathologists—"withdrawn or introverted personalities who prefer to stay in their own offices or X-ray rooms to keep away from people." † Like pathologists, radiologists are seen as being aloof, unsociable, and less confident and personable than most doctors, sometimes even unpleasant. "Every one of them seems cold," a senior said.

These reasons account for the antagonism that some feel toward the radiologist.‡ "They're basically lazy people—at least lazier than those in other fields," one said. "They do things at their own leisure. It's like a desk job with little responsibility, not even part of medical practice. They are just in it for the money."

This change of opinion, from initial admiration to antagonism, makes clear the values that emerge among medical students—that a good physician assumes primary care for patients and manifests dedication to their welfare by a willingness to work long hours and shoulder heavy responsi-

---

* Radiologists are described as being technically oriented by 10.2 percent of the freshmen, 15.8 percent of the sophomores, 3.4 percent of the juniors, and 20.0 percent of the seniors.

† Radiologists are seen as similar to pathologists by 10.2 percent of the freshmen, 12.3 percent of the sophomores, 36.2 percent of the juniors, and 21.8 percent of the seniors.

‡ Hostility against radiologists is openly expressed by freshmen, 3.4 percent; sophomores, 7.0 percent; juniors, 10.3 percent; and seniors, 14.5 percent.

bilities. In short, he or she is out on "the front lines" in the war against disease and death.

Neurologist

Four out of ten freshmen cannot see any distinguishing traits among neurologists. And although the noncommittal responses decline with increasing exposure to these practitioners, for some unknown reason uncertainty increases again in the senior year.*

As previously noted, medical specialists are sometimes attributed personality traits characteristic of their patients. True to form, neurologists, those who treat disorders of the brain and nervous system, are described in cerebral terms as "brainy." † They are seen as "super-intellectual persons, really brilliant people who find great enjoyment in intellectual exercises."

Firsthand exposure to these specialists does not dispel the "brainy" image. In fact, a steadily increasing number of students each year note their logical and analytical qualities, describing them as "inquisitive persons who like to play complicated mental games, work puzzles, and solve problems." By the senior year nearly six out of ten students describe neurology as "the ultimate in logic and medicine." ‡ "Their diagnoses are tricky," one said. "It's kind of like crossing wires and circuits and trying to put all of the facts together. They look for systems and try to work out a pattern."

To some the neurologist is "a scientist interested in the hairiest medical problems," to others "a detective tracking down clues to uncover complex mysteries." Still others see simply "a precision-oriented nitpicker" who takes delight in memorizing large quantities of minute detail.§ Almost all agree, however, that neurologists are "thinking people who are fascinated with complexities." "The neurologist would be overjoyed," one said, "if heaven consisted of nothing but jigsaw puzzles that could be worked on all of the time."

Recognition as an intellectual, students say, gives the neurologist much satisfaction, for these egotistical doctors take pride in their brilliance. Viewing themselves as "the cream of the crop," they regard their specialty

---

* In regard to classifying neurologists, "no opinion" is expressed by 40.7 percent of the freshmen, 36.8 percent of the sophomores, 12.1 percent of the juniors, and 27.3 percent of the seniors.

† Neurologists are described as "brainy" by 18.6 percent of the freshmen, 24.6 percent of the sophomores, 13.8 percent of the juniors, and 18.2 percent of the seniors.

‡ Those who perceive neurologists as being logical and analytical are: freshmen, 23.7 percent; sophomores, 42.1 percent; juniors, 48.3 percent; and seniors, 56.4 percent.

§ "Detailed-oriented and perfectionistic" are adjectives used to describe neurologists by 8.5 percent of the freshmen, 5.3 percent of the sophomores, 6.9 percent of the juniors, and 10.9 percent of the seniors.

as the quintessence of medicine. "They really take a lot of pride in their brains," a junior remarked. "They pump up their egos all the time by trying to impress others with their knowledge. They want their colleagues to view them as superintellects; esteem is very important to them." *

That neurologists sometimes promote this "brainy" image at the expense of others is indicated by a third-year student: "When we are in a clinical conference, the neurologists just can't wait until the one who is presenting a patient finishes so they can start clawing for blood. Everything has to be very precise and they leave little leeway for error. If you make a mistake—well, you're just an idiot."

Aside from intellectual considerations, some students regard neurologists as clinically and emotionally detached.† This is because a large share of their patients have problems not readily amenable to clinical intervention—such as strokes, brain tumors, or other neurological lesions. Although the neurologists may say what is wrong with such patients, sometimes not much can be done to help them. "Some patients are just told what they have and are separated from their money with 'Sorry, I can't help you,' " one said. "It really seems weird," another said. "How can anyone choose to go into a field where so many patients can't be helped?"

Only an unusual type of personality, students conclude, can work in a "clinically fruitless field" where there is infrequent satisfaction in the form of cures. Those who choose this specialty, they say, should not be types who are easily depressed or require immediate rewards. Neurologists generally seem to be emotionally withdrawn from their patients. "Their bedside manner is very impersonal," one senior said, "and they don't lose any sleep over clinical failures. They're cold but not inhuman." But in defense of the neurologist, a classmate remarked, "They have to be emotionally detached if they are to constantly confront diseases they can't cure."

As students learn more about the various branches of medicine, they increasingly compare neurologists with other specialists‡—to psychiatrists (very academically minded), to pathologists (academically and diagnostically inclined, and shielded from outside confrontations with patients), and to surgeons (compulsive, perfectionistic, and egotistical). But by far the greatest number of comments compare neurologists and internists. This is not surprising since neurology is, in fact, an offshoot of internal medicine. Specialists in both fields seem to have similar kinds of logical,

---

* The egotism of neurologists is mentioned by: freshmen, 11.9 percent; sophomores, 7.0 percent; juniors, 12.1 percent; and seniors, 9.1 percent.

† Neurologists are viewed as clinically and emotionally detached by 15.3 percent of the freshmen, 21.1 percent of the sophomores, 27.6 percent of the juniors, and 21.8 percent of the seniors.

‡ A few students see neurologists as similar to other specialists: freshmen, 10.2 percent; sophomores, 12.3 percent; juniors, 15.5 percent; and seniors, 21.8 percent.

analytical minds and an academic orientation; and both types "think a lot" and enjoy solving problems.

Dermatologist

Few freshmen have any idea as to the type of person who selects dermatology as a career. When queried, over 45 percent replied "I don't know." And by the senior year more than 30 percent still have no idea why this specialty is chosen.*

Among those having an opinion, the main view is that dermatologists like an easy life embellished with lots of practical advantages.† Dermatology is considered an easy specialty for these reasons:

a. It is clean: "It has none of the bloodiness or gory parts of medicine."
b. It is simple: "They can see the problem, recognize it, and make a snap, surface-level diagnosis. There is no need to comprehend the whole person."
c. It is delineated: "They deal with concrete and visible problems in narrowly restricted areas."

In addition, the dermatologist, in comparison to other specialists, reportedly experiences little pressure or responsibility. There are few demanding emergency-type situations that have grave life-or-death consequences. "Dermatologists deal with people who are not really sick," one commented. "They just help them with their discomforts." A dermatologist is quoted by a clinician as saying: "Whenever I hear a siren go by at 3 o'clock in the morning, I just roll over and go back to sleep, knowing full well that I won't be called to the hospital."

A steadily increasing number of students cite such practical advantages as the principal motivation for entering dermatology. By the senior year, three-fourths of the class describe this specialty as "a good field in which to get rich." "Dermatologists rarely cure patients," one said, "so they come back time after time, paying money for each visit; there's a perpetual supply and the hours are great!" These specialists, students note, live in big houses, drive luxury cars, take long vacations, and avidly participate in a variety of personal hobbies and outside interests. In short, dermatology is "a luxury-type medicine."

For the above reasons, students often doubt the motivation and dedica-

---

* Throughout the entire four years, an unusually large number reply "I don't know" when asked to describe the type of person who goes into dermatology: freshmen, 45.8 percent; sophomores, 52.6 percent; juniors, 41.4 percent; and seniors, 30.9 percent.

† More than in any other specialty, practical advantages are seen as motivating a career choice in dermatology. Those who mention this factor include 45.8 percent of the freshmen, 50.9 percent of the sophomores, 51.7 percent of the juniors, and 74.5 percent of the seniors.

tion of these practitioners. "They're not true go-getters who are really in there pitching for the patient," one said. "They are people who are looking for simple problems and a soft life." Instead of working hard in medicine, up to the standard of other physicians, "their idea of good practice is to treat skin rashes of rich women who live in the country-club area and to spend a lot of time hunting, golfing, and leading a full social life."

It is not surprising, then, that dermatologists, like radiologists, are sometimes described as "medical cop-outs"—practitioners who are neither dedicated nor clinically involved in primary patient care. In this view, dermatology is peripheral to medical practice, "sort of like the skin is to the body, rather superficial and outside the mainstream." "To settle for dermatology," said one senior, "is tantamount to leaving the medical profession—like selling one's medical birthright for a mess of dermatological pottage!" "I can't imagine why anyone would go all the way through medical school and then end up being a dermatologist," another commented. "I guess they're sorry they went into medicine and they're trying to get away from it. It's the easy way out."

A few students state the extreme view that dermatology is a "quackery —a racket" and its practitioners are "weird, shifty-eyed crooks" or "frustrated witch doctors."* Fortunately such views are balanced by a few who regard this specialty as a more complicated field than most realize and its practitioners as intelligent and knowledgeable clinicians who perform an important role.†

Anesthesiologist

Initially the anesthesiologist is more of an enigma to medical students than any other specialist, even more so than the dermatologist.‡ When asked to describe these practitioners, almost two-thirds of the freshmen say they have no idea whatsoever; and even in the senior year, more than a fourth of the class still have no description to offer. Among those having an opinion, little group consensus exists.

Upon learning that this specialty involves the application of physiology and pharmacology, students then begin to identify anesthesiologists in terms of these academic specialists—"Ph.D.-inclined people having more

---

* Those few who typify dermatologists as having the negative traits described include: freshmen, 8.5 percent; sophomores, 3.5 percent; juniors, 1.7 percent; and seniors, 5.5 percent.

† Dermatologists are described as knowledgeable and competent by 1.7 percent of the freshmen, 5.3 percent of the sophomores, 5.2 percent of the juniors, and 7.3 percent of the seniors.

‡ "No opinion" regarding the work of the anesthesiologist is held by 62.7 percent of the freshmen, 47.4 percent of the sophomores, 39.7 percent of the juniors, and 27.3 percent of the seniors.

of an exact science approach than a clinical one." Realizing that the anesthesiologist's main contact with patients is to put other doctors' patients to sleep, underclassmen tend to regard them as being more paramedical than medical. "They're high-class technicians," one said, "the kind of people that like to turn knobs and run machinery." * "Anesthesiology is the farthest thing out of actual medical practice," a classmate added. "It attracts those who just don't seem to make it anywhere else in medicine."

Such disparaging comments, although fairly common among underclassmen, cease altogether in the senior year when students experience a brief clerkship in this specialty. This experience fosters an awareness of this field's knowledgeable, capable, and highly skilled individuals.† "I used to think all they did was put people to sleep," one said, "but now I see them as real lifesavers. In fact, if I were in a pinch and someone in my family needed assistance fast, that's who I'd call."

A few seniors even go so far as to describe anesthesiology as "the most exact art in medicine." This acknowledgment came when one student first performed the anesthesiologist's role with animals:

> When I became the anesthesiologist, I learned how much of an art it is just to keep a rabbit alive. One little drop too much and it would be cyanosed. When I tried to bring it back, it would be jumping on the table. To keep it in that extremely narrow zone was quite an effort.

This student then concluded, "When I consider a person doing this with a human being—keeping him from responding to the surgeon's knives, yet keeping him from dying—I realize that person really has to have a lot on the ball!"

Physicians in other fields who lack primary patient contact are usually described as being shy, withdrawn, inhibited, and cold. And during the first three years, these labels are attributed to anesthesiologists.‡ But, after having gained firsthand exposure, a few seniors enthusiastically describe them as warm, friendly, outgoing personalities.§ They also see them as level-headed and having a high tolerance for stress. "They'd have to be," one said, "in order to put up with all of the crap from the surgeons."

---

* Anesthesiologists are seen as pharmacologically and technically oriented: freshmen, 5.1 percent; sophomores, 17.5 percent; juniors, 25.9 percent; and seniors, 29.1 percent.

† Although no freshmen view anesthesiologists as knowledgeable, capable, and highly skilled, this trend reverses in the ensuing years; 7.0 percent of the sophomores, 12.1 percent of the juniors, and 20.0 percent of the seniors see them as possessing these qualities.

‡ Anesthesiologists are seen as having negative traits only during the first three years (freshmen, 6.8 percent; sophomores, 10.5 percent; and juniors, 15.5 percent). No seniors mention this view.

§ Pleasing personalities are attributed to anesthesiologists by 3.4 percent of the freshmen, 8.8 percent of the sophomores, 8.6 percent of the juniors, and 10.9 percent of the seniors.

In the final year, almost one-fourth of the class compare anesthesiologists with surgeons;* that is, they are seen as having the surgeon's enjoyment of the excitement and drama of the operating room—the emergency, life-or-death atmosphere—but they do not like to cut. They would rather "avoid the blood-and-guts aspect by alleviating pain on the sidelines."

As with many other specialties, self-interest is also seen as playing a part in attracting people to this field.† An increasing number of students make this observation; in the senior year, nearly 30 percent of the class describe these doctors as persons who want an easy workload, good hours, few demands, plenty of money, and ample time for family and personal life.

SUMMING UP

Traditionally, doctors have been placed on a pedestal and attributed almost superhuman qualities of professional and personal excellence. And medical recruits often reflect these lay attitudes. Even when able to differentiate between personality types in the various specialties, they are still romantic in their views. But with greater exposure to the inner world of medical practice, students, like their mentors, develop critical insights about the various specialists.

Although some entering students already know what specialty they want, deciding on a branch of medicine is, for most of them, a complex decision that takes years of thoughtful consideration. A candidate must weigh personal interests and abilities against clinical opportunities. And, as this chapter's lead-in quote suggests, practitioners in each field also influence their thinking. If all specialties seemed equally attractive, the decision processes would be formidable. So, students narrow down the field by focusing on idiosyncratic features of each specialty and its practitioners.

Few, if any, obstetrical patients, for example, would agree that their male doctors have unusual sexual concerns. In fact, women who read drafts of this chapter were angered at the suggestion that obstetricians might have such problems. Psychologically speaking, a female patient cannot afford to regard her male doctor in this negative way; and, because of this practitioner's key role in seeing her through one of life's most meaningful moments, the birth of her child, she holds the obstetrician in high

---

* Anesthesiologists are seen as being similar to surgeons by: freshmen, 3.4 percent; sophomores, 5.3 percent; juniors, 10.3 percent; and seniors, 21.8 percent.

† Self-interest is perceived as a motivator in selecting the field of anesthesiology by: freshmen, 11.9 percent; sophomores, 14.0 percent; juniors, 10.3 percent; and seniors, 29.1 percent.

esteem. The medical student, however, is searching for a medical specialty rather than a physician to deliver future offspring; so the student casts aside this doctor's "halo" and focuses instead on the idiosyncracies. As mentioned, exaggerating the negative features helps undergraduates narrow down the field. This process no doubt prompts students to portray surgeons as "sublimating sadists who like to cut" or the pediatrician as the "high school Harry who has trouble getting along with people his own size."

Some specialty areas are, of course, more easily characterized than others. Most students have at one time or another been treated by a general practitioner and a pediatrician, so their initial impressions of these doctors are quite clear. Others, however, such as neurologists, dermatologists, and radiologists, project an unclear image due to lack of prior familiarity.

Lacking better ideas, students sometimes attribute to such specialists characterizations that are typical of the patients they serve. Thus, neurologists are seen as brainy, psychiatrists as crazy, pathologists as ghoulish, and dermatologists as superficial.

Finally, it is significant that the most consistently critical comments are made about specialists who avoid "front line" contact with patients, because such specialists presumably lack dedication for primary patient welfare. In these cases the negative appellations "lazy" and "mercenary" sometimes remain with those who choose "easy specialties."

Most admired are doctors who are willing to devote long hours of hard work in face-to-face contact with patients. Dedication and self-sacrifice have propelled students thus far in their professional journeys, and in medical school these values remain the criteria by which practitioners are judged. For this reason, most students eventually select those specialties that keep them in the mainstream of clinical practice and offer the greatest probability of respect from their medical colleagues.

NOTES

1. Patricia L. Kendall (1971a, b) provides an excellent background concerning the trends, contributing factors, and consequences of medical specialization. For a review of the research that has been done on medical students selecting a specialty, see Rezler (1969), Held and Zimet (1975), and Gough (1975a, b). See also Knafl and Burkett (1975) for a study of professional socialization among 20 surgery residents.
2. See Hutchins (1962) and Boverman (1965) for other studies that show the change of career choice patterns both during and after medical school. See also Becker et al. (1961, p. 402).
3. In this regard, see Livingston and Zimet (1965).

4. See Kendall's (1971a, pp. 484–485) discussion on the influence of role models in medical specialty choices.

5. For additional understanding of students' views concerning prestige rankings of the various fields of practice, see Fish and Mount (1966).

6. For a comparison of perceptions of students in other medical education settings, Bruhn and Parsons offer two studies (1964 and 1965) of different-year medical students' perceptions about the medical specialties. The forced-choice study (1964) reveals choices similar to those obtained in the open-ended questions used in this study.

10. Self-Attitudes

At first I felt awfully out of place with my little black bag and stetho-scope. I was always embarrassed and wanted to tell patients, "I am only a student." But now it's beginning to feel natural because people don't look at me askance as I go by. (A senior)

A FAMILIAR BEHAVIORAL SCIENCE THEOREM IS: When individuals define things or situations as real, these definitions become real in their conse-quences (Thomas, 1928). When one perceives himself or herself in a certain way (a bad person, for example), that self-definition becomes realized through the natural tendency to adopt the expected role. A person who feels inept in a particular activity will, in all likelihood, avoid that activity and thereby fail to develop the needed skills that invite success. Thus, a self-fulfilling prophecy is established.[1]

An effective way to initiate a desired behavior is to help that person first develop the appropriate self-attitude, that is, encourage the feeling of success and comfort in performing the prescribed role. Good scholarship, for example, does not spring naturally from those who regard themselves as bad students. But when unproductive students start thinking of them-selves as intelligent and scholarly, their behavior will naturally change in that direction, too. For as we view ourselves, so do we act.

Obviously, the successful practice of medicine requires the attainment of a professional identity. An effective physician must not only have mas-tered the required knowledge and skills, but must also have gained the self-confidence necessary to apply this professional training. To a very large extent, professional behavior reflects self-attitudes.

How medical school experiences affect the self-attitudes of prospective physicians is discussed in this chapter. First, the overall impact of medical education on the self-esteem of students is examined, and then the per-sonality changes that the latter see in themselves as a result of medical education are scrutinized. Finally, the emerging self-image is explored—how and when students start thinking of themselves as physicians and begin feeling confident in the performance of the doctor's role.

MEDICAL SCHOOL EFFECTS ON SELF-ESTEEM

On the college campus, premedical students are generally regarded with high esteem, not only because of their academic achievement but also for their prestigious career ambitions. Winning a competitive place in medical school is a personal victory for a college student, followed by plaudits from family, friends, and fellow students. In this network of significant others, who provide the social looking-glass whereby self-attitudes are formed, it would seem that he or she had arrived.

Ego-Deflating Effects of Medical School

In reality, however, entrance into medical school brings a precipitous drop in status. One's new reference group now consists of classmates, clinicians, and, to some extent, experienced hospital aides, all of whom regard beginning medical students as unproven underlings. When asked to describe where they fit in the social structure of the teaching hospital, most freshmen (88 percent) perceive themselves as being very low; some even rate themselves as being "on the very bottom rung of the ladder—the lowest of the low." [2]

Lacking medical experience and knowledge, the initiate must start anew to build status and the respect of associates. But this is much easier said than achieved. As previously indicated, competition for grades is keen. Everywhere a beginning student turns, there are others who seem smarter and more capable. "In medical school," one said, "you move up into another league as far as intelligence and competition are concerned and you find that you are no longer on top of the pile. When you are constantly confronted with others who are smarter, you can't think of yourself as 'it' anymore."

Students have ample reasons for self doubts, for it is virtually impossible to grasp and retain the overwhelming amount of material they are held accountable for. As previously pointed out, it is not unusual for beginning students to feel inadequate—in sharp contrast with earlier self-attitudes. "I was pretty cocky when I came here," a freshman said; "I thought I had it licked. I did so well in college I thought it would just take a minor adjustment and everything would be great. But it hasn't been that way at all; my self-confidence has really taken a beating." [3]

Struggling against formidable odds, students come face to face with personal shortcomings. "Your limitations are slapped right in front of you," one said, "and you feel small, inadequate, and unsure of yourself." For these reasons, one-third of the class during the freshman and sophomore years report that medical school has had a negative, humbling effect upon their self-esteem.*

Ego-Enhancing Effects of Medical School

Despite these ego-deflating experiences, nearly one-third of the freshman class view medical school as affecting their self-esteem in a positive, uplifting way. And this number increases progressively during each year of school. By the time they become seniors, more than three-fourths of the class acknowledge that medical training has enhanced their self-esteem.

The prestige of the medical profession has great potential for cultivating favorable self-images. To be accepted as a potential member of this elite profession makes students feel "set apart as someone special." Although this "exceptional" feeling fades in the day-to-day grind of the preclinical years, it is reinforced whenever students leave the confines of the medical center for the outside world. "When you are in med school you feel that you are at the bottom," a freshman explained; "but whenever you leave and go home, your status is definitely higher. People really respect you and are interested in what you are doing." A senior underscored this principle: "Anybody striving to be a doctor has immediate respect; this can't help but improve your self-image when it's shown you every time you turn around."

Not all ego rewards, however, come from outside sources. Simply being able to endure the difficulties gives medical students an intrinsic sense of accomplishment and self-esteem. Those who worry about their capacity to achieve are especially encouraged by sheer survival, their demonstrated ability to put up with the ordeal. "Medical school is a great challenge," one said, "but I'm making it! It's not an easy task, and only a select number of people get through. So it's really building my confidence and ego-strength."

As students progress toward their goal—heading, as one said, "for some place I like to be headed"—personal satisfaction and self-esteem are enhanced. This feeling of self-fulfillment is captured by the sophomore who pointed out, "Having the goal of wanting to be a good physician and feeling that I am progressing toward that goal gives me the positive feeling that I'm where I am supposed to be."

Self-esteem is especially bolstered in the junior and senior years by

* When asked, "How have medical school experiences affected your self-image?" negative effects were reported by 34.6 percent of the freshmen, 33.3 percent of the sophomores, 15.5 percent of the juniors, and 18.2 percent of the seniors. Positive effects were reported by 30.5 percent of the freshmen, 52.6 percent of the sophomores, 57.2 percent of the juniors, and 76.4 percent of the seniors. The remainder indicated "no change."

awareness of increased clinical knowledge and confidence. "I'm worth more now," one explained, "because I'm getting more intelligent each year and learning new skills; I like myself better because I'm getting somewhere."

The "badges of office" worn around the hospital further boost the ego of junior and senior medical students. One who struts around in a white coat conspicuously displaying a stethoscope is more readily regarded as a high-status person. "When patients call you 'doctor' and act respectful," one student observed, "it is pretty ego-satisfying."

The clinical responsibilities increasingly given to students during the last years of school intensify self-esteem by building feelings of independence and competence. One said:

> You feel that your training is finally beginning to bear fruit and that all of your efforts for the last seven or eight years have not been in vain. Rather than thinking of yourself as a perpetual student you now begin to see yourself as a trained professional, capable of doing something useful in the world.

Increased self-esteem in the clinical years also results from more personalized relationships with attending physicians and house staff. In the classroom setting, preclinical students get lost in the crowd. But in the hospital, a student is no longer simply one face among many. "Nearly everyone knows my name now," a junior marveled. Such one-to-one interaction provides a more direct exchange of ideas with those emulated; and this does far more for one's self-esteem than simply "sitting in a classroom and listening to somebody spout off at you for an hour."

Nonetheless, a few thorns still exist among the clinical roses. Although the number whose egos are deflated by medical school experiences decreases by one-half during the clinical years, one out of six upperclassmen still feels a little "let down." Although superior to freshmen and sophomores, they still feel as if they are "low on the totem pole," especially when first going on the hospital floors. There is a new set of superiors to please, and subservience to house staff and attending physicians sometimes makes them feel like "incompetent nobodies." Being dependent on nurses and other allied health workers to find their way around the wards also contributes to feelings of insignificance and helplessness.

Finally, dependence on family members for financial support does little to promote feelings of self-respect. "As long as you're not able to pay your own way," a senior volunteered, "your self-image isn't so great; and being a student when you are 24 or 25 years old does nothing for your ego, either." In balance, though, the positive, uplifting effects of medical training clearly outweigh these negative feelings. So, as graduation approaches, the typical feeling is, as one put it, "I look at myself and feel that I have improved a great deal."

SELF-PERCEIVED CHANGES DURING MEDICAL SCHOOL

The obvious changes occurring among students between their entrance into medical school as trainees and their departure as doctors years later are clearly visible to any observer. And these transformations do not escape the notice of participants. Even as freshmen, more than half the class report significant differences in themselves and their classmates. And those who regard their medical school exposure as too slight to have brought about much alteration frequently say they expect to change.

Following the freshman year, three out of four students view themselves as having changed noticeably; the remainder, when probed, usually acknowledge a lesser degree of change. One such junior said, "There have been no 90-degree turns; but I'm still developing on the same curve." *

Fortunately, most students perceive themselves as changing in a positive rather than a negative manner. This finding is demonstrated not only by student comments but also by results of the *Adjective Check List* (Gough and Heilbrun, 1965). This paper-and-pencil test gives subjects an opportunity to check adjectives (cheerful, tense, etc.) from a list of 300 that best describe themselves. Completed by students during their first week at medical school and again at the end of the senior year, this self-descriptive check list, as well as the interview data, shows pronounced shifts in self-attitudes, mostly in a constructive direction.

Acquiring Greater Maturity

The first change usually noticed by students about themselves is their maturation. They are more responsible, serious-minded, and disciplined. Rather than behaving impulsively as they were once prone to do, they begin to see themselves becoming more cautious and careful.† Commenting on the impulsiveness of beginning students, a third-year student observed: "I shudder to think that I was ever like that. They leap first and look later."

Even in the freshman year, some students perceive themselves as having matured. This developmental trend is made clear through comparisons with college students. After spending some time with one applicant, a freshman remarked, "I didn't realize how much I had matured until

---

* Of the freshmen, 44.1 percent perceive no significant changes in themselves or their classmates, but the number drops to 26.3 percent in the sophomore year. In the final two years the proportion who fail to note changes are 17.2 percent (junior year) and 25.4 percent (senior year).

† *Adjective Check List* (Gough and Heilbrun, 1965) data show that whereas only 20.7 percent of the entering freshmen describe themselves as being cautious, the proportion jumps to 75.6 percent in the senior year.

I listened to him talk and watched his actions. I couldn't believe that's the way I used to be."

As students progress through school, they tend to view themselves as more "grown up" or "settled down"; that is, more sober, subdued, and sedate. "I still like to joke around," one observed, "but it isn't continuous like before; I keep it under control now."

Kicking up their heels with the gang is a declining behavior, no doubt due to the fact that many students are marrying and assuming family responsibilities. But increasing maturity is also related to their training and work, particularly to the massiveness of future responsibilities in caring for patients. "You kind of march along day after day just trying to survive," one said, "and then suddenly all that responsibility for patients looms up before you. You figure, 'Man, I've got to shape up!' You'd like to put the brakes on a little to slow things as you go down the stretch, but it's too late." For this reason, as a student indicates, "Everybody in the class has grown up a lot; we've probably matured more in four years than we normally would have in ten had we not been in medical school."

Gaining Confidence and Self-Reliance

From the perspective of incoming freshmen, fourth-year students seem somewhat larger than life. "They walk a little taller, have a firmer hand-shake, and are more sure of themselves," a freshman observed. "You just hope you're going to be like that when you are a senior." *

Confidence is enhanced by successfully meeting the imposing challenges of medical school. As previously discussed, mere survival is an accomplishment, something in which students can justifiably take pride. Faith in oneself grows when acquiring greater knowledge and learning that one can function under pressure. Confidence increases most, though, through the acquisition of clinical know-how. Until then, students are not sure of their ability to integrate and apply their newly acquired knowledge. A third-year student explains: "I've had to do things that I never thought I would be able to do; a few clinical successes and a few good diagnoses have really boosted my confidence."

While progressing through school, students increasingly view themselves as being more assertive, as taking an active rather than a passive role in their own education.† As underclassmen, they are told what they are supposed

---

* *Adjective Check List* (Gough and Heilbrun, 1965) data show that whereas 50 percent of the entering freshmen describe themselves as being self-confident, the proportion increases to 75.6 percent in the senior year.

† *Adjective Check List* (Gough and Heilbrun, 1965) data show that 27.6 percent of the entering freshmen describe themselves as being assertive. This proportion rises to 53.3 percent in the senior year.

to learn and are given frequent examinations to make sure they actually do it. But in the clinical years, students are given greater responsibility for their own education, and self-direction replaces external pressures. "You realize that it's all up to you," one said. "You've got to think things out for yourself and make your own decisions because nobody else is going to do it for you." These experiences enhance self-assurance and assertiveness. Even the quieter students seem to come out of their shells and demonstrate independence.

Feeling a Part of the Medical Profession

As grades and other situation-oriented goals give way to long-range career objectives, students become aware of their transition from learner to professional. Increasingly, medicine becomes central to their being rather than a distant dream for the future. "Instead of classes, grades, and homework," a sophomore succinctly states, "medicine becomes a way of life."

This shift is greatly enhanced when students begin regarding their mentors, not as adversaries, but as role models to be emulated. Related to this is a change of attitude about studying. After two years of studying for competitive purposes, students now do so to prepare themselves for their own futures. A third-year student underscores this point: "During the first couple of years, it's like college all over again—you take notes, study, and cram for exams; but gradually you find yourself studying not because you have to, but because you want to."

Opportunities to perform the doctor's role also hasten identification with the medical profession. When treating patients, it is easy to project oneself into the full doctor status. A senior makes this comment:

> As a freshman, I really didn't think of myself as being part of the medical profession—I didn't associate with other doctors as I do now. By the end of my time in medical school, though, I started looking at myself as a physician, although I'm not quite there yet.

The behavioral effect of this attitudinal transition is easily seen. For example, students are often surprised to see once lighthearted and frivolous classmates "shape up" into highly motivated clinicians who take their work very seriously. "I see people who weren't especially good students at first," one said, "who blossomed out and came into their own; they're really interested in their work now." In this regard, seniors, as compared to freshmen, are naturally seen as having clearer focus on their career goals, more devoted to medicine, and less interested in other things—even preoccupied with medicine to the point of excluding other matters. "Whenever I hear seniors talking in the student lounge," a freshman observed, "it's always about some patient or where they are going to do their internship or the like; I never hear them talk about tennis or anything like that. Medicine is their sole topic of conversation." From the freshman perspective, seniors not only seem completely absorbed in the medical milieu; they also act less like students and more like doctors—steady, calm, reliable, controlled, self-possessed, and dignified.

Becoming More Realistic

The shift from an idealistic to a more realistic appraisal of physicians, the medical profession, and oneself as a future doctor is noted by some students. "Exposure to the realities of medical school," one said, "dissolves a lot of romantic myths about medical school and physicians in general."

As previously discussed, a common idea among freshmen is the necessity of mastering all the assigned materials because, as one put it, "When you go up on the wards, you're going to have to have all the answers for everything; you can't make mistakes." But this unrealistic view is, students note, replaced with a more practical one as they gain experience.

A corollary misconception is that doctors are infallible. "Before I entered medical school," a sophomore commented, "I didn't see how a doctor could do anything wrong." But after exposure to the teaching hospital, this student and others realize the absurdity of these notions. Their moment of illumination comes when comparing the enormous amount of knowledge and wisdom expected of doctors with the fact that, in spite of their intelligence and dedication, they are only human. And they learn by firsthand experience that, as one expressed it, "Doctors are going to make mistakes and nothing can be done about it."

Intensified exposure to the medical world helps the future doctor shape a more realistic self-image. If that image had previously been one of superior intelligence, it is often replaced by one of humility. Willingness to accept criticism is another indication of a more reasonable self-appraisal. "I can admit it now when I'm wrong," a junior acknowledged. "Whenever someone used to point out one of my mistakes, I'd have a list of excuses a yard long. Now I say, 'You're right. I'll try to do better next time.' I've learned that admitting an error has the added benefit of causing the other person to back off, too."

Romantic notions about doctors "saving everybody" and "altering the course of the world" are scaled down to more realistic proportions in medical school. "Rather than imagining myself saving the world," a junior said, "I intend to help as many people as I can." Even this curtailed ambition appears naive and sentimental to some, such as the senior who said, "I'm more willing now to look at the profession realistically. I'm more inclined to consider it a business in which I will be meeting the needs of the public as well as looking after my own interests. I will be providing for my family just as a businessman does."

Being More Relaxed and Contented

As students proceed through school they increasingly describe themselves as more relaxed and happy with their lot in life. Those who initially viewed themselves as compulsively driven, nervous, and tense gradually see themselves as more calm and easygoing. Once the worry of academic failure is minimized, the "push-push syndrome," as one describes it, gives way to a "simmered down" attitude.* "I've become calmer this year," a sophomore commented. "I've got a year behind me and know that I can do it if I apply myself. I thought I had to study all the time or I would flunk out of school; but now I realize that I'm okay."

Finding more clinical relevance to their activities accounts in large part, students say, for their increasing contentment. "Last year everything was crammed down my throat," a sophomore explained, "and I couldn't see any value to it. But now that I'm closer to the third year, I'm much more enthusiastic and happy." Once in the clinical years, students view the work as more relevant to their career aspirations. Rather than being dependents who do work assigned by others, they now visualize themselves as career apprentices being prepared for independence. A third-year student underscores the change:

> When I came to medical school, I was really gung-ho—but then I got all bogged down in classroom stuff and lost my vision about what I was doing here. I really got fed up and was just about to throw in the towel. But when I got involved in clinical work at the end of the second year, I started finding myself.

Other Changes

The foregoing discussion of self-perceived changes during medical school is based primarily upon responses to the open-ended question, "Have you changed much since beginning medical school? If so, how?" Responses on the *Adjective Check List*, administered at the beginning of the freshman year and again at the end of the senior year, complement these results. Test responses reveal other pronounced changes as well. Findings show a changing self-perception among students as being more

---

* *Adjective Check List* (Gough and Heilbrun, 1965) data indicate that whereas 31 percent of the entering freshmen view themselves as being calm, in the senior year 57.8 percent have this self-attitude.

outgoing, stubborn, optimistic, sensitive, and farsighted; and less quiet, nervous, trusting, and moderate.*

To recapitulate, most medical students view themselves as changing noticeably as a direct result of medical school experiences. Happily, these changes are, in the student view, in a constructive and positive direction. Despite the struggles and vicissitudes of medical school training, the result is generally a favorable one as far as self-concept is concerned.

IDENTIFYING WITH THE DOCTOR'S STATUS

Coming to regard oneself as a doctor, of course, does not happen quickly but requires time and a constant variety of career-oriented experiences. Although this professional "coming of age" is no doubt formally indicated when the newly minted doctor first signs his or her name followed by "M.D.," the actual process of becoming one is so gradual as to be almost imperceptible. There are few milestones to mark the change. Countless experiences blend together to enmesh a student in the process until at last the dream of being a doctor becomes reality.

During the yearly interviews, students are asked to indicate on a seven-point scale, one end of which is labeled "layman" and the other "doctor," where they currently view themselves to be in this transition. The results are shown in Fig. 10–1.† Judging from the freshman responses, simply getting into medical school does much to promote a professional self-concept, since it sets students apart from laymen. Each year thereafter, an increasing number see themselves as progressively gaining the "doctor" status. But, it should be noted, seniors do not yet view themselves as having "arrived." Viewing oneself as a doctor apparently involves more than just graduating from medical school. The following factors are contributing influences.

Acquiring Knowledge and Clinical Skills

The evolutionary path to becoming a doctor requires clinical proficiency based upon knowledge. As knowledge increases and ability to

---

* The percentage changes shown for each self-descriptive adjective from the freshman to the senior year are as follows: (1) outgoing, 31.0–55.6 percent; (2) stubborn, 27.6–51.1 percent; (3) optimistic, 50.0–73.3 percent; (4) sensitive, 56.9–80.0 percent; (5) farsighted, 55.2–75.6 percent; (6) quiet, 58.6–33.3 percent; (7) nervous, 39.7–15.6 percent; (8) trusting, 63.8–42.2 percent; and (9) moderate, 79.3–57.8 percent.

† The percentage of students in each year whose scale scores are 6 or 7 (that is, at the "doctor" end of the scale) is as follows: freshmen, 1.7; sophomores, 5.3; juniors, 13.8; and seniors, 45.4. By contrast, the percentage of those having scores of 1 or 2 (the "layman" end of the scale) is: freshmen, 32.2; sophomores, 12.3; juniors, 1.7; and seniors, 0.

FIGURE 10-1. Professional Self-Image During Medical School

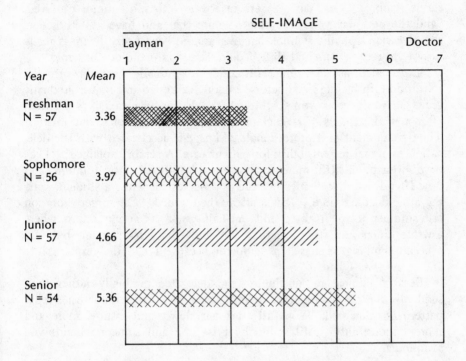

diagnose and handle patients improves, so does the image of oneself as a physician.

Because competition with classmates is keen, students sometimes fail to perceive how much they have learned until it is brought to their attention by outsiders. When associating only with other medical personnel, it is assumed that their own knowledge is common knowledge. But, during home visits, casual conversations on medical topics are clearly beyond the comprehension of laymen. "When you are always around the hospital," one said, "you have the feeling that everybody else knows what you know. But when you throw standard hospital terms around home, nobody knows what you are talking about. It really surprises me and makes me realize that I'm gradually making a transition."

Playing the Doctor's Role

Being constantly exposed to the medical environment encourages identification with the doctor's status. "You are just around the hospital so much for so many years," a senior points out, "that you gradually become part of it in your thinking." A professional identity is enhanced when the student is cast in the physician's role and given the proper status symbols. "One day you are in street clothes," a junior observed, "and the next day you're wearing a white coat and have a stethoscope, the physician's phallic symbol, hanging around your neck. There is really no way to escape a mental shift. You're thrust into the doctor's role."

Expected to act like physicians, students gradually "just slip into the role and begin feeling like doctors." As one expressed it, "It just gradually grows on you because you go through the doctor's routine so much that, after a while, things start clicking for you and it becomes automatic." The development of a professional self-image is accelerated with the delegation of actual responsibility for patient care. A senior explained: "They have given me a little more responsibility on my pediatric rotation, and now I tend to think of myself more as a doctor than just a student walking around doing time." This student then added, "On surgery rotation last summer, I spent three and one-half weeks as acting intern where I wrote orders and stuff like that. Not only did I learn a lot, but also I began thinking of myself as a doctor because I had the responsibility and knew that I had it."

Because clinical responsibilities are delegated gradually rather than suddenly, the development of a professional self-image follows a similar pattern. As one said, "You just start out slowly and assume more and more responsibility—until suddenly it is June and someone hands you a diploma."

Being Viewed by Others as a Doctor

That self-attitudes are shaped by interpersonal encounters is a well-documented principle. Self-views result from imagining how others view oneself. This social looking-glass phenomenon contributes substantially to the development of a professional self-image; for it is predictable that medical students will begin thinking of themselves as physicians when called "doctor" by patients and accepted by them as having clinical competence.

As previously discussed, many students initially feel uncomfortable in passing themselves off as doctors. "At the beginning of my first clinical rotation I was kind of embarrassed when patients called me 'doctor,'" one said, "I felt like I was cheating them and ought to tell them the truth." The first experience of being called "doctor" brings an urge "to chuckle at the remark." But when exposed to repeated usage, students gradually become accustomed to this prestigious title and begin thinking of themselves in this way. As they gain confidence, some clarify their status as students, not doctors. When a patient expresses surprise, the student's professional self-image is bolstered. "It really made my day," a junior reported in describing such an experience.

The self-image of a physician is enhanced when hospital personnel also use the doctor's title in addressing clinical students. Although interns and residents may, when speaking privately, call a student by his first name, the "doctor" title is routinely used around patients. Similarly, telephone operators consistently page third- and fourth-year students as "Dr. _____." "At first," a junior remarked, "it really feels weird to hear yourself being paged as a doctor; but later on you get used to it." The dual status occupied by clinical students—doctor and student—is clearly indicated by this senior: "It really gives you a big head when you hear yourself paged; but your ego soon gets deflated, because it isn't long before you're emptying a bedpan for somebody."

Professional self-concepts are nurtured most by the accepting and approving attitudes of attending doctors and house staff, who, with the passage of time, increasingly regard clinical students as physicians-to-be, apprentice members of the medical profession. Recognition by others outside the medical environment also reinforces the student's identification with the doctor's status. Even during the preclinical years, neighbors and acquaintances call medical students "doc" and request medical advice. "Your friends and family start asking you questions about various things," one said. "I have found myself looking into their ears, feeling their necks, etc., thinking they might have 'mono' or something."

In short, the social mirror in which students view themselves increasingly reflects a doctor's image. Consequently, they gradually internalize the doctor's status and come to regard themselves as regarded by others. This process is succinctly expressed by one senior who said, "People look at me as a doctor, so I am."

PERFORMING THE DOCTOR'S ROLE CONFIDENTLY

It is one thing to regard oneself as a doctor or a doctor-to-be (that is, to identify with the doctor's status), and quite another to feel competent to perform the doctor's role. Although freshmen may feel like apprentice doctors, they lack confidence in their ability to diagnose and treat patients. (Compare Figs. 10–1 and 10–2.) Although self-assurance increases gradually during the subsequent years of medical school, relatively few seniors express more than a moderate degree of confidence. Even the most self-assured seniors qualify their responses by pointing out a variety of conditions necessary to feel competent.* A large majority believe that full

* The percentage of students in each year whose scale scores are 6 or 7 (that is, at the "high confidence" end of the scale) is as follows: freshmen, 1.7; sophomores, 1.8; juniors, 5.4; and seniors, 15.6. By contrast, the percentage of those having scores of

FIGURE 10-2.   Self-Confidence Regarding Independent Performance of the Doctor's Role

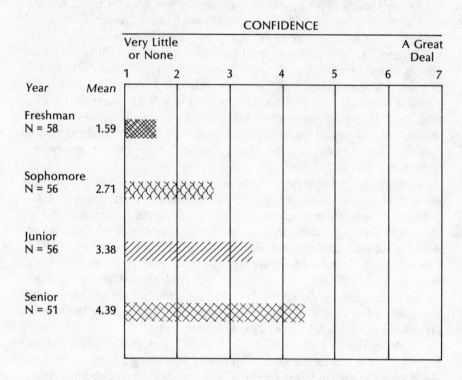

confidence does not come until internship or residency, or perhaps even later. "I doubt that I'll ever feel totally confident about all diseases," a senior commented. "Even big-wheel attendings [faculty physicians] don't feel that way about all of them. But I should feel pretty competent about handling the routine medical problems by the end of my internship."

Barriers to Self-Confidence

Developing confidence to perform the doctor's role competently depends, of course, upon wide exposure to practical clinical problems and ample opportunity to exercise personal responsibility. Although the medical school curriculum is designed to provide these, the teaching experience, in the judgment of students, falls short in some respects.

Because freshmen and sophomores spend most of their time in class-

1 or 2 (the "little or no confidence" end of the scale) is: freshmen, 84.5; sophomores, 50.0; juniors, 28.5; and seniors, 5.8.

rooms and laboratories, their clinical experience is extremely limited; and even during the last two years, students sometimes complain about inadequate exposure to patients. The field of medicine is so vast and the problems so varied and complicated that the exposure seems too limited in scope and depth.

As noted in Chapter 6, emphasis on the exotic rather than common medical problems can impede self-confidence. "Actually I think a person who has never been to medical school may feel more confident than I do," a sophomore commented. "An ordinary person knows more about common medical problems just from experience; in medical school we concentrate on rare things." Because the emphasis is on exotic diseases, students worry about their ability to diagnose commonplace maladies. "I saw my first strep throat yesterday," a junior remarked. "As common as this may be, I couldn't diagnose it. What popped into my mind was some strange syndrome studied in pathology. I just don't remember the common things because they aren't stressed."

Also undermining confidence is suspicion about the worth of classroom knowledge. "Many of the 'absolutes' we've picked up in the classroom" a sophomore said, "are not that absolute at the bedside." Word filters down from upperclassmen that "diseases don't look at all like you think they will." To illustrate this a junior pointed out, "We've had several lectures on pneumonococcus, the organism that causes pneumonia. We learned all about the symptoms, treatments, etc., but when I saw an actual case of pneumonia I didn't know what it was. Yet I supposedly had all this background and training. But you just don't learn this kind of thing from books."

Armed with book knowledge of medicine and little practical experience, is, preclinical students point out, like learning to drive a car by reading a driver's manual without adequate opportunity to sit behind the wheel. Confronting patients rather than books, undergraduates say, is the only way to build confidence. But they soon learn that seeing patients is not a panacea for self-doubts. For one thing, the abrupt change from the theoretical, book-oriented approach to the practical, problem-solving approach of the clinical years necessitates a readjustment in thinking. The logic of the textbook approach involves reasoning from the disease processes to the symptoms; but the practical approach reasons from the symptoms to the disease. So, it takes time to reorient one's thinking. "This new approach in reasoning just hasn't jelled yet," a junior complained.

Moreover, clinical students typically feel they are not given adequate opportunity to exercise independent judgment. Rarely, if ever, are they first in line to see patients; instead they stand in the shadows of house officers and attending physicians, waiting their turn. The dilemma is graphically portrayed by this senior:

By the time I get to a patient, they have already taken a battery of lab tests and have a pat story all worked out. When I come on the floors they tell me, "We've got a patient with Parkinson's disease in room 207 and a case of leukemia in 305." So, the diagnosis is already made for me! I have to practically hold my hands over my ears when I walk down the corridor to keep them from telling me. Even if I get by the nurses, the patient will pipe up and say, "Doctor So-and-So says I've got such-and-such a disease."

For these reasons, the clinical student still tends to feel, as one expressed it, "in the dark about my own competence."

Emerging Confidence

Despite these obstacles, expressions of self-doubt decrease in frequency as students progress toward graduation. Although seniors acknowledge there is still much to learn, they typically express optimism about being on the right track and eventually "getting there." With obvious pleasure, one commented, "I'm catching on quicker than I thought I would. I can at least get my diagnoses in the right ball park. I'm on my way!" [4]

Even so, students have learned that they must rely heavily on the use of reference books to deal with specific problems. Without these props, there is little feeling of confidence. And most come to realize that, because the field of medical knowledge is so vast, they will still need to rely on reference books even after entering practice. Experience has shown that a little learning illuminates vast areas of yet unexplored and unknown medical terrain.

For this reason, students increasingly come to realize that a good doctor never becomes completely self-assured; some self-doubt is, in fact, a healthy thing: "I'd be leery of myself," one said, "if I ever end up thinking I can't make a mistake." So, although the successful doctor has no self-doubt about the right and responsibility to perform the doctor's role, a wise one still maintains enough perspective to recognize limitations. In other words, good doctors do not "arrive"; they are constantly developing.

SUMMING UP

Learning to identify with the doctor's status and to feel comfortable while performing the medical role involves a subtle interpersonal process, one which depends, in large part, on the attitudes of others. Their feedback contributes to shaping self-attitudes.

Successful applicants to medical school initially experience high status, of an idealistic sort, since their intimate associates—family members and friends—now regard them as prospective doctors, members of an elite group that possesses great prestige. And these attitudes are reflected in the self-esteem of recruits.

Upon arrival in medical school, however, students experience a sharp decline in status. This is because almost everyone else in this new social network has higher status and is more knowledgeable and sophisticated about medical matters. In the hospital hierarchy, the entering medical student is just one of the many nameless beginners at the bottom of the pecking order.

But status within this relatively confining environment gradually comes to prospective doctors who prove themselves capable of successfully handling the divers vicissitudes of medical training. By advancing through school and overcoming the many challenging obstacles, students increasingly come to regard themselves as doctors rather than students and gain greater confidence in their ability to play the doctor's role. Slowly, through absorbing hospital routine until it becomes part of them, they begin to discard the student image as the moth discards the cocoon. Not only do they now possess greater knowledge and clinical skills, but also they can display the doctor's regalia and thus come to be viewed by others as physicians. Being called "doctor" by patients and staff helps students view themselves as physicians. Such a social looking-glass enhances the development of a professional self-image.

Despite the initial damage to their egos when they arrive at medical school, students clearly experience an ego boost whenever they encounter outsiders. All that is necessary to restore prospective doctors to their high status is to leave the medical school environment and again bask in the sunshine of admiration radiating from friends, family, and others. Such experiences cause students to reflect on their progress and cause them to feel pride in the achievement of worthwhile goals.

Clearly, the uplifting effects of medical school greatly outweigh the negative ones. Despite frequent complaints about aversive aspects of medical training, most students experience feelings of self-development and view themselves as changing in a positive direction. But graduation from medical school does not guarantee psychological fulfillment, for there is still much to be learned and many skills to be developed. Fortunately, graduate training lies ahead, where professional self-attitudes can be further developed.

NOTES

1. When discussing the concept of "self-fulfilling prophecy," I acknowledge the classical writings of Robert Merton in his book *Social Theory and Social Structure* (1957). Elsewhere I have elaborated on this principle as it ap-

plies to school behavior (Coombs and Davies, 1966), to interpersonal attraction (Coombs, 1969), and to sex role behavior (Coombs, 1968b).

2. Such responses are given to the question, "How high or low are freshman
students on the status ladder of the teaching hospital?" See the discussion
in Coombs and Boyle (1971b, pp. 103–108).

3. For a report on the negative impact of the first year on students' self-images,
see Pearl P. Rosenberg (1971, pp. 214–215).

4. Huntington (1957) also reports a steady rise in self-confidence in the image
of self as a doctor, rather than a student, during the four years of medical
education.

11. Personal Attributes and Values

When my life is over, I want to have accomplished something worthwhile; something more significant than "This is Joe Blow—born February 21 and died April 8." Like Snoopy in the Charlie Brown cartoon, I want people to say more about me after I'm gone than "He was a good guy; he chased sticks." (A sophomore)

THE IMPACT OF MEDICAL TRAINING, of course, depends in large measure upon the personality characteristics and basic values brought to medical school by participants. These personality features constitute the raw material of professional socialization. Presumably, these materials can be shaped and polished. After all, human personality is malleable, but just how malleable remains to be seen.

This chapter addresses the question of change by first describing the personality traits and basic value orientations of medical recruits at the outset of their training and then tracing alterations during the ensuing years of medical socialization. Do medical school experiences change basic aspirations and values? How are religious and political views affected? Are cynicism, humanitarianism, and other personality qualities influenced favorably or adversely by medical training? Answers to such questions help clarify the generalized impact of medical socialization.

PERSONALITY TRAITS

To learn how personality characteristics are affected by medical training, I administered a comprehensive psychological test, the *California Psychological Inventory* (Gough, 1967), to each student, first upon entering medical school and then again in the final weeks of medical school.[1] This 480-item test includes 18 scales, each of which covers one important facet of interpersonal psychology. To enhance clinical interpretation, scale scores are plotted on a profile sheet that groups them into four broad categories:

a. Measures of Poise, Ascendancy, and Self-Assurance.[2]
b. Measures of Socialization, Maturity, and Responsibility.[3]
c. Measures of Achievement Potential and Intellectual Efficiency.[4]
d. Measures of Intellectual and Interest Modes.[5]

Subjects can then be compared with college and national norms for the CPI, which are based upon thousands of cases.

Since profile interpretation is an art derived not only from general psychological sophistication but also from practical working knowledge of the test instrument, I enlisted the aid of Harrison G. Gough, who developed the CPI, and his colleague Wallace B. Hall at the Institute of Personality Assessment and Research, University of California at Berkeley. Each independently assessed the mean personality profiles of entering freshmen and graduating seniors. They did this by the Q-sort method.

This method consists of sorting cards (called a Q-deck), each of which contains a descriptive personality statement, into one of seven piles according to the degree to which the statement does or does not characterize the CPI profile.[6]

According to these expert raters, the most striking personality characteristics of the entering freshman are, in order of typicality:*

a. honest and direct in behavior; mature and realistic in outlook;
b. well-organized, capable, patient, and industrious; values achievement;
c. independent; intelligent and self-reliant; values achievement;
d. efficient; able to mobilize personal resources quickly and effectively;
e. quick and alert in manner; likes the new and different; impatient and critical of delay or hesitation;
f. verbally fluent; expresses self easily and with clarity.

By contrast, personality traits that are strikingly uncharacteristic of this typical entering freshman are (with the most uncharacteristic listed first):

a. easily embarrassed; feels inferior and inadequate;
b. lazy, indifferent about duties and obligations; generally undependable and immature;
c. restless and changeable; thinks and behaves differently from others;
d. undependable; poorly motivated; has difficulty in working toward prescribed goals;

* I have used here only those items where the two raters were in close agreement. In general, the two sortings correlated 0.75 on the freshman profile and 0.57 on the senior profile.

e. poorly organized; unable to concentrate attention and effort in intellectual problems;

f. submissive; gives in easily; lacking in self-confidence;

g. worried and preoccupied; tense, nervous, and generally upset;

h. coarse and vulgar; inclined to behave in a crude and impolite fashion.

When comparing freshman with senior profiles, the similarity is striking. The senior profile is slightly higher (more favorable) of the two, but there is little substantial difference. So it is not surprising that the Q-sort ratings of freshman and senior profiles are similar. Only two descriptive statements were rated by the judges as varying by more than one value.

In the senior year profile, the most characteristic features of the representative student, given in sequence of typicality, are:

a. independent; intelligent and self-reliant; values achievement;

b. conscientious; serious-minded;

c. forceful and self-assured in manner;

d. ambitious; likely to succeed in most things undertaken;

e. poised and self-confident; not troubled by pressure or criticism.

By contrast, the most uncharacteristic features of the typical graduating senior, in order of significance, are:

a. dull; lacks ability and understanding;

b. submissive; gives in easily; lacks self-confidence;

c. awkward and ill-at-ease socially; shy and inhibited with others;

d. unimaginative and literal-minded; slow and deliberate; lacks zest and enthusiasm;

e. easily embarrassed; feels inferior and inadequate;

f. unassuming, inhibited, and inattentive; bland and colorless in behavior;

g. unambitious; commonplace and conventional in thinking and behavior.

In summary, then, CPI results show that medical school training has a favorable rather than a detrimental effect upon personality development, but that the overall change is not profound. Medical students apparently leave school much as they entered, functioning at a high level of social and intellectual effectiveness.[7]

BASIC VALUES AND ASPIRATIONS

As this chapter's lead-in quotation suggests, medical students aspire to higher than ordinary goals. They want to accomplish important things.

To identify these personal values and aspirations and to trace changes, I asked students each year to name that which was of greatest importance in their lives and what they wanted most to achieve. I also asked for their views as to whether medical training had altered these basic values and aspirations. Only one in ten freshmen noted significant personal changes in basic values and aspirations; but by the senior year this number increased to nearly four in ten.*

Career Success

The most important ambition among freshman medical students, outweighing all others, is to attain professional competence and achievement. Seven out of ten freshmen name career success as being the most important thing in life—and this pronounced majority remains high throughout medical school. By the senior year, 78 percent still feel career success to be of greatest value.†

Translated into practical terms, success means making it through medical school, passing national boards, and getting the M.D. degree. But it also means arriving at one's own image of what a good physician should be—knowledgeable, competent, and concerned for patients. In aspiring to become experts in their field, these students want respect and admiration from fellow doctors and patients. In pursuit of this goal, as a senior acknowledged, "Medicine becomes a way of life; everything else is secondary."

Family Well-Being

The importance of a successful marriage and family life is also valued highly. Nearly half of the freshman class state this; and by the senior year the proportion increases to seven in ten.‡ Some think it important

---

* The percentage each year who responded affirmatively to my question "Has medical training altered your basic aspirations and view of what is of greatest value?" is as follows: freshmen, 11.9; sophomores, 12.3; juniors, 34.5; and seniors, 38.2.

† The percentages giving "professional competence and achievement" as their response to the multiple-answer question, "What is the most important thing in your life?" are as follows: freshmen, 72.4; sophomores, 68.4; juniors, 82.8; and seniors, 78.2. The question "What do you hope to achieve?" yielded a similar response from 58.6 percent of the freshmen, 68.4 percent of the sophomores, 70.7 percent of the juniors, and 58.6 percent of the seniors.

‡ The percentages replying "successful marriage and/or family life" when asked, "What is the most important thing in your life?" are as follows: freshmen, 48.3; sophomores, 54.4; juniors, 56.9; and seniors, 69.1. The percentages giving a similar response to the question "What do you hope most to achieve?" are: freshmen, 34.5; sophomores, 31.6; juniors, 44.8; and seniors, 43.6.

to establish and maintain a healthy marriage and family life to enhance career success. For instance, one said, "I can be a better doctor if I have a good family." Others, however, hold the view that, rather than being only a means to an end, the family has first priority. "There isn't any sense working hard and making a lot of money," one explained, "if you don't have a family to enjoy it with." But no matter which view takes precedence, these students find, as they learn more about the formidable demands medicine makes upon them, that considerable effort and thoughtful planning will be required to keep their family relationships healthy.

Self-Fulfillment and Personal Happiness

Finding peace of mind and happiness is the acknowledged ambition of one out of five freshmen. But during the ensuing years, this number declines to one in ten.* Happiness, they say, consists of finding oneself— "figuring out who I am, what I am doing here, and where I am going"— and then developing a philosophy of life that points out clear directions and purposes for living. To such introspective students, justifying one's own existence is of utmost importance. Fortunately, such fulfillment comes from having worthy work to do and then realizing the satisfaction that comes from doing it well. Obviously, the doctor's career affords ample opportunities to actualize desired achievements. And, judging from the declining number who mention these goals, self-fulfillment is in large measure realized as graduation becomes a reality. This, no doubt, explains the decreasing preoccupation with this goal.

Service to Others

The importance of serving others is also stressed by one in five freshmen. These students aspire to contribute to the world by helping other people. The altruistic motivations of one freshman, for example, were stimulated by feelings of ineptness while waiting helplessly for an ambulance to come to the aid of a child injured by an automobile. "I told myself that if I could save one kid like that, a medical education would be worth all the trouble." But as students advance through medical school and become preoccupied with their own needs, altruistic concerns come less readily to mind. By the senior year, only one in ten mentions service as being of greatest value—a decline of ten percent since the freshman

* The percentages replying "self-fulfillment and personal happiness" when asked, "What is the most important thing in your life?" are as follows: freshmen, 22.4; sophomores, 19.3; juniors, 24.1; and seniors, 10.9. The percentages giving this type of response when asked "What do you hope most to achieve?" are: freshmen, 24.1; sophomores, 33.3; juniors, 25.8; and seniors, 18.2.

year.* For some, coming face to face with the poor and the sick, those they once aspired to help, only makes them feel inept and uncomfortable. Other seniors acknowledge that their own struggles and poverty stricken conditions over the past few years have increased their interest in self-survival and in earning a good living. This raises the question as to whether humanitarian motives dwindle during medical school. This topic is now explored in greater depth.

CYNICISM AND HUMANITARIANISM

The question of whether medical school conditions students to become cynical and dehumanized has been debated since 1955 when Eron first reported results from two paper-and-pencil tests that showed cynicism increasing and humanitarianism decreasing as students progress through school. Since then, these findings have been confirmed by some researchers but disputed by others.[8] In general, my results do not support the Eron findings, for when the same psychological tests were administered to the study population, first before entering school and then again during each year of school, no appreciable change was noted.† Judging from these results, students left medical school no more cynical and dehumanized than when they entered; and this interpretation is reinforced by results of other test data. For example, the number of graduating seniors who describe themselves on Gough and Heilbrun's *Adjective Check List* (1965) as being "idealistic," "cynical," or "hard-hearted" is about the same as during the first week of medical school.‡ However, in comparing freshman and senior scores on the benevolence scale of the Gordon *Survey of Interpersonal Values* (1960), a moderate decline is noted; but the difference is not statistically significant.§ Also, no change was found between

---

* The percentages replying "to be of service to others" when asked "What is the most important thing in your life?" are as follows: freshmen, 22.3; sophomores, 12.3; juniors, 12.0; and seniors, 10.9. The percentages giving a similar response to the question "What do you hope most to achieve?" are: freshmen, 25.9; sophomores, 26.3; juniors, 15.5; and seniors, 12.7. (Compare ranking motives in Table 11–1.)

† Mean scores on the cynicism scale are as follows: freshmen before entering medical school, −40.7; freshmen, −44.5; sophomores, −39.0; juniors, −39.5; and seniors, −40.8. (A low score indicates cynicism.) Mean scores on the humanitarianism scale are: entering freshmen, 29.9; freshmen, 31.7; sophomores, 29.4; juniors, 26.1; and seniors, 27.8. (A high score indicates humanitarianism). There are no statistically significant changes here.

‡ The percentages of students who indicate "idealistic" increased from 58.6 at the beginning of the freshman year to 60.0 at the end of the senior year; the percentages who indicate "cynical" increased from 25.9 to 31.1; and the percentages who indicate "hard-hearted" decreased from 5.1 to 2.2.

§ Benevolence on the Gordon scale is defined as "doing things for other people, sharing with others, helping the unfortunate, being generous." In other words, a benevolent per-

freshman and senior scores on the social scale of the Allport, Vernon, and Lindzey *Study of Values* (1960). This scale measures the extent to which a person sees love as the only suitable form of human relationship. It shows entering medical students to be the same as the national norm for this scale. And, as students proceed through medical school, they become no less kind, sympathetic, or unselfish, etc.

In fact, as results of the Chapin *Social Insight Test* (1967) indicate, medical students become significantly more, not less, insightful about others and their feelings.[9] Moreover, as CPI data show, graduating seniors are significantly more tolerant of others—more accepting and nonjudgmental and less wary and suspicious—than when they were freshmen.[10]

Other data also contradict the Eron hypothesis. For example, when students were asked to rank several possible motivations for selecting a medical career, "service to people" was consistently ranked as a main attraction. Note in Table 11-1 how this is ranked first among the other possible motives during each of the first three years and then slips to second place during the senior year.*

Yet when asked for their own opinion as to whether medical students become cynical and dehumanized, the majority agree they do. Those expressing such a view number 76 percent in the first year and 81 percent

TABLE 11-1. Personal motives for becoming a physician.

	MEAN RANKING BY YEAR[a]				
MOTIVES	Pre-freshman	Fresh-man	Sopho-more	Junior	Senior
Service to people	1	1	1	1	2
Scientific interest	2	2	2.5	3	5
Professional prestige	3	3	5	4	3
Financial rewards	4	5	4	5	4
Independence	5	4	2.5	2	1
Attractive working conditions	6	6	6	6	6
Desire to work with hands	7	7	7	7	7

[a] 1 = most important; 7 = least important.

son is one who indicates a desire "to work for the good of society, help the poor and the needy, go out of the way to help others." Results are as follows: prefreshman mean score, 18.8 ± 5.10; senior mean score, 17.07 ± 5.68 ($t = 1.7412$; $0.05 < p. < 0.10$).

* The question that produced these responses was included in a mailed questionnaire sent to newly accepted students during the summer preceding the freshman year. It read: "What reasons motivate most physicians to choose medicine as a career?" The instruction asked respondents to rank the seven suggested reasons by writing from "1" (by the most typical reason) to "7" (by the least typical reason).

during the second year; then in the final years, the number drops to 55 percent and 56 percent, respectively. On the surface, these results seem to contradict results of the previously mentioned paper-and-pencil tests. But when the content of student comments is analyzed, it is clear that, by agreeing, students are not admitting to becoming cynical or dehumanized, at least in a generalized sense. Instead, they seize upon this question as an opportunity to criticize the medical teaching establishment. Having become disillusioned with medical education, students vent their criticism not on trainees per se, but upon deficiencies in the system that tend to dehumanize and promote cynicism.

Nature of Student Cynicism

Student expectations of medical school tend to be very idealistic. Traditionally, doctors have been regarded as super-heroes, and television programs perpetuate their romantic image. None of this, of course, escapes the notice of medical aspirants. But romantic illusions cannot sustain students through the day-to-day struggles of medical training. When they come face to face with the harsh realities of medical school, idealism and enthusiasm can rapidly wane.

Several weeks before the freshman year, soon after acceptance notifications had been sent, I mailed a questionnaire to each recruit. The format included a long list of descriptive statements about medical school with instructions to indicate those that best described personal expectations. When this test was later administered during the first week of class and then again in each succeeding year, the large gap between initial expectations and medical school realities became clear. For example, one statement read, "There is little time wasted in the medical curriculum." Expectations were clearly revealed by the fact that seven out of ten recently accepted applicants (73 percent) agreed with the statement. By the end of the first year, however, the number dropped to less than two in ten (17 percent); and a year later only 4 percent agreed.[11]

Interview questions also revealed considerable disillusionment about medical school.[12] I asked:

a. Has medical school been what you expected?
b. What did you expect?
c. What has been the biggest source of disappointment or disillusionment this year?

As previously mentioned, disillusionment was so great among some students that it expressed itself in unconcealed bitterness. Listed here are the main themes expressed by students when describing their disappointments about medical school:

Expectation: To enjoy the recognition and respect due one who occupies the hard-earned status of apprentice physician.

Reality: Granted less autonomy and personal freedom than had been experienced in college.

Result: "When you're treated like a baby, you get pretty cynical."

Expectation: Everything will be really exciting now; it's really important to be learning the physician's role from first-rate clinicians.

Reality: Little or no contact with patients; stuck in the classroom listening to professors who, in many cases, have had little clinical experience; forced to memorize large quantities of seemingly irrelevant materials.

Result: "After you beat your brains out for one test after another, you decide you don't really care. Cynicism is an escape from the frustration you feel, a byproduct of academic stress."

Expectation: Doctors are humanists; they have a cure for everything.

Reality: Not all doctors are motivated by benevolence; and only so much can be done to help patients.

Result: "My pink balloon about doctors burst after seeing all the self-interest involved. Seeing patients serving the needs of the teaching program rather than vice versa and noticing negligence tends to make me cynical."

Not all cynicism, however, is directed toward medical mentors. In some cases, like the following, patients are singled out as objects of cynicism. But such comments are relatively scarce and are not expressed with the same fervor of the foregoing themes.

Expectation: Patients are motivated, cooperative, and appreciative.

Reality: Some patients are uncooperative, and many are unapprecia-tive. Every patient is a potential protagonist in a lawsuit.

Result: "Some patients really leave a bad taste in your mouth and make you feel like saying, 'To hell with everybody! I'm going to stick up for myself.' "

Clearly, disillusionment can foster cynicism among medical recruits; but there is little evidence that this sour outlook becomes internalized as a generalized personality trait. Cynicism is primarily directed to the medical training establishment, especially the laboratory and classroom. Self-reported cynicism subsides markedly during the clinical years, when medical realities more nearly match student expectations. But for those who become cynical about patients, the impact can be more pervasive.

When personally involved with medical students on a heart-to-heart basis, as I have been, one sees through the defensive armor of their personal and professional pride. Such glimpses, I submit, do not reflect a generalized cynicism. Instead, one cannot help being impressed with their basic idealism—not the unrealistic "pink balloon" variety so typical of medical aspirants, but an idealism tempered by reality and an honest recognition of one's own needs as well as those of others.

Nature of Emotional Detachment

When contrasting entering recruits with graduating seniors, it is easy to conclude that medical training has a dehumanizing effect, for new recruits react to emotionally stressful situations—suffering and death, for example—essentially like laymen. But after four years of medical school training, these same individuals respond with detached objectivity and unruffled calm.

Considerable emotion is expected and tolerated in crisis situations. But clinicians must frequently confront such situations and maintain composure. The training for such a role requires not only acquired technical skills but also an emotional capability to respond with what Lief and Fox (1963) have called "detached concern." Concerning the social role expected of medical personnel, Merton (1957, p. 74) has said, "The physician must be emotionally detached in his attitudes toward patients, keeping 'his emotions on ice' and not becoming 'overly identified' with patients. But he must avoid becoming callous through excessive detachment and should have compassionate concern for the patient."

The process by which students learn to conceal their emotions typically begins during the first week of school when freshmen are escorted to the anatomy lab and told, "Okay! Everybody in the lab and grease up your cadaver." A room full of dead bodies is, of course, not an appealing sight, and the prospect of carving up a dead human being hardly appeals to humanistic ideals. The result is, as one student said, "You become somewhat dehumanized right off the bat."

In such a setting there is little consideration of personal feelings, and students must conceal any revulsion or fear in order not to appear weak or lacking in clinical fortitude. So they cope with inner anxieties by depersonalizing the cadaver—concentrating not on its humanness but on the details of dissection. (Refer to Chapter 6.) After awhile they become so desensitized, they can eat their lunches around the corpse. "It's just a thing on the table like any other object," students come to think. "We even make jokes about it." They realize, of course, that outsiders might be offended by such an attitude. But, as one acknowledged, "If we thought of it as a person, we couldn't stand it emotionally."

Basic-science courses provide the terminology and technical knowledge necessary for dealing with illness on an intellectual rather than an emotional basis. Hours of looking at slides of people who have various illnesses at progressive stages, discussed in scientific terminology, gradually desensitizes students to diseases. After awhile, blood, gore, and other aversive symbols, which normally elicit uncomfortable feelings, are viewed with calm, objective rationality.

When students leave the lecture room and laboratory for the hospital floors, they are exposed to pain, suffering, despair, and death. Here they must distance themselves personally from the living as well as the dead. To maintain equanimity and protect themselves from the discomfort of such stressful human encounters, students maintain the same protective shield that served them so well in dealing with dead bodies. By adopting a detached scientific attitude, just as they did with their cadavers, they can avoid personal identification with patients. Thus, students focus on the technical aspects of their work rather than on individuals per se. Losing oneself in the pathological details—thinking about diseased tissue— is less personally involving than pondering about the patient as a suffering human being. In this way, patients can become medical entities, objects of scientific interest.

Initially, such distancing bothers students. Not only are they critical of their impersonal clinical mentors, but also they worry about their own evolving attitudes. One student uneasily admitted, "Sometimes when I see a patient I get excited because he has a particular disease I can learn from. 'Oh boy,' I think, 'I saw a case of ——.' But then I remember that I am forgetting about the poor soul who has it."

If "the case" is particularly interesting a student will often invite a classmate to come around and inspect it. But among many students there is disquiet about being insensitive to the human aspects of interesting cases. This can be detected from the following quotation:

> We had a lady in OB the other night who was five weeks past term and carrying a dead baby. We were pretty sure the baby was dead, malformed, and without a brain because the X ray showed that the skull was deformed. I stayed up all night until she delivered just so I could see the baby. It was the best part of my day. A lot of other students came by to look at it, too.

Then this student added:

> If the patient knew that I stayed up all night just to see this deformed baby, she would feel bad and think I was inhuman—some kind of animal. I felt sorry for her, but it was so rare and had so much pathology involved that it was a great learning experience—one that was worth going out of my way to see.

The question is, then, how dehumanized do graduating seniors become? Clearly, medical training has altered their overt responses to emotionally stressful situations. Yet, concern for patients is still regarded as a high ideal. (Refer to Chapter 7.) Cold impersonal relations with patients are unanimously seen as being incompatible with good medical care. Even so, necessity dictates a certain degree of detachment if clinicians are to control their own emotions. "You can't go home and weep about everything," one said. "If you die with every patient, you'll be dying a thousand deaths."

Those who work in clinical settings must acquire the mechanisms that help them function effectively to serve the interests of those patients whose lives, in many cases, literally lie in their hands. Yet, in order to perform this vital function they must, paradoxically, resist the demands such cases make on their own feelings. But despite this "defensive insensitivity," they do remain susceptible to the pathos of the dramas occurring around them. The experiences do not destroy their capacity to feel or to empathize; they simply alert them to the necessity of managing feelings both in their own interest and that of their patients.[13]

RELIGIOUS VALUES

Before entering college, all but a few students recall having personal religious views; 86 percent professed belief in a Supreme Being. By the time they entered medical school, however, the number of believers had decreased to 74 percent. And by the senior year the number had dropped to 64 percent.* This decline in religious values during medical school is mirrored by results of the Allport, Vernon, and Lindzey *Study of Values* (1960), completed at the beginning of the freshman year and again at the end of the senior year.[14] This scale indicates a statistically significant decrease in religious outlook.

Interviews also confirm this decline among some, but not all, students. When asked "Has medical school affected your religious views in any way?" 73 percent of the freshmen said there had been no effect. But by the senior year only half of the class held this view. Twenty-six percent of the graduating seniors reported their interest in religion had diminished over the four years. Yet, by contrast, 14 percent of the seniors found that medical school had enhanced rather than diminished their religiosity.†

---

* Information on religious views was obtained by asking students each year to state whether they regard themselves to be a believer, an agnostic, or an atheist. They were also asked to recall which position they held prior to entering college. Results show that most unbelievers were agnostic; only two students classified themselves as atheists, and one of them decided in his senior year to be a believer. According to the latter, however, medical school played no part in his conversion. "I just happened to be here when I said to myself, 'Well, maybe there is a God'; but medical school per se has not had much effect on me."

† The remaining 10 percent are uncertain how medical school affected their religious views.

Why Religious Interest Diminishes

Several explanations can be offered for the decrease in religious commitment among some students. The high-pressure schedule, especially during basic-science years, leaves little time for participating in organized religious activities.* On weekends, instead of attending a church or synagogue, students usually study for pending examinations (many are scheduled for Monday morning) or else catch up on badly needed sleep or recreation. One conscientious freshman stopped attending Sunday services since while there she either fell asleep or worried about her studies. Such students simply drift away from organized religion. "Duties have kept me so busy," one said, "I haven't had time to think much about religion; I've gotten out of the habit and become more neutral."

Another reason for decreased religious awareness is that, as one said, "Religion is so rarely mentioned in medical school, you tend not to think about it." [15] Moreover, when religion is brought up, it is likely to be a negative reference. "There isn't much emphasis on religion throughout the medical community," a senior commented. "In fact, it is often looked down upon."

The scientific orientation of the medical curriculum generally encourages naturalistic rather than supernatural explanations; and as students gain ability to explain critical life events in terms of natural law, they often discard earlier religious ideas. "Medical school has removed some of the mysticism about disease and miracles," a senior explained. "I just haven't been able to integrate my ideas about God and religion with what I have learned in science." This transition from religious to naturalistic explanations is illustrated by the sophomore who said, "Realizing how marvelously well-patterned everything is, I used to think, 'There's got to be a God.' But then, I began to think, 'It could be due to natural laws.'"

Accepting naturalistic explanations of such fundamental questions as the creation of the universe and the nature of man can lead to feelings of self-reliance and confidence in one's growing intellectual powers and independence—pride in "having thrown off one's crutches." "Through increased objectivity and intellectual growth," a senior said, "I have become more comfortable without religion; I just don't have the same religious need that I once did."

Hospitals bring students into close contact with tragic events that cause people pain and suffering. Consequently, it is sometimes difficult to accept the idea of a controlling God who permits such personal indignities. It is much easier for many students to accept the idea, as one put

---

* About one in ten students never attended religious services; about one-third rarely attended (i.e., one to five times a year); and about 40 percent attended at least once a month (with about a fourth of these attending weekly). The remainder did not respond. Attendance figures remain about the same during all four years.

it, that "death is not a supernatural thing; people die from disease processes."

Personal glimpses of hypocrisy and religious fanaticism among some patients can also adversely affect student religiosity. As student clinicians discover in their work-ups, ostensibly devout patients do not always practice what they profess. "Digging back into their histories," one explained, "you find out that they don't really practice what they preach. The whole thing seems so hypocritical."

Faith healing, a common practice among some religious groups, also causes students to look negatively upon religion. "I've seen too many people screwed up by religion," a senior commented. "They go to faith healers for cancer and keep going back until it is too late for doctors to help them." This case is illustrative: "I had a patient with a solitary lung lesion that was probably malignant," a senior reported. "It was in an area that is easily accessible and there is a very low mortality associated with the operation. He was young and could probably have lived a normal life for many years. But after his minister spoke to him, he just said, 'No, if God wants me to have lung cancer, I will have it.'" Although this patient had a family, he refused to have any treatment; instead, he chose to just go home and die. From a clinical perspective, his religion was personally detrimental.

How Religious Beliefs Are Sustained or Strengthened

As previously mentioned, a minority find that medical school experiences have reinforced rather than diminished religious beliefs. Witnessing the comfort and strength that some patients derive from their faith during personal crises gives these students a greater appreciation for the value of religious beliefs: "I can see the great importance of religion in the lives of the mortally ill," one said. "Now I have more respect and don't treat religion as lightly as I once did."

The intricate wonders of the human body can also enhance religious feelings. "Anybody who dissects the human body can't help but see the fantastic organization, the ingenuity of design, the beauty of the whole thing," a junior explained. "Literally billions of cells are working together in concert, each with certain functions. The wonder of how it all works together makes me think there must be a God."

Witnessing the powers of the human body to recover, after medical science has seemingly failed, can cause students to reason, "Maybe there is something else—a higher power." "Some patients miraculously bounce back when you don't expect them to live," a senior observed. "When their recovery can't be explained rationally on medical grounds, you realize that other forces have pulled them through." Believing students feel that "it is incredibly egotistical for doctors to take credit for such events and to regard themselves as having ultimate control." One stated, "The more one learns about disease processes and the nature of life, the clearer it becomes that powers greater than humans possess are at work in medicine."

POLITICAL VALUES

Interest in power and political matters increases significantly during the four years of medical school. This is indicated by results of the All-port, Vernon, and Lindzey *Study of Values* (1960). Political interest is broadly defined here as "being interested in power"; such a person is "a leader, competitive and struggle-oriented, and interested in influence and renown." [16]

Not all classmates, however, have the same political views, especially concerning the proper role of government in medicine. The prospects of government involvement in their future medical career distresses some freshmen (about one-fourth of the class), but others (another fourth) favor such involvement. The majority, however, are ambivalent, seeing both good and bad features of each view. By the senior year, though, the class is nearly equally divided in thirds—those who oppose, those who favor, and those who are "torn between arguments of the head and of the heart."*

Conservative View

Generally speaking, politically conservative students oppose in principle any form of government action that "encroaches on private enterprise." "Socialized medicine," they feel, "is an evil to be avoided at all costs." "I've always been in favor of private enterprise," one said, "and dislike the socialist form of government where everybody expects a certain grade of medical care whether it can be paid for or not. It's not right to expect the government to supply on demand what everybody needs."

If changes are needed in the established system of medical care, these

---

* A balance between "ayes" and "nays" for governmental involvement is maintained during all four years of school. During the fourth year, however, opinions jell; the number who either oppose or approve increases, and the number who are ambivalent decreases correspondingly. Percentages are as follows: 23.7 freshmen approve, 22.0 oppose, and 44.1 are ambivalent; 22.8 sophomores approve, the same number oppose, and 47.4 are ambivalent; in the junior year, 20.7 approve, 19.0 oppose, and 53.4 are ambivalent; but the senior year evens out with 30.9 approving, 29.1 opposing, and 32.7 ambivalent. The remainder expressed no opinion.

students feel that such reform rightfully belongs to those most informed and best qualified—the medical profession. "Let all of us stick to what we know best," one commented.

Conservative students feel that it is the doctor's right to practice one's own brand of medicine and to set fees without outside influences, and this preference increases markedly during medical training. Since the prospect of working independently is undoubtedly one feature that makes medicine attractive in the first place, the idea of becoming a civil servant is abhorrent to many. "I don't want anyone telling me how many patients I should see or how much I should charge," one emphasized. "I don't want to answer to some government official."

As supportive evidence, students point out that in countries where government-sponsored medical programs have been established, the doctor's work declines and the profession loses its glamour and prestige. "It's just not right," one argued, "for government to put doctors on the same status level as everyone else; doctors are professionals." In this regard, a classmate added, "It used to be that everyone with anything on the ball went into medicine or law, but if medicine becomes socialized, I don't think you'll get many more topnotch people."

Liberal View

In contrast to their politically conservative classmates, liberally oriented students maintain that health is not a privilege but a basic human right: All people are entitled to good health regardless of their station in life.

Because they see many who, for one reason or another, are not receiving adequate medical care, these students are more sympathetic toward governmental participation, although they usually agree that bureaucratic governmental management is often clumsy, ineffective, and wasteful. "A person can't afford to get sick nowadays," a junior pointed out. "Medical care is pricing itself out of the ordinary individual's reach. And those who need care the most, the poor and the aged, aren't getting it."

Politically liberal students criticize the medical profession for being more concerned about protecting the status quo than in dealing with the national health problem. "The profession has really dropped the ball," one said, "and it's high time that somebody did something to guarantee medical care for all people." The American Medical Association in particular is viewed as being unresponsive to social needs, stubbornly refusing to concede that problems exist, and sluggish in instituting changes. It is described by liberal students as "a conservative, ultra-rightist organization," and "an outmoded, out-of-date, horse-and-buggy group that impedes progress." Its leadership is portrayed by these students as being "backward, archaic, old deadwood fuddyduddies who don't know what the hell they are doing to the profession." In this view, these "old guards" who hold on to the old ways despite changing societal needs are not representative of the younger doctor, at least not the liberally oriented ones.

Medical School Influences upon Political Views

Reflecting back on the four years of medical school, seniors generally view themselves and their classmates as becoming more conservative. When asked "Politically speaking, do students tend to become more liberal or conservative in medical school?" 73 percent replied "more conservative." Only a minority (16 percent) thought the change was in the liberal direction.

Why Conservatism Increases

Medicine is viewed by one student as "a profession where you're molded to the status quo." Most faculty members seem to be politically conservative, and there is a lot of adverse talk about socialized medicine.[17] Regular exposure to such views no doubt influences student attitudes, and the authoritative regimentation allows relatively little opportunity for dissent or deviation. Power rests with the faculty members, and both they and the students know it well. Consequently, getting through medical school is largely a matter of conforming to what the faculty wishes. "It's a matter of survival," one said. "If you don't conform, you're out."

But increasing conservatism also results from a mounting preoccupation with one's own needs and interests. Although a student may begin medical school with dreams of social justice and medical reform, after four years of sacrifice and struggle, that same student has a personal stake in the established system, and this stake appears less secure when liberals try to initiate changes. "When we first began," one said, "there was a lot of talk about organizing ourselves and going into the ghettos to work. But after a while we started questioning how this would affect us as doctors. The talk changed to 'I don't want to practice in a ghetto; I want a nice office, a good practice, and a comfortable life.' "

Family responsibilities also contribute toward conservatism. With marriage and parenthood, income and security assume greater importance. One student observed, "I've seen how some who get married suddenly become less eager to save the world." Age and experience also seem to strengthen a conservative view. Students advancing through medical school start thinking more like older persons. This point is made clear by a senior's statement: "Four years ago I was unable to really understand how my father felt about student demonstrations on the campus, but now I understand a little better." By growing older and gaining an investment in the established system, students tend to become less enthusiastic about changing the status quo.

How Liberalism Is Fostered

Despite these trends, some entrenched liberals (16 percent of the class) maintain the view that they and their classmates become more liberal during medical school. Among those who do, some comment only vaguely about the national trend toward liberalism. Others note the disparity between their views and those of their instructors and have simply tried to resist conservative indoctrination. Those who as freshmen expressed dissatisfaction with social conditions and government policies sometimes point out that medical school has reinforced their desire to do something about the unequal distribution of medical care to the poor. As one expressed it, "Exposure to patients from a wide variety of backgrounds and to classmates from a cross-section of the nation can't help but stretch the mental processes, freeing one from local parochial biases and, in general, liberalizing the mind politically and in other ways."

SUMMING UP

Considering the huge personal investment of time, money, and energy expended by medical students in gaining mastery of medicine, it is understandable that their personal values and attributes should both reflect and be shaped by their medical training experiences. Indeed, who else but those urgently seeking career success would endure the personal hardships and sacrifice necessary to become medical school graduates? Prospective doctors seem propelled by an inner need for career attainment—a desire to succeed, to achieve occupational prominence.

This is not surprising, since personal worthiness in our work-oriented society, especially for males, has traditionally been conferred by occupational attainment. Individuals meeting for the first time typically try to identify each other's status. This exchange often takes place by one asking, "What do you do?" or, more obliquely, "What brought you here [to this community]?" Answers to such inquiries fix the other's place in the occupational status structure. Ensuing responses, then, can be tendered according to status. To be recognized and treated as an able and important person is, of course, essential for the ego. Medical students seem urgently compelled to fill this need.

Fortunately, students' career aspirations serve them well during the stresses and adversities of medical school. Rather than quitting when things get rough, medical aspirants press forward in pursuit of their goal—

the M.D. degree. This promises a lifetime of admiration from others and the hopes of respectful recognition from medical colleagues.

Other qualities also make recruits admirably suited for the competitive demands of medical school. Judging from the variety of personality test scores, medical students are well endowed with desirable characteristics. They are intelligent, resourceful, serious-minded, self-assured, and so on— qualities that enhance success in any setting. Such personality traits, of course, served them well in college competition and are polished even more by the medical school experience.

One wonders, though, whether total absorption in career development to the relative exclusion of outside interests is a healthy thing. Does one pay a price in other ways for such dedication and zeal? Popular opinion has it that medical students become cynical and dehumanized. It is easy to see how this conclusion is reached, since enthusiastic idealists often turn into complaining and bickering critics upon entering medical school. Noting that once tenderhearted young men and women can find excite-ment upon observing a case of tetanus, for example, makes one wonder what happened to their benevolence. It is important to realize, though, that the doctor's role requires a certain amount of emotional distancing. Although clinicians must have empathy for patients, they cannot identify with them too closely in their pain and suffering if objectivity is to be maintained. No matter how sympathetic a clinician may be, emotional detachment is a major factor in performing the expected role.

Although some cynicism may develop among disillusioned students, especially toward the medical teaching establishment, my findings do not support the view that such an attitude becomes generalized as a personality trait. The data do show, though, that students tend to become less re-ligiously inclined and more politically interested. For although many retain their previous religious and political orientations, the tendency is, generally speaking, to become more naturalistic, secular, and politically conservative.

NOTES

1. For related reading pertaining to the use of CPI with medical personnel, see Gough, Fox, and Hall (1972) and Gough and Hall (1973).
2. These scales—"Dominance," "Capacity for Status," "Sociability," "Social Presence," "Self-Acceptance," and "Sense of Well-Being"—share a com-mon emphasis on feelings of interpersonal and intrapersonal adequacy. On these scales the study population is shown to function well in poise, ascendancy, and self-assurance. And, during its sojourn in medical school, there is a favorable increase in these qualities as measured. Three of the scales show the difference between incoming freshmen and graduating

seniors to be statistically significant (beyond the 0.05 level). These were as follows:

Dominance—Factors of leadership, ability, dominance, persistence, and social initiative are assessed. In this regard, our entering freshmen scored above the national norm but differed little from a college student norm. In other words, entering medical students tend to be independent and self-reliant rather than retiring, inhibited, and unassuming. And, according to test results, these characteristics became even more prominent during the four years of medical school (t, derived from a difference-of-means test $= 1.9087$; $p < 0.05$).

Capacity for Status—This scale measures the personal qualities and attributes that typically underlie and lead to status—such as being ambitious, resourceful, and ascendant and as having personal scope, communication skill, and breadth of interest. In this regard, incoming freshmen scored slightly above the national norm and slightly below the college student norm. During the four years of medical school these students increased significantly in the qualities that lead to high status ($t = 2.1625$; $p < 0.025$).

Social Presence—This scale assesses factors such as poise, spontaneity, and self-confidence in personal and social interaction. Generally speaking, these qualities were possessed by entering freshmen more than the proverbial man-in-the-street but slightly less than the typical college student. However, during medical school training there was a pronounced increase in these characteristics, surpassing the college norm. That is, as students progressed through medical school, they became less vacillating and uncertain in their decisions and more vigorous, imaginative, clever, and spontaneous ($t = 2.2134$; $p < 0.025$).

Increases were noted on other scales of this cluster, but the differences are not statistically significant.

Sociability—Individuals with outgoing, sociable, participative temperaments are identified by this scale. Those who score high tend to be outgoing, enterprising, competitive, and forward. By contrast, low scorers tend to be awkward, conventional, quiet, submissive, and unassuming. They are also more detached and passive in attitude and are easily suggestible. Upon entering medical school, freshmen scored slightly above both the national and the college norms. Qualities of sociability increased slightly during medical school, but, as mentioned, the difference is not statistically significant.

Self-Acceptance—Sense of personal worth, self-acceptance, and capacity for independent thinking are measured by this scale. In this regard, entering freshmen were markedly above the national and college student norms. Rather than being passive, self-abasing, and given to feelings of guilt or self-blame, they are generally more outspoken, aggressive, and persuasive. This is because they are confident and self-assured. But little measurable change in these qualities was noted during the period of their medical training.

Sense of Well-Being—This scale identifies persons who minimize their worries and complaints and who are relatively free from self-doubt and disillusionment. Entering freshmen scored the same as the national and college norms; although there was a slight increase in these personality characteristics during the ensuing four years, the difference is not statistically significant.

3. These scales—"Responsibility," "Socialization," "Self-Control," "Tolerance," and "Good Impression"—are principally concerned with social norms and values and the disposition to observe or reject such values. They show medical students, in general, to be similar to norms established for these scales. The only significant increase during the four years in training is in the "Tolerance" scale, which is described first; descriptions of the remaining scales follow.

Tolerance—Persons with permissive, accepting, and nonjudgmental social beliefs and attitudes are identified by this scale. A high scorer is not suspicious, wary, or overly judgmental in attitudes. Entering freshmen scored above the national norm but below the college norm. When the senior year was reached, though, there was a statistically significant increase $(t = 2.0816; p < 0.025)$.

Good Impression—This scale identifies persons capable of creating a favorable impression, who are concerned about how others react to them. High scorers place unusual and perhaps undue emphasis on winning the approval of others. By contrast, those who score low tend to be cool, aloof, and distant in their relationships with others. In this regard, both freshmen and senior scores are somewhat below the college and national norms. There was, however, a slight, but statistically insignificant, increase during medical school.

Responsibility—Persons of conscientious, responsible, and dependable disposition and temperament are identified by this scale. In this regard, entering freshmen scored slightly above the national and college norms. After four years of medical school, there was a slight decrease in these qualities.

Socialization—This scale appraises the degree to which cultural mandates concerning constraint, control, and self-denial have been internalized as self-governing agents. High scorers are typically seen as being diligent and dependable individuals, but also as conventional and lacking in initiative and the capacity to break with outmoded tradition. Low scorers are freer in the expression of impulse and less bound by tradition. Our findings show that entering freshmen scored above both the national and the college norms; there was a slight, though statistically insignificant, decrease during medical school.

Self-Control—This scale assesses the degree and adequacy of self-regulation and self-control and freedom from impulsivity and self-centeredness. Entering freshmen scored below both the national and the college norms on this scale. Their score increased slightly during the medical school training—up to the level of the national norm but still below the college norm—but the difference is not significant.

4. These scales—"Achievement via Conformance," "Achievement via In-

dependence," and "Intellectual Efficiency"—are grouped together because of their common bearing on matters of academic and intellectual endeavors. They show entering medical students to be well adapted in achievement and intellectual efficiency. During the four years of medical training achievement scores showed little change, but intellectual efficiency increased considerably, and therefore is first of the three to be described below.

Intellectual Efficiency—The degree of personal and intellectual efficiency attained by an individual is indicated by this scale. One who scores high is seen as being intelligent, efficient, clear-thinking, planful, thorough, and resourceful. Being alert and well-informed, this person places a high value on cognitive and intellectual matters. Freshmen scored higher than the national norm but about the same as the college norm. After four years of medical training there was a marked increase in these qualities; and this difference is statistically significant at the 0.01 level ($t = 2.5753; p < 0.01$).

Achievement via Conformance—This scale identifies those factors of interest and motivation that facilitate achievement in any setting where conformance is a positive behavior. Rather than being easily disorganized when under stress, high scorers tend to be persistent and industrious, and they value intellectual activity and achievement. They are also capable, cooperative, and sincere rather than coarse, stubborn, awkward, and insecure. In other words, they have personality qualities that help them to achieve by "fitting in." In this regard, entering freshmen scored slightly above the national norm and the same as the college norm. During medical school there was no change whatsoever.

Achievement via Independence—This scale assesses those personality factors that aid achievement, such as being independent and self-reliant instead of submissive and compliant; being forceful, strong, demanding, and foresighted rather than inhibited, anxious, and cautious; and having superior intellectual ability and judgment. On these qualities our freshmen scored markedly above the national norm but similar to the college norm. There was only a slight increase during medical school training.

5. This cluster of scales—"Psychological Mindedness," "Flexibility," and "Femininity"—reflects attitudes toward life that have broad and far-reaching significance. They, like the previous scales, showed that entering freshmen are not lacking in favorable personality qualities, and that they maintain, and very slightly enhance, these traits throughout medical school; but none showed statistically significant change. These scales are described briefly here.

Psychological Mindedness—This scale measures the degree to which an individual is interested in and responsive to the inner needs, motives, and experiences of others. High scorers tend to be observant, perceptive, and resourceful and are verbally fluent, socially ascendant, and not overly conforming and conventional. On these traits our freshmen scored higher than either the national or college norms. There was a slight improvement during medical school.

Flexibility—The degree of flexibility and adaptability of a person's thinking and social behavior are reflected in this scale. Rather than being guarded and rigid in manner or formal or pedantic in thought, high scorers are informal, adventurous, confident, and assertive. Not overly deferential to authority or tradition, they tend to be concerned with personal pleasure and diversion. Although scoring above the national norm, our freshmen medical students scored the same as the college norm; and there was only a slight increase in these qualities as students progressed through medical school.

Femininity—This scale assesses the masculinity or femininity of interests. That is, high scores indicate more interest traditionally associated with femininity (i.e., being appreciative, patient, helpful, moderate; and as being respectful and accepting of others and behaving in a conscientious and sympathetic way). Low scores indicate more "masculine" traits (i.e., hard-headed, active, robust, and restless; blunt and direct in thinking and action; and impatient with delay, indecision, and reflection). Our freshman students equaled both the national and college norms on these qualities. There was a slight trend toward the feminine traits during the four years of medical school.

6. These statements are from a 50-item deck called the "Interpersonal Q-Deck" used at the Institute of Personality Assessment and Research at the University of California, Berkeley. The scale logic of the descriptive personality statement is as follows:

Descriptive Personality Statement	Scale Value	Number of Cards in Category
1. Very characteristic of this person	7	3
2. Characteristic of this person	6	6
3. Somewhat characteristic of this person	5	10
4. Neutral or middle category	4	12
5. Somewhat uncharacteristic of this person	3	10
6. Uncharacteristic of this person	2	6
7. Very uncharacteristic of this person	1	3

The set of Q-items contains about an equal number of favorable and unfavorable descriptions. Thus, the clustering of favorable comments about the two profiles is a function of the profiles, not a predetermined result of using a Q-deck of laudatory remarks. For more detailed information about this technique, see Block (1961).

7. For further discussion of personality qualities among medical students, see Levitt (1966) and Lief (1971).

8. See Chapter 1 for a review of the literature on this debatable topic.

9. *The Social Insight Test*, developed by F. Stuart Chapin (1967), presents 25 problem situations in which individuals are trying to avoid embarrassment or to achieve some satisfaction as an offset to frustration. "Social insight" is defined as the ability to "see into" such problematic situations. To measure this, subjects are asked to consider each situation and select one of four alternative choices that presents the most appropriate, intel-

ligent, or logical comment on the situation. This is a sample situation from the test:

A weakly child was overprotected by his parents and other adult relatives, who were the only persons with whom he came into frequent contact. On entering school, he was ignored or rebuffed by his classmates. To this situation he responded by: (a) avoiding other children and spending his time daydreaming; (b) fighting with and bullying other children; (c) trying to attract attention by competing in games played by the group of children; (d) attempting to get other children to accept him by persistently "hanging around" or "tagging along" with them.

The prefreshman mean score on this test was 22.56 (standard deviation = 5.642) as compared to the senior mean of 26.89 (s.d. = 4.113; $t = 4.3451$; $p < 0.001$).

10. Refer to Note 3 in this chapter.

11. The gap between expectations and medical school realities is indicated by student responses to other statements such as those listed below.

   a. "Medical faculty members place considerably more importance on helping students than performing their own research and other activities": Agreeing responses came from 66.1 percent of prefreshmen, dropped to 16.2 percent in the freshman year, and then remained between 22 and 23 percent during subsequent years.

   b. "Much of the subject matter taught in medical school is irrelevant to the practice of medicine": Only 20.4 percent of the students disagreed prior to medical school enrollment, but the number increased to 44.8 percent in the freshman year, and to 63.2 percent in the sophomore year. In the final two years, the percentages were 63.6 and 53.5, respectively.

   c. "Everything that happens to a student in medical school will be important in learning to be a physician": Only 15.3 percent of the prefreshmen disagreed; but in successive years, the percentages increased to 44.9, 57.1, 63.7, and 60.4, respectively.

   d. "Teaching in medical school is generally superior to college teaching": Only 11.9 percent of the students disagreed before beginning training; but the number increased to 43.1 percent in the freshman year, 57.1 percent in the sophomore year, 61.4 percent in the junior year, and 58.2 percent in the senior year.

12. For a report of these results see Coombs and Boyle (1971b).

13. Because there are so few outlets for students to air and examine their feelings, it is possible for them to lose touch with their emotions. The system as it presently exists glorifies science and intellectual rationality. The subjective features of medical education and practice, if discussed at all, are usually covered on an intellectual level. So, unless students have informal channels to "unload," personal feelings are routinely suppressed. Because of this, it seems to me, some clinicians are needlessly hampered in their ability to provide healing aid spiritually or humanistically, as well as technically. How can a doctor allay the fears and anxieties of others if his or her own feelings have never been resolved?

14. For the purpose of the *Study of Values* test (Allport, Vernon, and Lind-

zey, 1960), religious persons are defined as those who are mystically oriented and who "seek to comprehend the cosmos as a whole, relating themselves to its embracing totality." Respondents are forced to choose between religious values and political, economic, aesthetic, and theoretical values. Sample questions are as follows:

"Which of the following branches of study do you expect ultimately will prove more important for mankind: (a) mathematics; (b) theology?

Would you consider it more important for your child to secure training in (a) religion; (b) athletics?"

On the religious scales, the entering-freshman mean (38.69 ± 11.075) is below the national norm for this test (41.01). The senior mean (34.10 ± 10.273) is even further below the national norm. When entering-freshman and senior means are compared by this t test, the difference is found to be significant at the 0.05 level.

15. To note how little interest apparently exists on the topic of religion, one need only to review the literature—or more accurately, the near absence of literature—on this subject. I have found only one article on the topic (Knight, 1961).

16. Sample questions on the Allport, Vernon, and Lindzey (1960) political scale are:

    Assuming that you are a person with the necessary ability and that the salary for each of the following occupations is the same, would you rather be a (a) mathematician, (b) sales manager, (c) clergyman, (d) politician?

    To what extent do the following famous persons interest you: (a) Florence Nightingale, (b) Napoleon, (c) Henry Ford, (d) Galileo?

    If you should see the following news item with headlines of equal size in your morning newspaper, which would you read more attentively: (a) *Supreme Court Decision Reported*, or (b) *New Scientific Theory Announced?*

Entering freshmen had a mean score of 38.51 ± 5.002. At the end of the senior year, the mean score was 41.70 ± 4.762. (A high score indicates political interest.) Utilizing the t test, this difference was found to be significant at the 0.01 level ($t = 3.1121$).

17. For an interesting though somewhat outdated article upon the influence of institutionally defined ideology, see Libo (1957). However, Goldman and Ebbert (1973) predict, on the basis of survey data, that future medical school graduates, contrary to existing stereotypes, will not become more conservative after leaving school.

12. Culmination

Becoming a doctor is a gradual process. It's a culmination of many small decisions and experiences throughout the years. You just get involved in the med school machinery and the first thing you know you are there. You wake up one day and realize you are a doctor after all. (A senior)

IN SUMMARY, medical school as a socializing system is similar in many respects to other institutions whose primary function is to change people. Like other professional schools or rehabilitation programs, for example, there is a formalized point of entry and one of exit; in between, participants experience an interlocking chain of challenging learning experiences designed to prepare them for future roles. Mastery of medicine is, of course, the goal pursued by all who aspire to become doctors.

SOCIALIZING NETWORK

The "med school machinery" referred to above conveys the impression of a processing system akin to factories where things are assembled. The initial materials are moved along in conveyor-belt-like fashion until they are shaped into finished products, products that are more marketable and socially attractive.

The many similarities between medical school and a factory lend themselves to ready comparison. Both processing systems have procedural steps designed to turn out specified products according to goals predetermined by management. In this vein, a sophomore said, "Because the faculty holds an iron hand over us, we all march through medical school in step. The program is so rigid everybody has to follow the same course; it's stifling." [1]

But because the raw materials of these two processing systems differ so markedly, the analogy must end there; for medical recruits are not inert matter to be molded willy-nilly by management and staff. Clearly, medical socialization is a dynamic process, not a passive one. Students react to the formal system as free-willed individuals and thereby become agents of change themselves. They create, as Homans (1950) indicates, an "internal social system," an informal network of shared interpersonal expectations that help make the "external system," the formalized experience, more manageable and tolerable.

Two aspects of the socializing experience make this possible. First, it is serial. That is, medical recruits can learn and benefit from the experiences of more advanced students, those who have only recently survived that which is soon to be encountered by the newcomers. Second, the experience is a collective one. Because individuals are processed in cohorts, they experience the same vicissitudes and adversities and can, therefore, work out collective solutions to their common problems.

For example, informal conduct norms quickly form among classmates to help minimize or curtail anxiety. This phenomenon may be illustrated by an incident I recorded as a field note. When discussing with a freshman an upcoming final examination in one of his minor courses, I offered to let him borrow my portable typewriter since it was a take-home examination. He thanked me but refused, saying that his classmates would be down on him if he were to type the test. He explained that there was an unwritten rule that no student would knock himself or herself out for that course. So much pressure came from other courses that, in order to reduce anxiety, classmates had informally agreed to a low level of performance in this particular course. "After all," he said, "they can't flunk the entire freshman class."

Although classmates and more advanced students may informally serve as mentors and role models for one another, the faculty is, of course, formally charged with the tutorial responsibility. Traditionally, the latter is organized according to specialization into a variety of departments, each of which competes for status as reflected by allocations of space, financial resources, and curriculum time. These departments also vie for scientific and clinical preeminence among their student clientele. So it is insulting, for example, when students study notes from another class while sitting through a lecture, for such treatment confers low status upon the department of that discipline and offends the professional pride of its staff. Proper respect can usually be ensured by inundating students with assigned materials and holding them accountable for this information by means of frequent tests.

Perhaps the most common faculty distinction affecting professional socialization is the difference between the Ph.D. professors, who are generally more theoretically and research-oriented, and the M.D. professors, who typically, as clinicians, think and work on substantive rather than academic problems. Since there is a natural tendency for like to beget like, medical students, who spend much of their first two years learning from basic scientists, often feel they are treated more like graduate students than prospective doctors; and this both irritates and frustrates them. When grievances are made known to academically inclined mentors, antagonistic relationships can result, the implications of which can significantly affect student adjustment. This basic feature of social structure accounts for much of the disillusionment and disenchantment experienced by students.

Another distinctive feature of the socializing network is that the *anticipated* status of the medical student (that is, the full-fledged physician's status) exceeds the *present* status of nurses and technicians. Whereas students are acutely aware that these clinical helpers must eventually follow their medical orders, as physicians-in-training students are in many ways subordinate. Nurses, for example, have considerable informal authority on the hospital floors and can easily deflate the ego of a haughty student. However, as students gain practical knowledge and begin asserting themselves, their status relationships with allied health workers change in their own favor.

Clearly, the socializing network is a dynamic entity, one characterized by continual jockeying for status and professional recognition. Recruits, as fledgling medical students, have very low status in the medical school hierarchy—"the very bottom rung of the ladder." But during the next four years, they struggle successfully for status. In their own minds at least, if not in fact, students surpass not only nurses and technicians but also Ph.D. professors, whom they can dismiss as "frustrated med school rejects." But such status one-upmanship is achieved with physician colleagues only by demonstrating professional dedication and clinical competence. Toward this end medical school graduates strive throughout their professional futures.

MEDICAL SCHOOL RECRUITS

Medical school is distinctive among people-changing institutions in the high motivation of its recruits and their willingness to accept formal goals set by others. By any standards of comparison, student-doctors possess an extraordinary degree of personal commitment to master medicine, an objective that for many stems from childhood as a life goal. Such singleness of mind is evident from the fact that many have not even considered the possibility of an alternate career.

Willingness to sacrifice in order to enhance success typifies medical recruits. Just gaining access to the training institution usually requires years of struggle and deprivation. Aspirants must not only have competed successfully for the best grades, but must also be willing to set aside personal pleasures and to shoulder heavy financial burdens. Less motivated candidates have typically fallen by the wayside in the natural selection process that occurs in high school and college competition.

Since the number of aspirants far exceeds the available openings, screening committees rigorously scrutinize candidates through achievement records, recommendations, and personal interviews. This process enhances a uniformity of motivation and social type among recruits.

Traditionally, the predominant social type accepted for medical training has consisted of young Caucasian males from stable middle-class families. Presumably such individuals were favored because they displayed the proper attitudes and mannerisms valued by screening committees who, aside from their ages, were of similar type. Medical school, it seems, like other social systems, tends to attract those who already share the attitudes and traits of incumbents.

Recently, however, the traditional screening system has been altered to include more women and ethnic minorities. But, unfortunately, at the time I began this study, only a few token members of the latter groups were admitted, so the generalizations contained herein are delimited primarily to the traditional group. Nonetheless, whatever social categories are represented by recruits, all seem to share a common motivation and commitment to the mastery of medicine.[2] Unlike participants in many other change institutions, few, if any, medical recruits need motivating; this is a salient principle. Clearly, professional socialization in medical school does not begin from scratch. Unlike socializing systems that purportedly try to change deficient personality traits, medical recruits, of whatever social type, reflect enthusiastic motivation, especially at the outset.

SOCIALIZING PROCESS

Professional socialization in medical school involves a series of challenging learning experiences that equip recruits with the necessary knowledge, technical skills, behavioral traits, and attitudes expected of the accomplished physician. As in most teaching institutions, the educational program consists of stages in which different role-demands are imposed at progressive times. The expectation is that the prospective doctor's response to earlier demands will result in the ability to meet and fulfill later ones.

The curriculum ensures an upward status passage—from lowly freshman to progressively higher stages of sophomore, junior, and senior—as students demonstrate abilities to successfully master the developmental tasks of each sequential level. By "developmental task" I mean a task that arises at a certain period, the successful accomplishment of which leads to personal satisfaction and success with later tasks; whereas failure in such a task leads to disappointment, disapproval by associates, and difficulty with later tasks (Havighurst, 1953).

As Duvall (1957) has pointed out, victory in mastering a given developmental task involves four interrelated psychosocial aspects. First, recruits must perceive new possibilities for themselves. This is accomplished by noting what is expected by others and by observing what is accomplished by those who are more advanced.

Second, participants must be motivated enough to be willing to work and struggle to achieve the next developmental step. The goal, of course, must be attainable. This does not imply that recruits should never experience failure or criticism, but that the problem should, more often than not, be solvable. The reward must also be commensurate with the effort.

Third, students must successfully resolve competing demands, blending potentially incompatible norms into a functionally consistent and stable pattern of professional behavior; for example, they must struggle successfully for good grades without making classmates feel inferior. Merton (1957, pp. 73–75) has provided other examples of competing demands,[3] a few of which are paraphrased below:

a. Student-physicians should be interested in enlarging their medical responsibilities while advancing through medical school, but must not prematurely take a measure of responsibility for which they are not adequately prepared (or, at least, are not legally qualified to undertake).

b. Physicians must maintain a self-critical attitude and be disciplined in the scientific appraisal of evidence, but be decisive and not postpone decisions longer than the situation requires, even when the scientific evidence is inadequate.

c. Physicians must have a sense of autonomy, take the burden of responsibility, and act as the situation, in their best judgment requires, but autonomy must not be allowed to become complacency or smug self-assurance and must be coupled with a due sense of humility.

d. Physicians must have the kind of detailed knowledge that often requires specialized education, but must not become narrowly specialized; they should be well-rounded and broadly educated.

e. Physicians should have strong moral character with abiding commitments to basic moral values, but must avoid passing moral judgments on patients.

f. Physicians must provide adequate and unhurried medical care for each patient, but should not allow any patient to usurp their limited time at the expense of other patients.

g. Physicians should · institute all scientific tests needed to reach a sound diagnosis, but should be discriminating in the use of these tests, since these are often costly and may impose a sizable financial burden on patients.

h. Physicians should see to it that medical care is available for every patient whenever it is required, but doctors, too, have a right to a "normal life" which they share with their families.

i. Physicians must collaborate with others on the medical team rather than dominate them (nurses, social workers, technicians), but must have the final responsibility for the team and see to it that their associates meet high standards.

Fourth and finally, recruits form a new self-concept. By demonstrating successful mastery of a task, students not only gain intrinsic satisfaction, but also rise in status and otherwise gain favorable responses from others. This social looking glass makes them feel more able, more knowledgeable, and more professional—in short, more physician-like.

My thesis is that personal growth in medical school results from struggling successfully to master developmental tasks, many of which tax students' resources to the limit. In this view, challenging obstacles serve as catalysts for role-relevant development. First, recruits are exposed to formidable classroom-type problems. Here they must prove their mettle by mastering enormous amounts of material and by passing written examinations. During this early stage, they must also dissect dead humans dispassionately and handle contagious organisms without manifesting fear or squeamishness. Having conquered these and similar hurdles, students then encounter stressful interpersonal experiences, such as handling forbidden parts of others' bodies and discussing intimate aspects of sex and marriage. They also participate in autopsies and surgical procedures and confront a variety of acute crises, dealing as well with hopelessly ill and dying patients.

Every time a student, through struggling effort, advances to a new level, makes an intellectual discovery, sees a new connection, or understands a new idea, curiosity is nourished and capacity increased, and thus the student is prepared and motivated for further growth. The process is not unlike rock climbing. Although exhilarating plateaus are occasionally reached that dramatize progress, most of the journey involves a painfully slow and often discouraging inching upward. But each careful step serves as a foothold for future progress and enhances vision, perspective, and feelings of personal fulfillment. Eventually, gratified though weary participants reach their goal. But since higher peaks lie ahead in the journey (internship, residency, and so on), there is only limited time for celebrating.

Fortunately, the upward trek is accompanied by a curriculum guide that marks the route and by experienced instructors who impart necessary knowledge and skills through example and precept. Classmates can also be a source of support and comfort. Inspiration, too, comes from the realization that the goal is achievable, for many others traveling the same course have attained the summit.

STAGES OF PROFESSIONAL AFFECT

The technical knowledge and skill bases of professional development, openly recognized and valued as they are, typically progress predictably in accordance with formal plan. The curriculum is designed to enhance student success in these areas, and progress can be assessed easily through written or oral examinations. But the subjective aspects of professional development—the inner adjustments experienced by students in coping with stress—are rarely measured or even discusssed by the faculty. Little time is reserved for assisting the troubled student and spouse, if there is one, in adjusting feelings to the pressures and vicissitudes of the training experience except, of course, when developmental casualties become unmistakenly visible. Then, and usually only then, are faculty resources marshaled to help students deal with feelings that arise from the stressful experiences of medical training.

In the medical center milieu, rationality and restrained emotionality are highly valued; science reigns supreme. Rarely do professionals in this atmosphere reveal their inner feelings to others—the fears, anxieties, frustrations, and self-doubts that normally accompany stressful experiences. Good doctors, it seems, must be marvelously in control of their feelings at all times; even in the face of human tragedy they must remain calm and objective.

Although behavioral science courses, which are increasingly given time in the medical curriculum, have great potential for meeting the needs of students to ventilate and reflect upon the subjective features of medical education and practice, presentations usually follow the traditional model, with topics intellectualized in didactic presentations while students listen passively. Although feelings may cry for expression, the scientific and technological climate of the medical school as currently constituted requires one to keep such expression under control. So, unless students have an empathetic marital companion or an intimate friend who is willing to listen, they will in all likelihood suppress expression of personal feelings.

The result is that medical trainees typically evolve through fairly predictable develpmental stages in coping with their own feelings. Although these stages are not fixed or immutable, they characterize, I submit, the majority of recruits who experience the traditional system of medical training.

Since the ultimate challenge of the clinical role brings the emerging physician face to face with the intensely human drama of death and dying, I describe these stages in terms of this ubiquitous event.[4]

Stage 1—Idealizing a Doctor's Role

Initially, students have the same attitudes and feelings as the general public. Having little personal experience with suffering and dying, they are no more enlightened than laymen. They have not escaped the fears and phobias that beset other human beings. Dealing routinely with stressful human experiences requires coping skills that they have not yet developed.

At this preprofessional stage, personal identification with suffering patients is strong, and students are apt to find themselves participating imaginatively in the suffering involved. They have not yet evolved from the layman's attitude toward suffering and death. In time, they will acquire the equanimity of the veteran doctor, a fact many of them realize. Even this realization, though, does not always keep the transition from being painful. Intellectual understanding is one thing, but managing feelings is quite another.

When they first begin medical training, students find the approach of the case-hardened clinician to be offensive. In their idealistic view, the physician, like the proverbial country doctor, should be warm and compassionate. So it is disillusioning to witness the unfeeling way in which doctors typically handle patients—even though most students realize, at least on an intellectual level, that such detachment does not necessarily indicate a lack of concern and that a doctor's failure to become emotionally involved may be in the patient's best interest. Later on, in fact, students shed the typical layman's response and find themselves reacting much like their clinical mentors.

Stage 2—Desensitizing Death Symbols

From the beginning of medical training, students are desensitized to the symbols and conditions that surround death. They no longer react to blood, gore, corpses, and stench that normally disturb people. During the first days of school, they are escorted into the anatomy lab and introduced to a dead body that must be cut into and dissected in careful detail. As previously mentioned, the ability to undergo such experiences without revealing disgust or squeamishness is a valued characteristic at the medical center. So, pretending nonchalance, students remain "cool" and suppress openness about personal anxieties.

A number of coping mechanisms are utilized to manage feelings and thereby make the experience more tolerable.[5] Humor provides tension release and helps students forget the morose aspects of their introduction to anatomy. Inner relief is most typically derived, though, by losing oneself in the details of the dissection process and memorizing the scientific names of bones, muscles, nerves, and other body parts. In doing so, dissection becomes a mechanistic exercise rather than a humanistic experience.

Further desensitization occurs in the sophomore year when students are introduced to their first autopsy. This brings them closer to the subjective or personal aspects of death because only a few hours earlier the patient was living. And, because the body has not been treated in any way, it is easier to perceive it as a real person. Also, the attending physician is nearly always present, and this helps define the dead person as a patient rather than a mere specimen. Moreover, unlike the cadaver experience, students have knowledge of the patient's identity and medical history through reading the chart and listening to the doctor's report about the fatal illness.

In order to maintain equanimity and protect themselves from the discomfort of such a stressful experience, students, like their mentors, adopt detached scientific attitudes. Emotionality is avoided or suppressed by focusing on the technical aspects. Losing themselves in details of the autopsy helps prospective doctors maintain an "objective professional response." Thinking about diseased tissue is much less emotionally draining than pondering about the patient as a person.

The practice of dealing with illness and death on an intellectual rather than an emotional basis is well entrenched during the first two years of medical school when scientific terminology and textbook knowledge provide the substance of required basic-science courses. Through this means students come closer to the expected professional responses—calm objective rationality and fully controlled emotions. This desensitized condition prepares them for the face-to-face encounters they will have with living patients.

Stage 3—Objectifying and Combating Death

When the training scene shifts from the lecture room and laboratory to the hospital, students are exposed to some of life's most poignant dramas. The companions of death—pain, suffering, fear, and despair—are everywhere. Here students learn to distance themselves from the living as well as the dead.

The main depersonalizing technique, modeled effectively by the clinical staff, is to objectify death—in other words, deny the subjective features. Clinicians begin to view patients not as people with feelings, but as medical entities, specimens, or objects of scientific interest. By adopting a scientific frame of mind, utilized so effectively in their previous work with dead bodies, clinicians can effectively avoid the uncomfortable inner feelings that occur when they are exposed to sick and dying patients. This pose serves as a protective shield.

The dynamics by which clinicians dissociate themselves involve an intellectual dissection of the patient into parts and then concentration on and treatment of only the pathological parts rather than the "whole person." It is this orientation that expresses itself in such comments as "the liver in 724." For it is less stressful to concentrate on the anatomy and physiological processes than on a suffering human being. Thus, Mr. Brown becomes "a fractured femur" and Mrs. Jones "an ovarian cyst."

It must not be concluded, though, that doctors take their clinical responsibilities lightly. On the contrary, heavy demands are habitually made upon medical trainees to be exhaustively thorough in keeping people alive and well. When a patient stops breathing or his heart stops beating, extraordinary efforts are routinely made to revive him and prolong his life. First, an emergency announcement is made in code language over the hospital public address system ("Code Red, Room 227," for example). Every available physician is then expected to rush to the patient's bedside. Special emergency squads hurry through the halls, and the patient is hooked up to a variety of monitors and life-saving machinery. Not until every life-saving attempt has been exhausted do they let up. Such efforts are routine in the hospital setting.

Although verbal praise is rarely given for a job well done, medical staff members are fiercely critical of haphazard clinical performance. Clinical pathology conferences, called CPCs or "death rounds," provide a forum for this criticism. Whenever a patient dies, the attending staff, house staff, and others concerned gather in an auditorium to discuss the "case." Whoever was responsible for the patient presents the clinical history, and the pathology report is given. Everyone then discusses what should have been done differently so that death might have been avoided. Clearly, the assumption is that death is preventable and is not supposed to happen to patients of good physicians. At least, this is the idea that is handed down to medical trainees. No wonder a sense of personal defeat is felt each time a patient dies.

Stage 4—Questioning the Medical Teaching Model

With increasing experience, clinicians can come to question and ultimately reject the prevailing values espoused in medical training regarding death. This observation is reinforced by supplemental interviews with practicing physicians.[6] The medical teaching model, as these clinicians perceive it, tends to dehumanize the patient and make a mere technician of the physician. They see it as glorifying the science of medicine (a thorough knowledge of disease processes and a ready command of clinical techniques) at the expense of the art of medicine (an interpersonal ability to meet the patient's needs by relating warmly and meaningfully to him and his family). In the quest to master the science of medicine, the clinician can come to regard the patient as a diseased object rather than as a fellow human being. "I hate to admit it," one said, "but I had come to view the patient almost as an extension of the apparatus in the room."

The turning point comes when those who reach this stage can no longer bear the absurd extremes taken to fend off the death of a patient. "I've heard that no one dies with dignity in this hospital," one said. "There is always a crowd of people around frantically working over the patient and hooking him up to gadgets."

The extraordinary efforts to keep some patients alive, though doomed to a vegetable-like existence, are seen as "just so much medical pyrotechnics" designed to fulfill the physician's own needs rather than the patient's and his family's. Professional recognition and self-esteem come to a clinician who demonstrates technical mastery. But the reputation for being a compassionate and sympathetic clinician brings little cognizance from one's colleagues.

Doctors' egos are easily inflated when they are cast in the role of healer and master of death. Patients entrusting their lives to them naturally want to believe in their healing powers. Placed on a pedestal, one can easily feel omnipotent and become intoxicated with a sense of power.

But as clinicians who have reached this point see it, "the God complex" is incompatible with good medical practice. In their opinion, it is unrealistic to expect a cure for everybody and inappropriate in many situations to unnecessarily prolong life.

Those who have reached this plateau of insight perceive a good clinician to be one who has mastered the art as well as the science of medicine. Rather than being compulsively concerned with mastery over death, a good clinician considers the feelings of the patient and the family before all else.

Stage 5—Dealing with Personal Feelings

Up to this point, their experiences have conditioned clinicians to suppress personal anxieties.[7] Everyone knows that a good doctor is supposed to be calm, with personal feelings under control—someone on whom the family can rely for steady support and understanding. Clinicians who feel anxiety or fear in the face of death must carefully conceal these emotions. "I've had a lot of training in putting up a good front so that others can't see what I'm feeling inside," one said. "I've learned to keep this cool facade of being in control, but inside I'm feeling a lot of stress."

Until clinicians reach this level of self-examination, they often cope with impending death by utilizing avoidance as a technique. "I try to keep away from patients if I know what's coming up so as to reduce the emotional stress," a senior student confessed. Feelings of helplessness stimulated by hopelessly ill patients can be relieved by passing these patients off to someone else or appearing too busy to spend much time with them. "We ignore the patient because we are so fearful ourselves," one admitted.

Typically, every effort is made in the hospital setting to shield staff from mourning relatives. In the emergency room, quiet crying is tolerated, but if any kind of emotional outburst occurs, relatives are usually hustled off to the chapel or "meditation room" as fast as possible. "We isolate them so that their grief is not so obvious," one said. "It isn't done cruelly, but, frankly, the purpose is more to protect the emergency room staff than to help the family."

Physicians transcend this phase of avoidance as they begin to realize that how one feels inside is sometimes more important than what is actually said or done. Self-examination is stimulated when, in trying to be more than a mere technician, the doctor attempts to deal meaningfully with the feelings of patients and their families. If they are to be of true assistance to others in more than a technical sense, clinicians must come to grips with their deepest and darkest fears. How can they allay the terrors and anxieties of others if they have not resolved their own? Is it natural to expect comforting relief from one whose training has neglected methods of dealing realistically with such emotions?

Reflecting back upon their earlier training, clinicians at this stage fault their mentors for giving them so little help with the subjective aspects of clinical practice. "It's almost as though I've had to deal with this part of medical practice without being prepared for it," one said. When death and dying are discussed in medical school, if at all, the topic is intellectualized "in cookbook-like fashion, no different from learning to work up a case of hypertension." Another said, "We were never asked to express our feelings or discuss how we felt about death." And rarely do clinical mentors openly reveal their own feelings—the frustrations, anger, or feelings of helplessness that occur when a patient dies. So medical trainees are left to their own resources in resolving inner dilemmas on this sensitive topic.[8]

This unhappy state of affairs is mastered only when the clinician faces up to personal feelings and no longer utilizes the usual coping mechanisms for insulation from the daily stresses in the medical milieu. "I can speak for myself and possibly for a lot of other physicians," one practicing doctor said. "In my younger years, my professional self-image wouldn't permit me to be slowed down or have my efficiency reduced by my feelings. So I evolved into a condition of what I now call 'disembodied intelligence,' but now I'm trying to get more and more in touch with my own feelings, to recognize them and tolerate them and thereby be in a better position to help others with their feelings."

Once having reached this stage, the introspective clinician who has recognized personal feelings and limitations and has managed to reconcile them as well is uniquely capable of practicing compleat medicine. He or she alone has the personal ability and resources to bring technical knowledge and sympathetic care to suffering patients and their loved ones.

MEDICAL SCHOOL PRODUCT

Some years ago, Harold I. Lief and his colleagues (Lief, 1971) conducted a psychiatric assessment of 60 freshman medical students at Tulane University School of Medicine. Using personal interviews and a battery of psychological tests such as the Rorschach and the Miller Analogy tests, they classified students according to four personality types: mature, emergent, adjusted, and conflicted.

The *mature* student is characterized by a high level of competence; such students are effective in their human environment, fully functioning human beings. These six attributes characterize the mature student: intellectuality, close friendships, independence in value judgments, tolerance of ambiguity, breadth of interest, and sense of humor. Such a student is introspective and comfortable with his own feelings as well as those of others.

The *emergent* student is on the way to becoming a mature person but still has many traits of late adolescence. At times these students show mature capabilities, judgments, and behaviors, but at other times they are unpredictable and lack emotional control. They are not yet totally reliable or ready for major responsibility. Excessive deference or rebellion is typical as is overzealousness in trying to prove their adulthood. Because of inner confusion, these students vacillate in feelings and behavior. Such students are uncertain about themselves and the world around them; but they have much creative potential and will do well if helped to sort out their experiences and understand the underlying meanings behind them.

The *adjusted* student initially appears perfectly normal and healthy, totally adjusted. This individual is poised, well-mannered, and makes good impressions and friends with equal ease. On the surface, at least, this student has mastered the skills of social manipulation, of getting along with others. But on closer scrutiny, signs of emotional constriction are apparent. Although this student may talk freely about things or events, talking about personal feelings is difficult, for such a student lacks psychological-mindedness. This doctor-to-be is concrete rather than abstract, a technician rather than a meditator, an individual with only limited personal interests.

Finally, the *conflicted* student suffers from an emotional handicap, such as being obsessive–compulsive, paranoid, schizophrenic, having an "inadequate personality," or experiencing hysteria or anxiety reactions. Fortunately, most of these students, Lief says, are only moderately handicapped, so that serious impairment of their clinical functioning is improbable. The remarkable fact is, however, that almost seven out of ten students were diagnosed as "conflicted" (38 percent) * or "adjusted" (30 percent). The remainder, less than a third, were classified as "mature" (17 percent) or "emergent" (15 percent).

Unquestionably, the persistent pressures of medical education, both academic and clinical, the relative isolation from the outside world, and the personal loneliness that students often experience have great potential for reinforcing emotional constriction and contributing to narrowness of interest, especially among those so inclined at the outset. Lief's psychiatric analysis makes clear that most students would benefit greatly if the medical curriculum included regular structured opportunities for them to freely and openly discuss the subjective as well as the technical aspects of their experiences.[9] My own interviews and personal observations have clearly revealed the students' unmet need to air, to reflect upon, to emotionally explore, and sort out personal feelings as related to specified developmental tasks. This unfilled need adversely affects student adjustment in the medical school environment and, no doubt, also lowers the potential quality of patient care.

Although this seems a conspicuous deficiency in the existing education system, medical recruits typically emerge from medical school much more academically and clinically astute than when they entered. One wonders, though, how much more effective they might be if given the benefits of emotional exploration. Yet, despite the fact that they have survived numerous challenging vicissitudes, and have had little help feeling their way on this emotional battlefield, the accomplishment of four years' hard work has generally left them more capable, more mature, more confident, and self-fulfilled. Having finally achieved the doctor's status, these young physicians are ready for increased independence and greater clinical responsibilities. They are now prepared for the next stage of the professional journey—graduate medical training. Like butterflies recently freed of the caterpillar existence, exulting medical school graduates eagerly anticipate the future. For they have achieved a conspicuous accomplishment on the road to mastering medicine, one that has immediate relevance for society as well as for themselves.

---

* Of the 23 students classified as "conflicted," seven were diagnosed as obsessive–compulsive psychiatric character types, five as paranoid, five as schizophrenic, one as hysterical, two as having anxiety reactions, and three as "inadequate personalities." Eight of these students applied for and received psychotherapy. Three others eventually dropped out of school.

NOTES

1. This aspect of medical training is increasingly being altered in U.S. medical schools to allow more elective time and "multiple track" training (Pattishall, 1972).

2. For a discussion of commitment as related to personal change in adult life, see Becker (1964).

3. These selections are reprinted in their entirety and amplified in Merton (1976).

4. I have elaborated on these stages in more detail in an article entitled "Socialization for Death: The Physician's Role" (Coombs and Powers, 1975).

5. For further reading about the coping mechanisms utilized by clinicians to manage stress, see Coombs and Goldman (1973).

6. My insights about Stages 4 and 5 have been sharpened by interviews with 13 practicing physicians. Their ages ranged from 30 to 57 with a mean age of 41. Three were women, ten were men, and all but one, an anesthesiologist, were currently in psychiatric training or in the private practice of psychiatry. Eight were in general practice prior to beginning psychiatric training; among these the average length of general practice was 12 years, with a range of from 2 to 25 years. The anesthesiologist had practiced this specialty for 7 years. Two of those interviewed had been in the military service after interning, and the remaining two had gone directly into psychiatric training.

7. In the case of male physicians, handling of emotions can pose special problems, since the tendency to suppress personal feelings is prompted by the way male children are typically raised. (See Coombs, 1968b.)

8. Glaser and Strauss (1968) have pointed out: "The psychological aspects of dealing with the dying and their families are virtually absent from training. Hence, although physicians and nurses are highly skilled at handling the bodies of terminal patients, their behavior to them otherwise is actually outside the province of professional standards."

9. The School of Medicine at the University of Chicago has altered the traditional pattern by having students interview patients within six weeks after beginning the freshman year (*Los Angeles Times*, 1975). In the first weeks, actresses portraying patients with cancer and other maladies are brought into the classroom for simulated interviews. Here the patient "reveals" innermost feelings about pain and death. Such sessions help students recognize personal difficulties and provide opportunities to talk about sensitive topics like sex and bodily functions that are not normally discussed in polite society.

References

ADSETT, C. A. (1968). "Psychological health of medical students in relation to the medical education process." *Journal of Medical Education* **43** (Pt 1, June), 728–734.

ALLPORT, GORDON W., PHILIP E. VERNON, AND GARDNER LINDZEY (1960). *Study of Values: A Scale for Measuring the Dominant Interests in Personality*. 3rd edition (Boston: Houghton Mifflin Company).

ASSOCIATION OF AMERICAN MEDICAL COLLEGES (1974a). "Financing undergraduate medical education: A statement of policy." (Report of the Committee on the Financing of Medical Education, Charles C. Sprague, M.D., Chairman, Washington, D.C.)

—— (1974b). 1974–75 AAMC Curriculum Directory (Washington, D.C.).

—— (1974c). "Undergraduate medical education: Elements, objectives, costs." (A report by the Committee on the Financing of Medical Education.) *Journal of Medical Education* **49** (January), 97–128.

—— (1975). Medical School Admission Requirements, 1976–77, U.S.A. and Canada. 26th edition, pp. 33–42 (Washington, D.C.).

—— (1977). "Annual report for 1976: Education." *Journal of Medical Education* **52** (March), 262–264.

BARTON, DAVID (1972). "The need for including instruction on death and dying in the medical curriculum." *Journal of Medical Education* **47** (March), 169–175.

BECKER, HOWARD S. (1956). "Interviewing medical students." *American Journal of Sociology* **62** (September), 199–201.

—— (1964). "Personal change in adult life." *Sociometry* **27** (March), 40–53.

BECKER, HOWARD S., AND BLANCHE GEER (1958). "The fate of idealism in medical school." *American Sociological Review* **23** (February), 50–56.

BECKER, HOWARD S., BLANCHE GEER, EVERETT C. HUGHES, AND ANSELM L. STRAUSS (1961). *Boys in White: Student Culture in Medical School* (Chicago: University of Chicago Press).

BLAINE, GRAHAM B., AND CHARLES C. McARTHUR (1961) *Emotional Problems of the Student* (New York: Appleton-Century-Crofts).

269

BLOCK, JACK (1961). *The Q-Sort Method in Personality Assessment and Psychiatric Research* (Springfield, Illinois: Charles C Thomas).

BLOOM, SAMUEL W. (1963). "The process of becoming a physician." *The Annals of the American Academy of Political and Social Science* 346 (March), 77–87.

—— (1965). "The sociology of medical education." *The Milbank Memorial Fund Quarterly* 43 (April), 143–184.

—— (1971). "The medical center as a social system." In Robert H. Coombs and Clark E. Vincent (eds.), *Psychosocial Aspects of Medical Training* (Springfield, Illinois: Charles C Thomas), pp. 429–448.

—— (1973). *Power and Descent in the Medical School* (New York: The Free Press).

BLUMER, HERBERT (1962). "Society as symbolic interaction." In Arnold M. Rose (ed.), *Human Behavior and Social Processes* (Boston: Houghton Mifflin Company), pp. 179–192.

BOJAR, S. (1961). "Psychiatric problems of medical students." In G. B. Blaine and C. C. McArthur (eds.), *Emotional Problems of the Student* (New York: Appleton-Century-Crofts), pp. 218–219.

BOVERMAN, HAROLD (1965). "Senior student career choices in retrospect." *Journal of Medical Education* 40 (February), 161–165.

BOWERS, JOHN Z. (1968). "Special problems of women medical students." *Journal of Medical Education* 43 (May), 532–537.

BOYLE, BLAKE P., AND ROBERT H. COOMBS (1971). "Personality profiles related to emotional stress in the initial year of medical training." *Journal of Medical Education* 46 (October), 882–888.

BRIM, ORVILLE G., JR., AND STANTON WHEELER (1966). *Socialization After Childhood: Two Essays* (New York: John Wiley and Sons, Inc.).

BROWN, ROBERT S. (1970). "House staff attitudes toward teaching." *Journal of Medical Education* 45 (March), 156–159.

BRUHN, J. G., AND O. A. PARSONS (1964). "Medical student attitudes toward four medical specialties." *Journal of Medical Education* 39 (January), 40–49.

—— (1965). "Attitudes toward medical specialties: Two follow-up studies." *Journal of Medical Education* 40 (March), 273–280.

CAMPBELL, MARGARET A. (1974). *Why Would a Girl Go Into Medicine? Medical Education in the United States: A Guide for Women* (Old Westbury, New York: Feminist Press).

CAUGHEY, JOHN L. (1966). "More medical students: The need and available supply." *Journal of The American Medical Association* 198 (December 5), 1105–1107.

CEITHAML, JOSEPH (1965). "The financial state of the American medical student." *Journal of Medical Education* 40 (June), 497–505.

CHAPIN, F. STUART (1967). *The Social Insight Test* (Palo Alto, California: Consulting Psychologists Press, Inc.).

CHRISTIE, RICHARD, AND ROBERT K. MERTON (1958). "Procedures for the sociological study of the value climate of medical schools," in *The Ecology of the Medical Students* (A report of the Fifth Teaching Institute, Association of American Medical Colleges, Evanston, Illinois).

CLAUSEN, JOHN A. (ed.) (1968). *Socialization and Society* (Boston: Little, Brown and Company).

COBB, SIDNEY, AND JOHN R. P. FRENCH, JR. (1966). "Birth order among medical students." *Journal of The American Medical Association* 195 (January 24), 312–313.

COCHRANE, CARL M. (1971). "Successful medical trainees and practitioners." In Robert H. Coombs and Clark E. Vincent (eds.), *Psychosocial Aspects of Medical Training* (Springfield, Illinois: Charles C Thomas), pp. 168–190.

COHEN, E. D., AND S. P. KORPER (1976). "Women in medicine: A survey of professional activities, career interruptions, and conflict resolutions." (Trends in medical education and specialization.) *Connecticut Medicine* 40 (February), 103–110.

COOMBS, ROBERT H. (1966). "Value consensus and partner satisfaction among dating couples." *Journal of Marriage and the Family* 28 (May), 166–173.

—— (1968a). "Sex education for physicians: Is it adequate?" *The Family Coordinator* 17 (October), 271–277.

—— (1968b). "The socialization of male and female: Sex status and sex role." In Clark E. Vincent (ed), *Human Sexuality in Medical Education and Practice* (Springfield, Illinois: Charles C Thomas), pp. 249–284.

—— (1969). "Social participation, self-concept and interpersonal valuation." *Sociometry* 32 (September), 273–286.

—— (1971a). "Inhibition in verbal sexual communication." *Medical Aspects of Human Sexuality* V (April), 152–163.

—— (1971b). "The medical marriage." In Robert H. Coombs and Clark E. Vincent (eds.), *Psychosocial Aspects of Medical Training* (Springfield, Illinois: Charles C Thomas), pp. 133–167.

COOMBS, ROBERT H., AND BLAKE P. BOYLE (1971a). "Marriage as a buffer against emotional stress in medical training." *California Mental Health Research Digest* 9 (Spring and Summer), 59–65.

—— (1971b). "The transition to medical school: Expectations versus realities." In Robert H. Coombs and Clark E. Vincent (eds.), *Psychosocial Aspects of Medical Training* (Springfield, Illinois: Charles C Thomas), pp. 91–109.

COOMBS, ROBERT H., AND VERNON DAVIES (1966). "Self-conception and the relationship between high school and college scholastic achievement." *Sociology and Social Research* 50, no. 4 (July), 460–471.

COOMBS, ROBERT H., AND LAWRENCE J. GOLDMAN (1973). "Maintenance and discontinuity of coping mechanisms in an intensive care unit." *Social Problems* 20 (Winter), 342–355.

COOMBS, ROBERT H., LINCOLN J. FRY, AND PATRICIA G. LEWIS (eds.) (1976).

Socialization in Drug Abuse (Cambridge: Schenkman Publishing Company/Transaction Books).

COOMBS, ROBERT H., AND PAULINE S. POWERS (1975). "Socialization for death: The physician's role." *Urban Life* 4 (October), 250–271.

COOMBS, ROBERT H., AND LOUIS P. STEIN (1971). "Medical-student society and culture." In Robert H. Coombs and Clark E. Vincent (eds.), *Psychosocial Aspects of Medical Training* (Springfield, Illinois: Charles C Thomas), pp. 110–132.

COSER, ROSE LAUB (1962). *Life in the Ward* (Lansing: Michigan State University Press).

CROWLEY, ANNE E. (ed.) (1975a). *Medical Education in the United States, 1973–1974. Journal of The American Medical Association, Supplement* 231 (January–special issue).

—— (1975b). *Medical Education in the United States, 1974–1975 Journal of The American Medical Association* 234 (December 29–special issue).

"Datagram" (1971). "Trends in medical school tuition levels, 1952–53 to 1972–73." *Journal of Medical Education* 46 (February), 175–176.

—— (1972). "U.S. medical student enrollments, 1968–1969 through 1971–1972." *Journal of Medical Education* 47 (February), 150–153.

—— (1976a). "Medical student enrollment, 1971–72 through 1975–76." *Journal of Medical Education* 51 (February), 144–146.

—— (1976b). "Applicants for 1975–76 first-year medical school class." *Journal of Medical Education* 51 (October), 867–869.

—— (1977). "Medical school enrollment, 1972–73 through 1976–77." *Journal of Medical Education* 52 (February), 164–166.

DAVIS, MILTON S. (1971). "Variation in patients' compliance with doctors' orders: Medical practice and doctor-patient interaction." *Psychiatry in Medicine* 2 (January), 31–54.

DAVISON, WILBURT C. (1952). *The First Twenty Years: A History of Duke University School of Nursing and Health Service and Duke Hospital, 1930–1950* (Durham, North Carolina: Duke University).

DEBRABANDER, BERT, AND CARLOS A. LEON (1968). "A comparative study of attitudes among Columbian medical and nonmedical students." *Journal of Medical Education* 43 (August), 912–915.

DRESDEN, J. H., F. COLLINS, AND R. ROESSLER (1975). "Cognitive and noncognitive characteristics of minority medical school applicants." *Journal of the National Medical Association* 67 (July), 321–323.

DUBÉ, W. F. (1974a). "U.S. medical school enrollment, 1969–70 through 1973–74." In "Datagram," *Journal of Medical Education* 49 (March), 302–307.

—— (1974b). "Undergraduate origins of U.S. medical students." In "Datagram," *Journal of Medical Education* 49 (October), 1005–1010.

—— (1975). "U.S. medical school enrollment, 1970–71 through 1974–75." In "Datagram," *Journal of Medical Education* 50 (March), 303–306.

DUBÉ, W. F., AND DAVIS G. JOHNSON (1976). "Study of U.S. medical school applicants, 1974–75." *Journal of Medical Education* 51 (November), 877–896.

Durkheim, Emile (1938). *The Rules of Sociological Method* (Chicago: University of Chicago Press).

Duvall, Evelyn Mellis (1957). *Family Development* (Chicago: Lippincott).

Engel, George L. (1971). "Care and feeding of the medical student." *Journal of The American Medical Association* 215 (February), 1135–1141.

Erdmann, James B., Dale E. Mattson, Jack G. Hutton, Jr., and Winburn L. Wallace (1971). "The medical college admission test: Past, present, and future." *Journal of Medical Education* 46 (November), 937–946.

Eriksen, E. H. (1959). "Late adolescence." In D. H. Funkenstein (ed.), *The Student and Mental Health: An International View* (New York: World Federation for Mental Health).

Eron, Leonard D. (1955). "Effect of medical education on medical students' attitudes." *Journal of Medical Education* 30 (October), 559–566.

—— (1958). "Effect of medical education on attitudes: A follow-up study." *Journal of Medical Education* 33 (Pt 2) (October), 25–33.

Evans, D. A., and E. B. Jackson, Jr. (1976). "Deans of minority student affairs in medical schools." *Journal of Medical Education* 51 (March), 197–199.

Fish, D. G., and J. H. Mount (1966). "Canadian medical students' judgments of the prestige ascribed by the public to various fields of medical practice." *College of General Practice of Canada, Journal* (July), 1–8.

Fox, Renée (1959). *Experiment Perilous* (Glencoe, Illinois: The Free Press).

Funkenstein, Daniel H. (1961). "A study of college seniors who abandoned their plans for medicine." *Journal of Medical Education* 36 (August), 924–933.

—— (1968). "Implications of the rapid social changes in universities and medical schools for the education of future physicians." *Journal of Medical Education* 43 (April), 433–454.

Gaines, V. P. (1975). Letter: "Minority recruitment and retention." *Journal of Medical Education* 50 (April), 416–417.

Geertsma, Robert H., and Robert J. Stoller (1966). "Changes in medical students' conceptions of the ideal patient." *Journal of Medical Education* 41 (January), 45–48.

Glaser, Barney G., and Anselm L. Strauss (1968). *Time for Dying* (Chicago: Aldine Publishing Company).

Goffman, Erving (1961). *Asylums: Essays of the Social Situation of Mental Patients and Other Inmates* (Chicago: Aldine Publishing Company).

Goldhaber, Samuel Z. (1973). "Medical education: Harvard reverts to tradition." *Science* 181 (September 14), 1027–1032.

Goldman, Lee, and Arthur Ebbert, Jr. (1973). "The fate of medical student liberalism: A prediction." *Journal of Medical Education* 48 (December), 1095–1103.

GORDON, LEONARD V. (1960). *Survey of Interpersonal Values* (Chicago: Science Research Associates, Inc.).

GORDON, LEONARD V., AND IVAN N. MENSH (1962). "Values of medical students at different levels of training." *Journal of Educational Psychology* 53, 48–51.

GORDON, TRAVIS L. (1977). *Descriptive Study of Medical School Applicants, 1975–76*. (Prepared by the Association of American Medical Colleges for the Bureau of Health Manpower, Washington, D.C.)

GOSLIN, DAVID A. (ed.) (1969). *Handbook of Socialization Theory and Research* (Chicago: Rand McNally and Company).

GOUGH, HARRISON G. (1967). *California Psychological Inventory* (Palo Alto, California: Consulting Psychologists Press, Inc.).

―――― (1971). "The recruitment and selection of medical students." In Robert H. Coombs and Clark E. Vincent (eds.), *Psychosocial Aspects of Medical Training* (Springfield, Illinois: Charles C Thomas), pp. 5–43.

―――― (1975a). "Factorial study of medical specialty preferences." *British Journal of Medical Education* 9 (June), 78–85.

―――― (1975b). "Specialty preferences of physicians and medical students." *Journal of Medical Education* 50 (June), 581–588.

GOUGH, HARRISON G., RONALD E. FOX, AND WALLACE B. HALL (1972). "Personality inventory assessment of psychiatric residents." *Journal of Counseling Psychology* 19 (July), 269–274.

GOUGH, HARRISON G., AND WALLACE B. HALL (1973). "A prospective study of personality changes in students in medicine, dentistry, and nursing." *Research in Higher Education* 1 (2), 127–140.

―――― (1975). "An attempt to predict graduation from medical school." *Journal of Medical Education* 50 (October), 940–950.

GOUGH, HARRISON G., AND ALFRED R. HEILBRUN, JR. (1965). *Adjective Check List* (Palo Alto, California: Consulting Psychologists Press, Inc.).

GRAFF, HAROLD, AND WILLIAM GROSSMAN (1973). "Trends in accelerated medical programs." *Journal of Medical Education* 48 (March), 283–285.

GRAY, ROBERT M., AND W. R. ELTON NEWMAN (1961). "Anomia and cynical attitudes of medical students." *Utah Academic Proceedings* 28, 68–73.

GRAY, ROBERT M., PHILIP M. MOODY, AND W. R. ELTON NEWMAN (1965). "An analysis of physicians' attitudes of cynicism and humanitarianism before and after entering medical practice." *Journal of Medical Education* 40 (August), 760–766.

GROSS, W., AND S. CROVITZ (1975). "A comparison of medical students' attitudes toward women and women medical students." *Journal of Medical Education* 50 (April), 392–394.

HAVIGHURST, ROBERT J. (1953). *Human Development and Education* (New York: Longman, Green).

HELD, MARK L., AND CARL N. ZIMET (1975). "A longitudinal study of medical specialty choice and certainty level." *Journal of Medical Education* 50 (November), 1044–1051.

HILBERMAN, E., J. KONANE, AND M. PEREZ-REYES et al. (1975). "Support groups for women in medical school: A first-year program." *Journal of Medical Education* 50 (September), 867–875.

HOMANS, GEORGE C. (1950). *The Human Group* (New York: Harcourt Brace and World, Inc.).

HOROWITZ, MILTON J. (1964). *Educating Tomorrow's Doctors* (New York: Appleton-Century-Crofts).

HOUSER, HENRY PAUL (1965). "Value orientations and conflict potential: A study of medical academicians and medical practitioners." *Dissertation Abstracts* 25 (April), 6104.

HOWELL, M. C. (1974). "Sounding board: What medical schools teach about women." *New England Journal of Medicine* 291 (August 8), 304–307.

HOWELL, M. C., AND D. HIATT (1975). "Do student health services discriminate against women? A survey of services in the U.S. medical schools." *Journal of the American Colleges Health Association* 23 (June), 359–363.

HUBBARD, WILLIAM N., JR., AND ROBERT B. HOWARD (1967). "The educational environment in the large medical school." *Journal of Medical Education* 42 (July), 633–641.

HUNTER, R. C. A., R. H. PRINCE, AND A. E. SCHWARTZMAN (1961). "Comments on emotional disturbances in a medical undergraduate population." *Canadian Medical Association Journal* 85 (October), 989–992.

HUNTINGTON, M. J. (1957). "The development of a professional self-image." In Robert K. Merton, George G. Reader, and Patricia L. Kendall (eds.), *The Student-Physician: Introductory Studies in the Sociology of Medical Education* (Cambridge, Massachusetts: Harvard University Press), pp. 179–187.

HUTCHINS, EDWIN B. (n.d.). *Medical College Environment Index* (Technical Report No. L661. Evanston, Illinois: Division of Education, Association of American Medical Colleges).

—— (1962). *Career Choice Trends Within and Between Graduating Classes* (Technical Report No. L662. Evanston, Illinois: Office of Basic Research, Division of Education, Association of American Medical Colleges).

Institute of Medicine (1974). "Costs of education in the health professions, parts I and II." (Report of a study for U.S. Department of Health, Education, and Welfare, Bureau of Health Resources Development, Bethesda, Maryland, and National Academy of Sciences, Washington, D.C.)

JARECKY, ROY K., DAVIS G. JOHNSON, AND DALE E. MATTSON (1968). "The study of applicants, 1967–1968." *Journal of Medical Education* 43 (December), 1215–1228.

JASON, HILLIARD (1972). "The admissions process in medicine." *Journal of Medical Education* 47 (August), 663.

JOHNSON, DAVIS G. (1965). "The study of applicants, 1964–65." *Journal of Medical Education* 40 (Pt 1) (November), 1017–1030.

JOHNSON, DAVIS G., V. C. SMITH, JR., AND S. L. TARNOFF (1975). "Recruit-

ment and progress of minority medical school entrants, 1970–1972."
Journal of Medical Education 50 (July), 713–755.

KENDALL, PATRICIA L. (1965). "The relationship between medical educators
and medical practitioners." *Annals of The New York Academy of Sciences*
128 (September 27), 568–576 (article 2).

—— (1971a). "Medical specialization: Trends and contributing factors." In
Robert H. Coombs and Clark E. Vincent (eds.), *Psychosocial Aspects of
Medical Training* (Springfield, Illinois: Charles C Thomas), pp. 449–497.

—— (1971b). "Consequences of the trend toward specialization." In Robert
H. Coombs and Clark E. Vincent (eds.), *Psychosocial Aspects of Medical
Training* (Springfield, Illinois: Charles C Thomas), pp. 498–524.

KENNEDY, DANIEL B., AND AUGUST KERBER (1972). *Resocialization: An American Experiment* (New York: Behavioral Publications).

KERR, CLARK (1972). "Enlarging human capability: The central role of the
health sciences." *Journal of Medical Education* 47 (November), 843–850.

KNAFL, KATHLEEN, AND GARY BURKETT (1975). "Professional socialization in
a surgical specialty: Acquiring medical judgment." *Social Science and
Medicine* 9 (July) 397–404.

KNIGHT, JAMES A. (1961). "A study of religious beliefs and attitudes of senior
medical students." *Journal of Medical Education* 36 (November), 1557–
1564.

LESSER, MAY H. (1974). *The Art of Learning Medicine* (New York: Appleton-
Century-Crofts).

(Letter) (1974). "Sexism in medicine—How it functions." *New England
Journal of Medicine* 291 (November 21), 1141–1142.

LEVENSON, BERNARD (1968). "Panel studies." In David Sills (ed.), *International Encyclopedia of the Social Sciences* (New York: Macmillan Company and The Free Press), Vol. 2, p. 371.

LEVINE, DAVID M., CAROL S. WEISMAN, AND HENRY M. SEIDEL (1975).
"Career decisions of unaccepted applicants to medical school." *Journal of
The American Medical Association* 232 (June 16), 1141–1143.

LEVINSON, DANIEL J. (1967). "Medical education and the theory of adult
socialization." *Journal of Health and Social Behavior* 8 (December), 253–
264.

LEVITT, L. P. (1966). "The personality of the medical student." *The Chicago
Medical School Quarterly* 25 (Winter), 201–214.

LEVITT, MORTON, AND BEN RUBENSTEIN (1967). "Medical school faculty attitudes toward applicants and students with emotional problems." *Journal
of Medical Education* 42 (August), 742–751.

LEWIS, CHARLES E., AND BARBARA A. RESNIK (1966). "Relative orientations of
students of medicine and nursing to ambulatory patient care." *Journal of
Medical Education* 41 (February), 162–166.

LIBO, LESTER (1957). "Authoritarianism and attitudes toward socialized medicine among senior medical students." *Journal of Social Psychology* 46
(August), 133–136.

LIEF, HAROLD I. (1971). "Personality characteristics of medical students." In Robert H. Coombs and Clark E. Vincent (eds.), *Psychosocial Aspects of Medical Training* (Springfield, Illinois: Charles C Thomas), pp. 44–87.

LIEF, HAROLD I., AND RENÉE C. FOX (1963). Training for 'detached concern' in medical students. In H. I. Lief, V. Lief, and N. R. Lief (eds.), *The Psychological Basis of Medical Practice* (New York: Hoeber Medical Division, Harper and Row), pp. 12–35.

LIEF, HAROLD I., R. C. LANCASTER, AND V. SPRUIELL (1963). "Is 'self-kick' the answer?" *Journal of Medical Education* 38 (November), 971–973.

LIVINGSTON, PETER B., AND CARL N. ZIMET (1965). "Death anxiety, authoritarianism and choice of specialty in medical students." *Journal of Nervous and Mental Disease* 140 (March), 222–230.

Los Angeles Times (1975). "Doctors-to-be learn to talk to patients: Medical school program teaches how to deal with feelings." Pt. 1-A, p.1 (November 20).

Macy Foundation (1975). "Minority groups for medicine." (A Macy Foundation Study.) *Journal of the National Medical Association* 67 (March), 177.

MARSHALL, CARTER L., A. GLUCK, AND J. G. KOLLIN (1973). "Promotion of nonphysician faculty in American medical schools." *Journal of Medical Education* 48 (December), 1111–1115.

MARTIRE, JOSEPH R. (1969). "The crisis in American medical education: The student viewpoint." *Journal of Medical Education* 44 (November), 1070–1075.

MATTSON, DALE E., DAVIS G. JOHNSON, AND WILLIAM E. SEDLACEK (1968). "The study of applicants, 1966–67." *Journal of Medical Education* 43 (January), 1–13.

McCARTHY, E. B. (1975). "An approach to increasing opportunities for minority students to enter medical training: Summer programs in health sciences." *North Carolina Medical Journal* 36 (April), 226–229.

McDERMOTT, JOHN F., JR., W. F. CHAR, AND M. J. HANSEN (1973). "Motivation for medicine in the seventies." *American Journal of Psychiatry* 130 (March), 252–256.

McGUIRE, F. L. (1966). "Psycho-social studies of medical students: A critical review." *Journal of Medical Education* 41 (May), 424–445.

Medical World News (1974). "Soaring medical school costs." Pp. 27–35 (January 4).

MERTON, ROBERT K. (1957a). *Social Theory and Social Structure* (Glencoe, Illinois: The Free Press).

—— (1957b). "Some preliminaries to a sociology of medical education." In Robert K. Merton, George Reader, and Patricia L. Kendall (eds.), *The Student-Physician: Introductory Studies in the Sociology of Medical Education* (Cambridge, Massachusetts: Harvard University Press), pp. 3–79.

—— (1976). *Sociological Ambivalence and Other Essays* (New York: The Free Press).

MERTON, ROBERT K., AND ELINOR BARBER (1976). "Sociological ambivalence." In Robert K. Merton, *Sociological Ambivalence and Other Essays* (New York: The Free Press), pp. 3–31.

MERTON, ROBERT K., GEORGE READER, AND PATRICIA L. KENDALL (1957). *The Student-Physician: Introductory Studies in the Sociology of Medical Education* (Cambridge, Massachusetts: Harvard University Press).

MILLER, LOUISE B., AND EDMOND F. ERWIN (1959). "A Study of attitudes and anxiety in medical students." *Journal of Medical Education* 34 (November), 1089–1092.

NADELSON, C., AND M. NOTMAN (1974). "Success or failure: Women as medical school applicants." *Journal of the American Medical Women's Association* 29 (April), 167–172.

NELSON, BONNIE (1972). "Datagram: Medical college admission test." *Journal of Medical Education* 47 (September), 750–752.

New York Times (1966). "Medical revolution urged at Harvard." P.1, col. 3 (October 9).

NICHOLS, E. J., AND CHARLES D. SPIELBERGER (1967). "Effects of medical education on anxiety in students." *Mental Hygiene* 51 (January), 74–79.

OETGEN, WILLIAM J., AND MAX P. PEPPER (1972). "Medical school admissions committee members: A descriptive study." *Journal of Medical Education* 47 (December), 966–968.

OLESEN, VIRGINIA L., AND ELVI W. WHITTAKER (1968). *The Silent Dialogue: A Study in the Social Psychology of Professional Socialization* (San Francisco: Jossey-Bass, Inc.).

OLIN, HARRY S. (1972). "A proposed model to teach medical students the care of the dying patient." *Journal of Medical Education* 47 (July), 564–567.

ORWELL, GEORGE (1954). *A Collection of Essays* (Garden City, New York: Doubleday and Company, Inc.).

PATTISHALL, EVAN G., JR. (1972). "Curriculum trends in medical education and their implications for behavioral science." In American Sociological Association (Medical Sociology Council), *Study for Teaching Behavioral Sciences in Schools of Medicine, Volume III: Behavioral Science Perspectives in Medical Education*, Report No. HSM-110-69-211 (Rockville, Maryland: National Center for Health Services Research and Development), pp. 2–39.

PAULY, IRA B., AND STEVEN G. GOLDSTEIN (1970). "Physicians' perceptions of their education in human sexuality." *Journal of Medical Education* 45 (October), 745–753.

PITTS, FERRIS N., GEORGE WINOKUR, AND MARK A. STEWART (1961). "Psychiatric syndromes, anxiety symptoms and responses to stress in medical students." *American Journal of Psychiatry* 118 (October), 333–340.

POLLACK, SEYMOUR, AND PHIL R. MANNING (1967). "An experience in teaching the doctor-patient relationship to first-year medical students." *Journal of Medical Education* 42 (August), 770–774.

REEVES, JOHN M. (1964). "Cynicism in medical education: Review of the literature."*Medical Arts and Science* 18 (Third Quarter), 110–115.

REZLER, AGNES (1969). "Vocational choice in medicine." *Journal of Medical Education* 44 (April), 285–292.

RIS, H. W. (1974). "What do women want?" *Journal of the American Medical Women's Association* 29 (October), 446–447, 451, 453 *passim.*

ROCKOFF, MARK A. (1973). "Interactions between medical students and nursing personnel." *Journal of Medical Education* 48 (August), 725–731.

ROSENBERG, M., W. THIELENS, AND P. F. LAZARSFELD (1951). "The panel study." In M. Jahoda, M. Deutsch, and S. W. Cook (eds.), *Research Methods in Social Relations,* 1st edition (Hinsdale, Illinois: Dryden Press), Vol. 2.

ROSENBERG, PEARL P. (1971). "Students' perceptions and concerns during their first year in medical school." *Journal of Medical Education* 46 (March), 211–218.

ROSENBERG, PEARL P., AND RICHARD G. WEBER (1973). "The effect of curriculum change on the 'new medical student.' " *Journal of Medical Education* 48 (April), 366–368.

ROTHMAN, A. I. (1972). "Longitudinal study of medical students: Long-term versus short-term objectives." *Journal of Medical Education* 47 (November), 901–902.

ROUSSELOT, LOUIS M. (1973). "Federal efforts to influence physician education, specialization distribution projections and options." *American Journal of Medicine* 55 (August), 123–130.

SASLOW, G. (1956). "Symposium on the medical student: Psychiatric problems of medical students." *Journal of Medical Education* 31 (January), 27–33.

SCHACHTER, STANLEY (1963). "Birth order, eminence and higher education." *American Sociological Review* 28 (October), 757–768.

SCHUMACHER, DALE N. (1968). "Research in medical education: An analysis of student clinical activities." *Journal of Medical Education* 43 (March), 383–388.

SEDLACEK, WILLIAM E. (1967). "The study of applicants, 1965–1966." *Journal of Medical Education* 42 (January), 28–46.

SENIOR, BORIS, AND BEVERLY A. SMITH (1973). "The motivation of the patient as a neglected factor in therapy." *Journal of Medical Education* 48 (June), 589–591.

SHAPIRO, ALVIN P., ROBERT F. SCHUCK, STANLEY G. SCHULTZ, AND BRUCE N. BURNHILL (1974). "The impact of curricular change on performance on National Board examinations." *Journal of Medical Education* 49 (December), 1113–1118.

SHAVER, PHILLIP, JOHN R. P. FRENCH, JR., AND SIDNEY COBB (1970). "Birth order of medical students and the occupational ambitions of their parents." *International Journal of Psychology* 5, no. 3, 197–207.

SMITH, E. B. (1976). Editorial: "Decreasing numbers of black medical students." *Journal of the National Medical Association* 68 (January), 73.

SMITH, LOUIS C. REMUND, AND ANNA R. CROCKER (1970). "How medical students finance their education." (Publication of U.S. Department of Health, Education, and Welfare, Public Health Service 1336–1. Washington, D.C.: U.S. Government Printing Office.)

—— (1971). "How medical students finance their education." *Journal of Medical Education* 46 (July), 567–574.

SPIRO, H. M. (1975). "Myths and mirths: Women in medicine." *New England Journal of Medicine* 292 (February 13), 354–356.

STOLLER, ROBERT J., AND ROBERT H. GEERTSMA (1958). "Measurement of medical students' acceptance of emotionally ill patients." *Journal of Medical Education* 33 (August), 585–590.

STRECKER, E. A., K. APPEL, AND F. J. BRACELAND (1936). "Psychiatric studies in medical education." *American Journal of Psychiatry* 92 (January), 937–958.

STRITTER, FRANK T., JACK G. HUTTON, JR., AND W. F. DUBÉ (1970). "Study of U.S. medical school applicants, 1968–69." *Journal of Medical Education* 45 (April), 195–209.

——(1971). "Study of medical school applicants, 1969–70." *Journal of Medical Education* 46 (January), 25–41.

SVALASTOGA, KAARE (1970). "Longitudinal research designs." *International Journal of Comparative Sociology* 11 (December), 283–291.

THOMAS, W. I. (1928). *The Child in America* (New York: Alfred A. Knopf).

WALL, WILLIAM D., AND H. L. WILLIAMS (1970). *Longitudinal Studies and the Social Sciences* (London: Heinemann).

WAX, MURRAY (1962). "On public dissatisfaction with the medical profession: Personal observations." *Journal of Health and Human Behavior* 3 (Summer), 152–156.

WIENER, STANLEY L. (1974). "Ward rounds revisited—the validity of the data base." *Journal of Medical Education* 49 (April), 351–356.

WINGARD, JOHN R., AND JOHN W. WILLIAMSON (1973). "Grades as predictors of physician's career performance: An evaluative literature review." *Journal of Medical Education* 48 (April), 311–322.

WINNER, D. A. (1972). "The changing numbers of women students." Proceedings of the *Royal Society of Medicine* 68 (August), 499–502.

WOODS, S. M., J. NATTERSON, AND J. SILVERMAN (1966). "Medical students' disease: Hypochondriasis in medical education." *Journal of Medical Education* 41 (August), 785–790.

Name Index

Subject Index

AAMC: *see* Association of American Medical Colleges

AAMC Curriculum Directory, 109n, 165n

Academic background, 26–27

Achievement:
 via conformance, 249–50
 via independence, 249–50

Activism, 71, 74

Acute illness, 158–60, 163

Adjective Check List, 8–9, 215–16, 219, 234; *see also* Tests

Adults, 151–54, 163

Allied health workers, 41–42, 60–62, 139, 146, 149, 163, 256

AMA: *see* American Medical Association

Ambivalence, 243, 258–59

American Board of Family Medicine, 187

American Medical Association, 38n, 244–45

Anatomy, 42, 64, 87, 103, 113–14, 135n, 261

Anesthesiology/anesthesiologist, 93–94, 183, 206–8

Applications/admissions, 29–32

Association of American Medical Colleges, 4, 20n, 21n, 37n, 62n, 108, 109n, 269

Attitudes, 5, 11–12, 16–20, 113–14, 156, 163–64, 168fn, 169–70, 211–29, 247, 262–64; *see also* Self-attitudes

Attrition, 23, 20, 111, 133

Autopsies, 130, 259, 262

Avoidance, 131, 146–47, 158, 265; *see also* Coping

Basic scientists, 42–47, 62, 102, 106, 108, 255–56
 as role models, 62, 217

Behavioral sciences, 86, 89; *see also* Faculty

Biochemistry, 42, 85, 87–88

Biostatistics, 89

Birth order, 26, 35, 36n

Boys in White: Student Culture in Medical School, 17, 20

Cadavers, 112–14, 238–39, 262; *see also* Death

California Psychological Inventory, 8, 229–31, 235, 247n, 249n, 250n, 251n, 278n

California, University of, Berkeley, 230, 251n

Cardiology, 91

Career decision, 27–29

Career liabilities, 169, 172–74

Career motives, 168–69, 169fn

Career rewards, 169–72

Chaperon, 155; *see also* Nurses, Staff

Chicago, University of, School of Medicine, 165n, 268n

Children, 151–54, 163

Chronic illness, 127–31, 135n, 158–60, 163, 259–64

Classmates, 63–82; *see also* Study institution

288   *Subject Index*

Surgery/surgeons, 90–94, 106–7, 175, 183–84, 190–92, 209n, 222
Survey of Interpersonal Values, 8, 234

Terminal illness, 127–32, 135n, 163, 165n, 174, 259–64
Tests, psychological, 8–9, 20n, 215, 229, 234, 240, 243, 266
Transition, layman to doctor, 220–22, 224–27
Tulane University School of Medicine, 266

Urology, 91, 93–94, 184

Value homophily, 67
Values and aspirations, 231–35

Women, 12, 21n, 25, 36n, 38n, 133–34, 208, 257

Yale University, 86

610.7369
C775

106690

DATE DUE			
DEC 04 '80	DEC 12 '80		
NO 26 '90	NOV 26 '90		

DEMCO 38-297